Student Study Guide

to accompany

Kinn's **The Medical Assistant**

An Applied Learning Approach

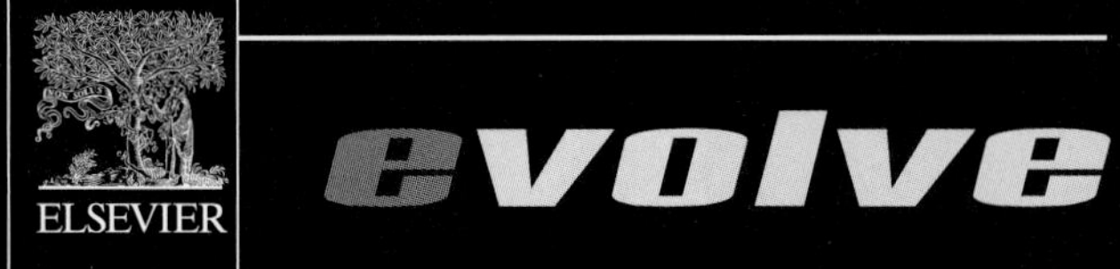

To access your Student Resources, visit the Web address belo

http://evolve.elsevier.com/Kinn/

- **Content Updates**
  The latest content updates from the authors of the textbook to keep you current wit recent developments in medical assisting, updated procedures, and more!

- **Online Quizzes**
  Quizzes for each chapter are set up for instant feedback, any time you want a little practice.

- **WebLinks**
  An exciting resource that lets you link to hundreds of websites carefully chosen to supplement the content of the textbook and student study guide. The WebLinks are regularly updated, with new ones added as they develop.

- **Chapter Resources**
  Additional materials, including chapter summaries and suggested readings, to enhance each chapter.

- **Study Tips**
  Get advice on how to maximize study time and review material for optimal results. Discover your individual learning style and find out how it applies to your ability to learn new material.

Student Study Guide

to accompany

Kinn's **The Medical Assistant**

An Applied Learning Approach

NINTH EDITION

Tammy B. Morton, MS, RN, CS, CMA

Formerly Department Head, Medical Assisting Program
TriCounty Technical College
Pendleton, South Carolina

SAUNDERS
An Imprint of Elsevier

SAUNDERS
An Imprint of Elsevier
11830 Westline Industrial Drive
St. Louis, Missouri 63146

Student Study Guide to Accompany
Kinn's The Medical Assistant: An Applied Learning Approach, 9th edition 1-4160-0116-6

This Study Guide is dedicated to
my family, friends, and former students
who have encouraged and supported me
throughout my teaching career

Many thanks to Karen Sorrow, Kathy Duncan, Mary Helper, Adrianne Cochran, Christine Ambrose, and Jeanne Genz for helping make the project a success.

Executive Editor: Adrianne Cochran
Developmental Editor: Christine Ambrose
Publishing Services Manager: Gayle May
Designer: Mark Oberkrom

Printed in the United States of America

CE/MV-B

Last digit is print number: 9 8 7 6 5 4 3

To the Student

This study guide was created to assist you in achieving the objectives of each chapter in *The Medical Assistant: An Applied Learning Approach* and in establishing a solid base of knowledge in medical assisting. Completing the exercises in each chapter in this guide will help to reinforce the material studied in the textbook and learned in class.

Study Hints for All Students

Ask Questions!

There are no stupid questions. If you do not know something or are not sure about it, you need to find out. Other people may be wondering the same thing but may be too shy to ask. The answer could mean life or death to your patient. That is certainly more important than feeling embarrassed about asking a question.

Chapter Objectives

At the beginning of each chapter in the textbook are learning objectives that you should have mastered when you finish studying that chapter. Write these objectives in your notebook, leaving a blank space after each. Fill in the answers as you find them while reading the chapter. Review to make sure your answers are correct and complete. Use these answers when you study for tests. This should also be done for separate course objectives that your instructor has listed in your class syllabus.

Vocabulary

At the beginning of each chapter in the textbook are vocabulary terms that you will encounter as you read the chapter. These vocabulary terms are in bold the first time they appear in the chapter.

Summary of Learning Objectives

Use the Summary of Learning Objectives at the end of each chapter in the textbook to help with review for exams.

Reading Hints

When reading each chapter in the textbook, look at the subject headings to learn what each section is about. Read first for the general meaning. Then reread parts you did not understand. It may help to read those parts aloud. Carefully read the information given in each table and study each figure and its legend.

Concepts

While studying, put difficult concepts into your own words to determine whether you understand them. Check this understanding with another student or the instructor. Write these concepts in your notebook.

Class Notes

When taking lecture notes in class, leave a large margin on the left side of each notebook page and write only on right-hand pages, leaving all left-hand pages blank. Look over your lecture notes soon after each class, while your memory is fresh. Fill in missing words; complete sentences and ideas; and underline key phrases, definitions, and concepts. At the top of each page, write the topic of that page. In the left margin, write the key word for that part of your notes. On the opposite left-hand page, write a summary or outline that combines material from both the textbook and the lecture. These can be your study notes for review.

Study Groups

Form a study group with some other students so you can help one another. Practice speaking and reading aloud. Ask questions about material you are not sure about. Work together to find answers.

References for Improving Study Skills

Good study skills are essential for achieving your goals in medical assisting. Time management, efficient use of study time, and a consistent approach to studying are all beneficial. There are various methods for reading a textbook and for taking class notes. Some methods that have proven helpful can be found in *Saunders Health Professional's Planner*.

Additional Study Hints for English as a Second Language (ESL) Students

Vocabulary

If you find a nontechnical word you do not know (e.g., drowsy), try to guess its meaning from the sentence (e.g., *With electrolyte imbalance, the patient may feel fatigued and drowsy*). If you are not sure of the meaning or if it seems particularly important, look it up in the dictionary.

Vocabulary Notebook

Keep a small alphabetized notebook or address book in your pocket or purse. Write down new nontechnical words you read or hear along with their meanings and pronunciations. Write each word under its initial letter so you can find it easily, as in a dictionary. For words you do not know or for words that have a different meaning in medical assisting, write down how they are used and how they sound. Look up their meanings in a dictionary or ask your instructor or first-language buddy. Then write the different meanings or usages that you have found in your book, including the medical assisting meaning. Continue to add new words as you discover them.

First-Language Buddy

ESL students should find a first-language buddy—another student who is a native speaker of English and who is willing to answer questions about word meanings, pronunciations, and culture. Maybe, in turn, your buddy would like to learn about your language and culture. This could be useful for his or her medical assisting experience as well.

Introduction

This student study guide is designed with Learning Style Icons to help you identify exercises that will appeal to your strengths and weaknesses. Over time you have developed a method for perceiving and processing information. This patient of behavior is called your learning style. There are many different ways of examining learning styles but professionals agree that success of students has more to do with their ability to "make sense" of the information rather than whether or not they are "smart". Education that is based on attention to individual learning styles is sensitive to the different ways students learn and approach new material with a wide variety of methods so that all students have the opportunity to learn. Determining your individual learning style and understanding how it applies to your ability to learn new material is the first step to becoming a successful student.

To learn new material, two things have to happen. First is your perception of the information. This is the method you have developed over time that helps you examine the material and recognize it as real. The next step is to process the information. Processing the information is how you internalize it and make it your own. Investigating various learning styles tells you how you can combine different methods of perceiving and processing information. In his book *Becoming a Master Student,* David Ellis discusses these different methods of information perception, processing, and learning.*

Information perception involves how you go about examining new material and making it real. There are two ways learners perceive new material. Some people are concrete perceivers who learn information through direct experience by doing, acting, sensing, or feeling. Concrete learners prefer to learn things that have a personal meaning or things they feel are relevant and important to them. Other learners are abstract perceivers who take in information through analysis, observation and reflection. Abstract learners like to think things through. They analyze the new material and build theories to help understand it. They prefer structured learning situations and use a step-by-step approach to problem solving.

Information processing is how you internalize the new information and make it your own. There are also two different methods for processing material. Active processors prefer to jump in and start doing things immediately. They make sense of the new material by immediately using it. They look for practical ways to apply the new material and typically don't mind taking risks to get the desired results. They learn best with practice and hands-on activities. Reflective processors, however, have to think about the information before they can internalize it. They prefer to observe and consider what is going on. The only way they can make sense of new material is to spend time thinking about it and learning a great deal of information about it before acting.

*Ellis D: Becoming a master student, ed 10, Boston, 2002, Houghton Mifflin.

None of us fall completely into one or the other of these categories. However, by being aware of how we generally prefer to first perceive information and then process it, we can be more sensitive to our learning style and approach new learning situations with a plan for learning the material in a way that best suits our learning preferences. Your preferred perceiving/processing learning profile will fall into one of the following stages.

Learners in Stage 1 have a concrete/reflective style. 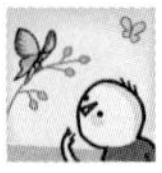 and 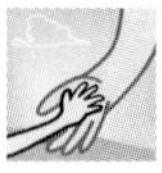 These students want to know the purpose of the information and have a personal connection to the content. They like to consider a situation from many different points of view, observe others, and plan before taking action. Their strengths are in understanding people, brainstorming, and recognizing and cretively solving problems. If you fall into this stage you enjou small group activities and learn well in study groups.

Stage 2 learners have an abstract/reflective style. 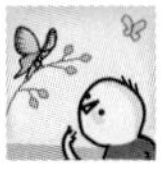 and 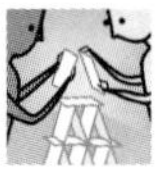 These students are eager to learn just for the sheer pleasure of learning rather than because the material relates to their personal lives. They like to learn lots of facts and arrange new material in a logical and clear manner. Stage 2 learners plan studying and like to create ways of thinking about the material but don't always make the connection with the practical application of the material. If you are a Stage 2 learner you prefer organized, logical presentations of material and, therefore, enjoy lectures and generally dislike group work. You also need time to process and think about the new material before applying it.

Learners in Stage 3 have an abstract/active style. 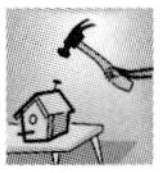 and 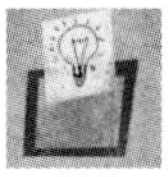 Learners with this combination of learning style want to experiment and test the knowledge they are learning. If you are a Stage 3 learner you want to know how techniques or ideas work buy you also want to practice what you are learning. Your strengths are in problem solving and making decisions but you may tend to lack focus and be hasty in your decision-making. You learn best with hands-on practice by doing experiments, projects, and lab activities. You also enjoy working alone or in small groups.

Stage 4 is made up of concrete/active learners. 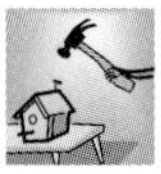 and 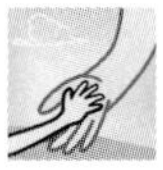 Students in this stage are concerned about how they can use what they learn to make a difference in their lives. If you fall into this stage, you like to relate new material to other areas of your life. You have leadership capabilities, can create on your feet, and are usually vocal in a group but you may have difficulty getting your work done completely and on time. Stage 4 learners enjoy teaching others and working in groups and learn best when they can apply the new information to real-world problems.

To get the most out of knowing your learning profile you need to apply this knowledge to how you approach learning. There are plusses and minuses to all four of the learning stages. When faced with a learning situation that does not match your learning preference, see how you can adapt your individual learning to make the best of the information. For example, if you are bored by lectures, look for an opportunity to apply the information being presented into a real-world problem you are facing in the classroom or at home. When learning new material, if you are an abstract perceiver, take time outside of class to think about the information so you are ready to process it into your learning system. If you benefit from learning in a group then make the effort to organize review sessions and study groups with other interested students. If you learn best by teaching others offer to assist your peers with their learning. Take time now to investigate your preferred method of learning and it will help you perceive and process information more effectively throughout your school career.

Debby Kennedy and Tammy Morton

Contents

Procedure Checklists

Student Study Guide

to accompany

Kinn's The Medical Assistant

An Applied Learning Approach

CHAPTER 1

Becoming a Successful Student

Part I. Vocabulary

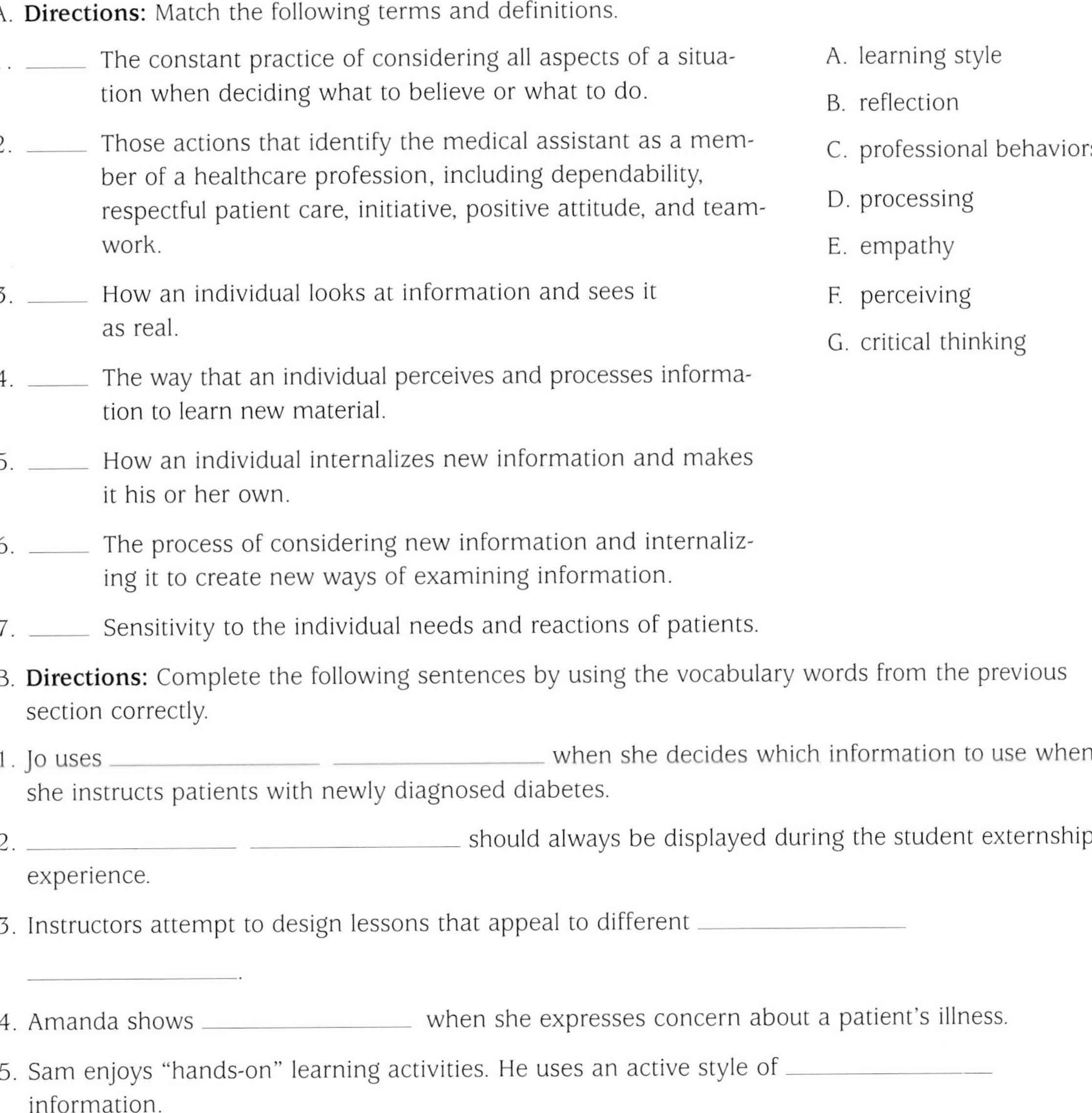

A. **Directions:** Match the following terms and definitions.

1. ______ The constant practice of considering all aspects of a situation when deciding what to believe or what to do.
2. ______ Those actions that identify the medical assistant as a member of a healthcare profession, including dependability, respectful patient care, initiative, positive attitude, and teamwork.
3. ______ How an individual looks at information and sees it as real.
4. ______ The way that an individual perceives and processes information to learn new material.
5. ______ How an individual internalizes new information and makes it his or her own.
6. ______ The process of considering new information and internalizing it to create new ways of examining information.
7. ______ Sensitivity to the individual needs and reactions of patients.

A. learning style
B. reflection
C. professional behaviors
D. processing
E. empathy
F. perceiving
G. critical thinking

B. **Directions:** Complete the following sentences by using the vocabulary words from the previous section correctly.

1. Jo uses ______________ ______________ when she decides which information to use when she instructs patients with newly diagnosed diabetes.
2. ______________ ______________ should always be displayed during the student externship experience.
3. Instructors attempt to design lessons that appeal to different ______________ ______________.
4. Amanda shows ______________ when she expresses concern about a patient's illness.
5. Sam enjoys "hands-on" learning activities. He uses an active style of ______________ information.
6. Concrete and abstract are two ways of ______________ new information.

Part II. Learning Style Inventory

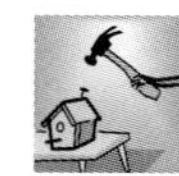

Directions: Using the descriptions of various learning styles from Chapter 1, insert the correct Learning Style Stage Number into the diagram below by correlating the processing and perceiving style. In his book, *Becoming a Master Student,* Ellis discusses these different methods of information perception, processing, and learning.*

	Processing	
Perceiving	Watching (Reflective)	Doing (Active)
Feeling (Concrete)	Stage ____________	Stage ____________
Thinking (Abstract)	Stage ____________	Stage ____________

Part III. Time Management

1. List five time management skills.
   a. ______________________________
   b. ______________________________
   c. ______________________________
   d. ______________________________
   e. ______________________________
2. Describe five strategies for breaking the cycle of procrastination.
   a. ______________________________
   b. ______________________________
   c. ______________________________
   d. ______________________________
   e. ______________________________

*Ellis D: Becoming a master student, ed 10, Boston, 2002, Houghton Mifflin.

Part IV. Conflict Resolution

Directions: Indicate which statements are true (T) and which statements are false (F).

1. _____ The best way to deal with conflict situations is through open, honest, assertive communication.
2. _____ The first step in conflict resolution is examination of pros and cons.
3. _____ Conflicts should be resolved immediately.
4. _____ Sometimes you will not be able to solve problems or a conflict may not be important enough for you to act to change it.
5. _____ It is best if you attempt to solve the conflict in a private place at a prescheduled time.
6. _____ You need to understand the problem and gather as much information about the situation as possible before you decide to act.
7. _____ As a future member of the healthcare team, you will frequently face problems and conflict.

Part V. Workplace Applications

Scenario: Connie is the manager of a busy family practice office. The insurance clerk has complained that the receptionist takes too many smoking breaks and accepts too many personal calls while at work.

Step One: Think about this situation and how you believe it should be handled. Record your ideas.

_____

_____

_____

_____

_____

Step Two: Pair up with a classmate and discuss your ideas. Record ideas on which you agree and compare them with those in the text.

_____

_____

_____

_____

_____

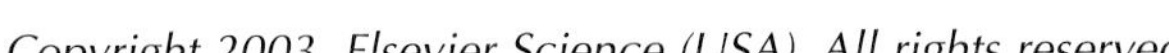

Step Three: Share your ideas with your classmates. Make notes of any ideas that you did not think of before.

Part VI. Study Skills

Examine your own note-taking ability. Review the note-taking strategies in Chapter 1, and record the ideas that you plan to incorporate into your academic goals for this term.

Directions: Complete the following success checklist.

	Yes	No
1. I am prepared for class.		
2. My notebook is organized.		
3. I read my assignments before coming to class.		
4. I attend all classes.		
5. I listen most of the time.		
6. I arrive early to class.		
7. I date notes in my notebook.		
8. I save all papers and course materials for review.		
9. I try to connect what I read in the text with what I learn in class.		
10. My schoolwork is a high priority.		

If you answered "No" to any of the items on the checklist, write a short plan for improvement in this area.

____

____

____

____

____

Part VII. Test-Taking Strategies

Directions: Complete the following sentences.

1. The first step of taking charge of your academic success is to

   ____

   ____.

2. Before you begin a test ____.

Chapter 1 Quiz

Name: ____________________

1. List three examples of professional behaviors.

   a. ____________

   b. ____________

   c. ____________

2. ____________ is showing sensitivity to the individual needs and reactions of patients.

3. The process of considering new information and internalizing it to create new ways of examining information is called ____________.

4. Initial confrontations regarding conflicts in the office should be done in ____________.

5. True or False: Concrete learners enjoy theories and facts.

   ____

6. True or False: Active learning involves "hands-on" experiences.

   ____

7. List Two ways to use effective time management.

   a. ____________

   b. ____________

8. Give an example of a mind map.

   ____

Chapter 2 Quiz

Name: ______________________________

1. Which agency evaluates the quality of laboratory reports?

   a. OSHA

   b. CLIA

   c. CDC

   ____

2. Name a professional who works under the supervision of a medical technologist.

   ____

3. What type of registered nurse has advanced training to diagnose and treat common illnesses?

   a. anesthetist

   b. practitioner

   c. dietician

   d. practical

   ____

4. True or False: An occupational therapist works to help patients regain functions that will improve their quality of life.

   ____

5. A ______________ treats life-threatening illnesses and supervises ambulance services.

6. ______________ therapists are trained to use oxygen therapy and measure lung capacity.

7. True or False: Chiropractors write prescriptions.

   ____

8. The credentials DDS and DMD are used by

   ______________.

9. The agency that inspects workplaces for safety is

   a. CDC

   b. OSHA

   c. DHHS

   ____

10. A way of prioritizing patients so that those with the most serious conditions receive care first is called

    a. case management

    b. accreditation

    c. triage

    ____

Part V. Professional Appearance

A. Working with a partner, write a dress code for an office.

B. Locate the closest professional chapter for medical assistants. Record the name of the group, the date, and the location of their next meeting in your area.

Part VI. Professional Organizations

Directions: Complete the following sentences.

1. Gail uses the CMA credential behind her name. It stands for ____________ ____________ ____________.
2. The CMA exam is offered by the ____________.
3. Tom is looking for an accredited medical assisting program. The two agencies that accredit programs are ____________ and ____________.
4. The American Medical Technologists offer the ____________ credential for graduates of accredited medical assisting programs who pass the exam.

Chapter 3 Quiz

Name: ______________________________

1. The first national organization formed for medical assistants was:

   a. CAAHEP

   b. ABHES

   c. AMT

   d. AAMA

   ____

2. True or False: Both men and women can be equally successful as medical assistants.

   ____

3. True or False: Medical assistants may perform electrocardiograms and prepare patients for x-ray examinations.

   ____

4. True or False: Individuals working in the medical assisting field have a mandatory retirement age.

   ____

5. True or False: Most medical assisting positions are in hospitals.

   ____

6. True or False: The medical assisting student should treat the externship experience as if it were a probationary period for an actual job.

   ____

7. Which credential is **NOT** offered by the AMT?

   a. COLT

   b. RMA

   c. CMA

   d. RPT

   ____

8. True or False: Medical assistants always wear white uniforms.

   ____

CHAPTER 4

Professional Behavior in the Workplace

Part I. Vocabulary

Directions: Fill in the blanks with the appropriate vocabulary terms.

1. The nurse manager presents an employee-of-the-month certificate at staff meetings to boost employee ________________.
2. Salaries are usually ________________ with education and experience.
3. ________________ means to intentionally put off doing something that should be done.
4. A medical assistant who is disrespectful to people in authority might be accused of ________________.
5. When an employee volunteers to help in other departments, this shows ________________.
6. Failure to follow preoperative instructions can be ________________ to the patient's health.
7. ________________ is characterized by conforming to ethical and technical standards.

Part II.

List the eight characteristics of the professional persona.

1. ________________
2. ________________
3. ________________
4. ________________
5. ________________
6. ________________
7. ________________
8. ________________

Part III.

List five deterrents to professionalism.

1. ______________________________

2. ______________________________

3. ______________________________

4. ______________________________

5. ______________________________

Which of these five deterrents do you think will be the most difficult for you to deal with in the medical office?

____

____

Why? ______________________________

____

____

____

Part IV.

Directions: Your text lists four professional attributes. Rate yourself in each of the four areas by circling the appropriate statement.

Teamwork:	I need to improve.	I'm about average.	I'm a team player.
Time Management:	I need to improve.	I'm about average.	I am very organized.
Prioritizing:	I need to improve.	I'm about average.	This is one of my strengths.
Goal-Setting:	I need to improve.	I'm about average.	I'm goal-oriented.

Part V.

1. Karen seems to have trouble remembering exact doses of medications that were verbally ordered by Dr. Ross. How can she avoid this problem in the future?

____

____

____

____

____

2. Karen works in the office lab. She is often asked questions about insurance and billing that she must refer to other personnel. How should Karen efficiently request information or assistance from other office personnel?

3. The office manager has asked Karen to make sure her blood pressures are documented more legibly on the patient records. Why is neatness so important?

4. Karen and her fiancé broke up last week. How should she deal with personal stressors while she is in the workplace?

5. A patient needs to be scheduled for an outpatient endoscopic exam. When Karen gave the instruction sheet to the patient, she suspected that the patient was embarrassed because he could not read. How could Karen handle this situation?

Chapter 4 Quiz

Name: ______________________________

1. Which of the following words is misspelled?

   a. Characteristic

   b. Compitence

   c. Commensurate

   ____

2. True or False: Office politics are always negative.

   ____

3. ______________ is to intentionally put off doing something that should be done.

   a. Initiative

   b. Procrastination

   c. Professionalism

   d. Discretion

4. True or False: Insubordination can be grounds for termination.

   ____

5. A ______________, by definition, is talk or widely disseminated opinion with no discernible source or a statement that is not known to be true.

6. ______________ is the process of working well with others to reach mutual goals.

7. True or False: Insubordination might be justified if you are asked to perform an illegal act.

   ____

8. Which of the following words is misspelled?

   a. Demeanor

   b. Discretion

   c. Disemminated

   d. Detrimental

   e. All are spelled correctly

   f. None are spelled correctly

   ____

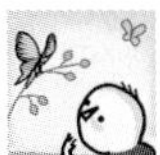

Part V.

Directions: Discuss the following scenarios as they relate to Maslow's hierarchy of needs.

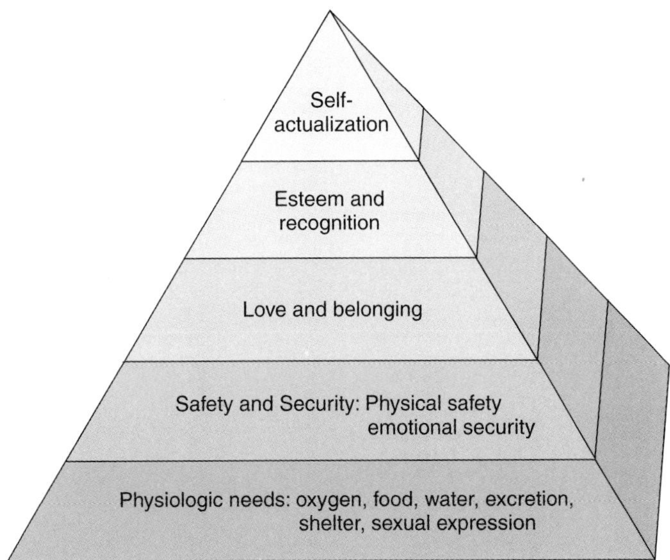

1. Kim is usually a good speller. However, her spelling grades have dropped since she was given a diagnosis of asthma.

2. In hazardous situations, paramedics are instructed to protect themselves before caring for patients.

3. Bill says that he could not pay attention during the staff meeting because he was distracted by the aroma from the large tray of pastries, which had been sent in by the sales representative from the drug company.

Chapter 5 Quiz

Name: ______________________________

1. Which of the following words is misspelled?

   a. Litigious

   b. Paraphrasing

   c. Sarcasm

   d. Vehemently

   ____

2. ______________ means easily aroused; tending to erupt in violence.

   a. Stereotype

   b. Vehemently

   c. Volatile

3. True or False: The description of the study of the phenomena of death and of psychological methods of coping with death is called *thanatology*.

   ____

4. True or False: According to Maslow, basic physiological needs must be met before higher level needs can be addressed.

   ____

5. ______________ -ended questions are more likely to provide more information.

6. ______________ is a sharp and often satirical response or ironic utterance designed to cut or give pain.

7. True or False: An older child who starts sucking his or her thumb during a stressful period might be demonstrating regressive behavior.

   ____

8. Which of the following defense mechanisms results in the inability to remember a painful event?

   a. Denial

   b. Repression

   c. Regression

   d. Apathy

   ____

CHAPTER 6

Medicine and Ethics

Part I. Vocabulary

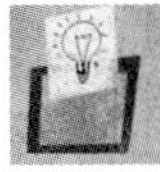

Directions: Match the following terms and definitions.

1. _____ Faithfulness to something to which one is bound by pledge or duty.
2. _____ The act of doing or producing good, especially performing acts of charity or kindness.
3. _____ The realm embracing property rights that belong to the community at large, are unprotected by copyright or patent, and are subject to appropriation by anyone.
4. _____ Refraining from the act of harming or committing evil.
5. _____ A devotion to, or conformity with, the truth.
6. _____ The act or practice of killing or permitting the death of hopelessly sick or injured individuals in a relatively painless way for reasons of mercy.
7. _____ Apportioning for a specific purpose or to particular persons or things.

A. euthanasia
B. allocating
C. veracity
D. fidelity
E. nonmaleficence
F. public domain
G. beneficence

Part II.

Directions: Label the following as nonmaleficence (N), veracity (V), fidelity (F), or beneficence (B).

1. ______________ Melissa offers free blood pressure checks at her office on Wednesday afternoons.
2. ______________ Dr. Parker insists that medical assistants check medications three times before administering them.
3. ______________ Geri notified the office manager that she dropped the microscope while cleaning it.
4. ______________ Joyce refuses to discuss office business with people outside work.

Part III. ______

A. **Directions:** List the five steps of ethical decision making.

a. ______

b. ______

c. ______

d. ______

e. ______

B. **Directions:** Indicate which statements are true (T) and which statements are false (F).

1. ______ A method of anonymous HIV testing in which a code is used instead of names to protect the confidentiality of the patient is illegal.

2. ______ Ramifications are consequences produced by a cause or following from a set of conditions.

3. ______ Clinical trials are research studies that test how well new medical treatments or other interventions work in the subjects, usually human beings.

Part IV. ______

Directions: Define each of the following ethical situations and describe some of the issues surrounding these topics.

Abortion

______

______

______

______

______

Abuse

______

______

______

______

______

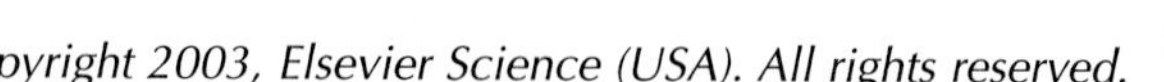

Allocation of Health Resources

Artificial Insemination

Surrogate Motherhood

Human Cloning

Genetic Counseling

Physician-Assisted Suicide

Withholding or Withdrawing Life-Prolonging Treatment

Organ Donation

Capital Punishment

HIV Testing

Human Genome

Fee-Splitting

Part V. Workplace Applications

Scenario: You notice a co-worker giving out drug samples to someone without the permission of the physician.

Step One: Think about this situation and how you believe it should be handled. Record your ideas.

Step Two: Pair up with a classmate and discuss your ideas. Record ideas on which you agree. List any new ideas. Note any items about which you disagree.

Step Three: Share your ideas with your classmates. Make notes of any ideas that you did not think of before.

Chapter 6 Quiz

Name: ______________________________

1. List four examples of ethical duties.

   a. ____________

   b. ____________

   c. ____________

   d. ____________

2. ____________ deals with courtesy, customs, and manners.

3. The CEJA is part of the ____________.

   a. AAMA

   b. AMA

   c. CMA

4. True or False: The access to genetic information prompts many concerns and presents ethical, legal, and moral questions.

   ____

5. True or False: The law requires that abuse be reported, and if a physician does not report abuse, his or her ethical standards have also been breached.

   ____

6. True or False: Confidentiality is one of the cardinal rules of the medical profession.

   ____

7. Define fee-splitting.

   ____

   ____

8. Define ghost surgery.

   ____

   ____

Chapter 7 Quiz

Name: ______________________________

1. A patient rolls up his sleeve for you to draw blood. Which type of consent is this?

   a. informed

   b. implied

   c. expressed

   ____

2. Name an agency that deals with administrative law.

   ____

3. In a medical malpractice suit, the doctor is usually the

   a. plaintiff

   b. attorney

   c. bailiff

   d. defendant

   ____

4. True or False: Consideration is an exchange of something of value, for example, money for the physician's time.

   ____

5. True or False: Schedule II drugs include narcotics and Ritalin.

   ____

6. A ______________ of limitations is a period after which a lawsuit cannot be filed.

7. True or False: Informed consent includes knowledge of alternate treatments and risks.

   ____

8. An ______________ ______________ is a person younger than 18 or 21 years who can legally give consent.

9. The agency that regulates controlled substances is the

   a. FDA

   b. OSHA

   c. HIPPA

   d. DEA

   ____

10. Medical licensure can be obtained through

    a. examination

    b. reciprocity

    c. endorsement

    d. all of the above

    ____

CHAPTER 8

Computers in the Medical Office

Part I. Vocabulary

Directions: Use the appropriate vocabulary term from the text to fill in the blank.

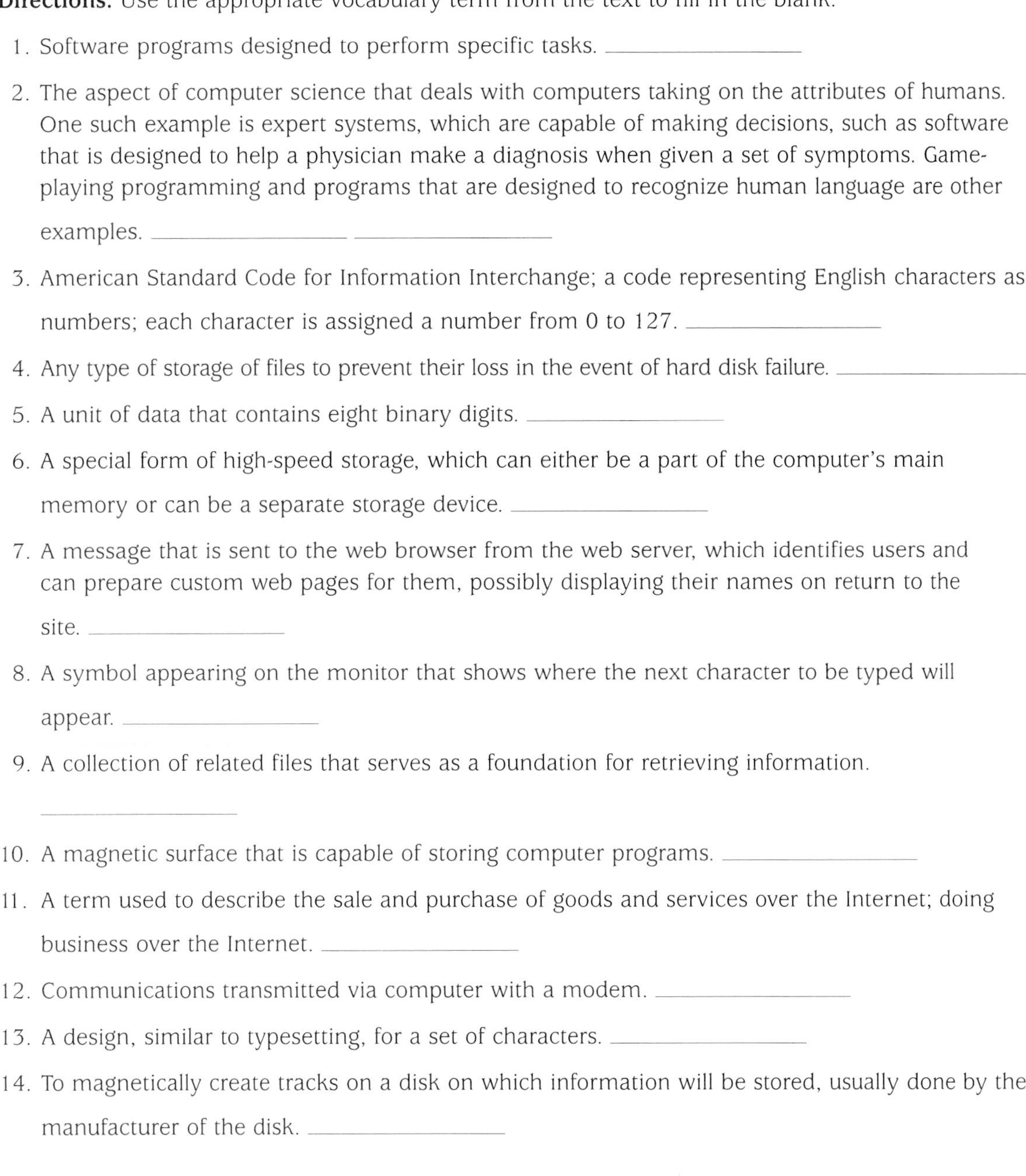

1. Software programs designed to perform specific tasks. ________________
2. The aspect of computer science that deals with computers taking on the attributes of humans. One such example is expert systems, which are capable of making decisions, such as software that is designed to help a physician make a diagnosis when given a set of symptoms. Game-playing programming and programs that are designed to recognize human language are other examples. ________________ ________________
3. American Standard Code for Information Interchange; a code representing English characters as numbers; each character is assigned a number from 0 to 127. ________________
4. Any type of storage of files to prevent their loss in the event of hard disk failure. ________________
5. A unit of data that contains eight binary digits. ________________
6. A special form of high-speed storage, which can either be a part of the computer's main memory or can be a separate storage device. ________________
7. A message that is sent to the web browser from the web server, which identifies users and can prepare custom web pages for them, possibly displaying their names on return to the site. ________________
8. A symbol appearing on the monitor that shows where the next character to be typed will appear. ________________
9. A collection of related files that serves as a foundation for retrieving information. ________________
10. A magnetic surface that is capable of storing computer programs. ________________
11. A term used to describe the sale and purchase of goods and services over the Internet; doing business over the Internet. ________________
12. Communications transmitted via computer with a modem. ________________
13. A design, similar to typesetting, for a set of characters. ________________
14. To magnetically create tracks on a disk on which information will be stored, usually done by the manufacturer of the disk. ________________

15. Approximately one billion bytes. ________________

16. The readable paper copy or printout of information. ________________

17. A common connection point for devices in a network containing multiple ports, often used to connect segments of a local area network (LAN). ________________

18. Abbreviation for hyper text markup language, which is the language used to create documents for use on the Internet. ________________

19. A picture, often on the desktop of a computer, which represents a program or object; by clicking on it, the user is directed to the program. ________________

20. Information entered into and used by the computer. ________________

21. An object-oriented high-level programming language commonly used and well-suited for the Internet. ________________

22. Approximately one million bytes. ________________

23. The measuring device for microprocessors, abbreviated MHz. ________________

24. A device that allows information to be transmitted over phone lines, at speeds measured in bits per second (bps); short for modulator-demodulator. ________________

25. The presentation of graphics, animation, video, sound, and text on a computer in an integrated way, or all at once. ________________

26. Information that is processed by the computer and transmitted to a monitor, printer, or other device. ________________

27. A device used to connect any number of local area networks (LANs), which communicate with other routers and determine the best route between any two hosts. ________________

28. A device that reads text or illustrations on a printed page and can translate the information on that page into a form that the computer can understand. ________________

29. Abbreviation for uniform resource locator; specifies the global address of documents or information on the Internet. ________________

30. An artificial environment presented to a computer user, which simulates a real environment; the user often wears special gloves, earphones, and goggles to enhance the experience.

    ________________ ________________

31. A small and portable disk drive that is primarily used for backing up information and archiving computer files. It will hold the equivalent of about 70 floppy disks. ________________

Part II.

A. **Directions:** Fill in the blanks.

1. ________________ is internal memory that contains a portion of the operating system and computer language. This is sometimes known as *main memory*.

2. ________________ can be thought of as an internal scratch pad for the computer. It contains the program instructions and the data that are currently being processed, and it is normally erased when the power is shut off.

B. Workplace Applications

Directions: Describe two different ways to perform each task in a word-processing program.

1. Open a file.

____

____

2. Save a file.

____

____

3. Print a file.

____

____

4. Save a file under a different name.

____

____

5. Exit a program.

____

____

6. Cut and paste text.

____

____

7. Center text.

____

____

8. Bold text.

____

____

9. Insert a table.

____

____

10. Undo a mistake.

____

____

Part III. ______

A. **Directions:** Label each of the following as Input, Output, or Storage.

1. Mouse ______
2. Keyboard ______
3. Printer ______
4. Scanner ______
5. DVD ______
6. CD-ROM ______
7. Zip disk ______
8. Touch screen ______
9. Floppy disk ______
10. Modem ______

B. **Directions:** List seven ways that computers assist workers in medical offices.

1. ______
2. ______
3. ______
4. ______
5. ______
6. ______
7. ______

Part IV. ______

A. **Directions:** Give examples of each of the following.

1. Input ______
2. Processing ______
3. Storage ______
4. Output ______

B. **Directions:** Use an Internet search to visit various websites within the following domains; record the name of the agency and the URLs for the sites you find.

1. .com (for commercial businesses) ______
2. .org (for organizations, usually nonprofit) ______
3. .edu (for educational institutions) ______

4. .gov (for governmental agencies) ______

5. .net (for network organizations) ______

C. Visit a local store that sells computers or use a newspaper to examine a particular computer that is being sold. Answer the following questions.

1. How much RAM and ROM does the system have? ______
2. What is the clock speed? ______
3. What type of data storage is available? ______
4. What is the baud rate of the modem? ______
5. What software comes with the system? ______
6. Is a printer included? If so, what type? ______
7. Document the name of the store and price of the system. ______

D. **Directions:** Examine the work setting below. Label the numbered items as lighting, work surface, mouse, monitors, keyboards, storage and files, or adjustable chairs.

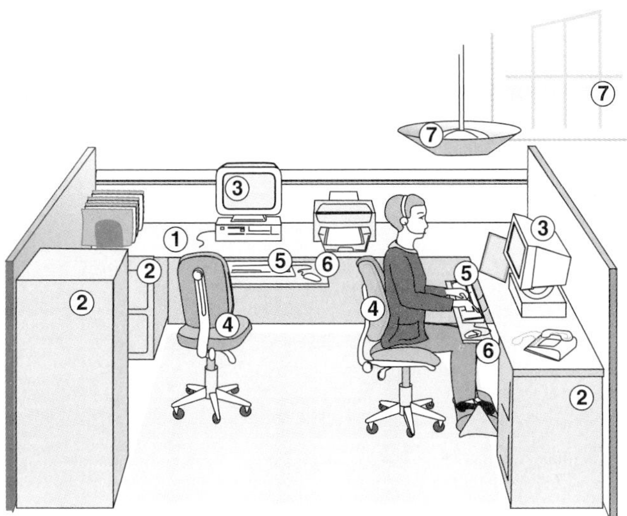

Ergonomic environment of an HIM department. (Redrawn from Gaylor L: The Administrative Dental Assistant, Philadelphia, WB, Saunders, 2000, p. 290.) (From Davis N, LaCour M: *Introduction to health information technology*, Philadelphia, 2002, WB Saunders.)

1. ______
2. ______
3. ______
4. ______
5. ______
6. ______
7. ______

Chapter 8 Quiz

Name: ____

1. The clock speed is measured in _______

2. True or False: A DSL modem can operate while the phone is in use. _____

3. What is a major advantage of a laser printer?

   ____

   ____

4. Name two pieces of hardware.

   a. ______________________________

   b. ______________________________

5. LAN stands for ______ - ______ ______.

6. What are applications?

   ____

   ____

7. A megabyte contains ________ of data.

8. True or False: A printer is an output device. ___________

9. A zip drive is a _________ device.

10. True or False: A mouse is an import device. ____________________________

Chapter 9 Quiz

Name: ____

1. The quality of being clear is ________.

2. When it is 8:00 am in Atlanta, it is __________ in Los Angeles.

3. True or False: Pagers are an example of a one-way communication device.

   ____

4. Telephone systems that are answered by a recorded voice with a series of options is called

   ____

   ____

   ________________________________.

5. Lunch hour and after-hours calls are frequently handled by an

   ________________________________.

6. Give some examples of emergency calls.

   a. ____________________________

   b. ____________________________

   c. ____________________________

7. A change in pitch is ______________.

8. Speech of an unvaried pitch is

   ______________________________.

9. True or False: To avoid being offensive is to be tactful. _________________

10. List two ways to deal with an angry caller.

    a. ____________________________

    b. ____________________________

Modified Wave Scheduling

Double Booking

Grouping Procedures

Advance Booking

Chapter 10 Quiz

Name: ____

1. A person who fails to keep an appointment is sometimes referred to as a ____________ - ______________ .

2. A returning patient is called ________ .

3. The process of establishing urgency is called __________________________ .

4. List two characteristics to consider when selecting an appointment book for a medical office.

   a. ____________________________

   b. ____________________________

5. True or False: One of the advantages of computerized scheduling is that more than one person can schedule at a time.

   ____

6. Having only walk-in appointments is called ________ ________ ________ .

7. Describe flexible office hours.

   ____

   ____

8. Scheduling three patients to arrive at the same time is ________________ scheduling.

9. Chronically late patients are scheduled at the ________ of the day.

10. Failed appointments should be ________________ in the medical record.

CHAPTER 11

Patient Reception and Processing

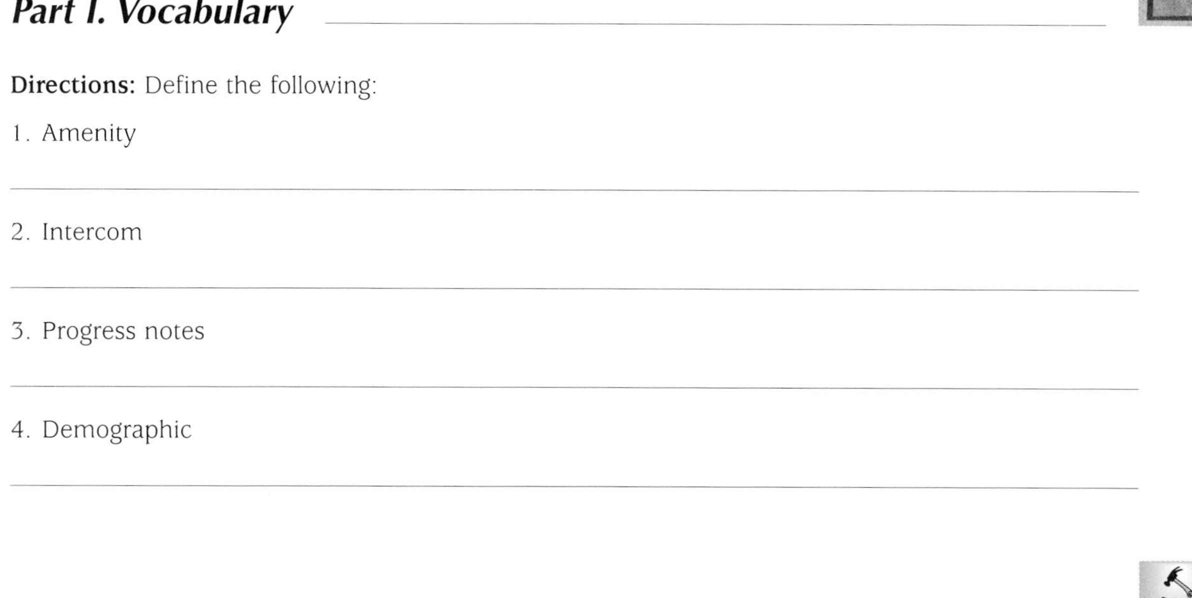

Part I. Vocabulary

Directions: Define the following:

1. Amenity

2. Intercom

3. Progress notes

4. Demographic

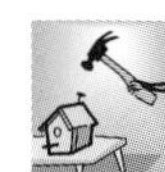

Part II.

Directions: Correct the misspelled words.

1. Fevrent
2. Flaged
3. Harmoneous
4. Immigrent
5. Perseption
6. Phonitec
7. Sequencially

Part III.

A. Visit several reception areas for local banks, hospitals, doctors' offices, or even your school. Record your impressions in the table below.

Location				
Cleanliness				
Colors				
Seating				
Lighting				
Comfort				
Amenities				
Noise				

B. Paige is getting ready for the next workday. What is the first step in preparing for patient arrival? What will she need to look at to complete this task?

____

____

____

____

C. What is a task that she could complete the evening before?

____

____

____

____

Part IV.

A. What are your thoughts and concerns regarding patient check-in?

B. On the blank letterhead provided on p. 72, design your own registration form.

C. List several routine tasks for closing an office.

D. How do you feel about asking for payments and copayments?

Blackburn Primary Care Associates
1990 Turquoise Drive
Blackburn, WI 54937
(555) 555-1234

E. With a partner, role play. Pretend you are interviewing a patient named Ivan Shapiro. Find out more about his chest pain, what medicines he is taking, and his past illnesses. Document his responses on the health history form provided.

Case One, Form 3

ANDRUS/CLINI-REC® HEALTH HISTORY QUESTIONNAIRE

Chart No. ________

Today's Date ________

Identification Information

Name Shapiro, Ivan — Date of Birth 3/6/45

Occupation Carpenter — Marital Status Married

PART A – PRESENT HEALTH HISTORY

I. CURRENT MEDICAL PROBLEMS

Please list the medical problems for which you came to see the doctor. About when did they begin?

Problems	Date Began
Chest pain when exercising	

What concerns you most about these problems?

If you are being treated for any other illness or medical problems by another physician, please describe the problems and write the name of the physician or medical facility treating you.

Illness or Medical Problem	Physician or Medical Facility	City

II. MEDICATIONS

Please list all medications you are now taking, including those you buy without a doctor's prescription (such as aspirin, cold tablets or vitamin supplements).

III. ALLERGIES AND SENSITIVITIES

List anything that you are allergic to such as certain foods, medications, dust, chemicals or soaps, household items, pollens, bee stings, etc., and indicate how each affects you.

Allergic To:	Effect	Allergic To:	Effect
Penicillin	Hives		

IV. GENERAL HEALTH, ATTITUDE AND HABITS

How is your overall health now?	Health now:	Poor __ Fair __ Good X Excellent __
How has it been most of your life?	Health has been:	Poor __ Fair __ Good X Excellent __
In the past year:		
Has your appetite changed?	Appetite:	Decreased __ Increased __ Stayed same X
Has your weight changed?	Weight:	Lost __ lbs. Gained 10 lbs. No change __
Are you thirsty much of the time?	Thirsty:	No X Yes __
Has your overall 'pep' changed?	Pep:	Decreased __ Increased __ Stayed same X
Do you usually have trouble sleeping?	Trouble sleeping:	No __ Yes X
How much do you exercise?	Exercise:	Little or none __ Less than I need __ All I need X
Do you smoke?	Smokes:	No X Yes __ If yes, how many years? __
How many each day?		__ Cigarettes __ Cigars __ Pipesfull
Have you ever smoked?	Smoked:	No __ Yes X If yes, how many years? 15
How many each day?		20 Cigarettes __ Cigars __ Pipesfull
Do you drink alcoholic beverages?	Alcohol:	No __ Yes X I drink __ Beers __ Glasses of wine __ Drinks of hard liquor - per day Socially
Have you ever had a problem with alcohol?	Prior problem:	No X Yes __
How much coffee or tea do you usually drink?	Coffee/Tea:	2 cups of coffee or tea a day
Do you regularly wear seatbelts?	Seatbelts:	No __ Yes X

DO YOU:	Rarely/Never	Occasionally	Frequently
Feel nervous?	X		
Feel depressed?	X		
Find it hard to make decisions?	X		
Lose your temper?		X	
Worry a lot?	X		
Tire easily?		X	
Have trouble relaxing?		X	
Have any sexual problems?	X		

DO YOU:	Rarely/Never	Occasionally	Frequently
Ever feel like committing suicide?	X		
Feel bored with your life?	X		
Use marijuana?	X		
Use "hard drugs"?	X		

Do you want to talk to the doctor about a personal matter? No X Yes __

STOCK NO. 19-742-4 8/95 Page 1

CONFIDENTIAL

Health history questionnaire

Case One, Form 3

PART A – PRESENT HEALTH HISTORY (continued)

IV. GENERAL HEALTH, ATTITUDE AND HABITS (continued)

Have you recently had any changes in your:	No	Yes	If yes, please explain:
Marital status?	X		
Job or work?		X	Self employed
Residence?		X	Moved from LA CA
Financial status?	X		
Are you having any legal problems or trouble with the law?	X		

PART B – PAST HISTORY

I. FAMILY HEALTH

Please give the following information about your immediate family:

Relationship	Age, if Living	Age At Death	State of Health Or Cause of Death
Father		78	Lung cancer
Mother		45	Heart disease
Brothers and Sisters	38		good
Spouse	51		good
Children	22		good
	25		good

Have any **blood relatives** had any of the following illnesses? If so, indicate relationship (mother, brother, etc.)

Illness	Family Members
Asthma	
Diabetes	
Cancer	Father
Blood Disease	
Glaucoma	
Epilepsy	
Rheumatoid Arthritis	Aunt
Tuberculosis	
Gout	
High Blood Pressure	Mother
Heart Disease	Mother
Mental Problems	
Suicide	
Stroke	Grandmother
Alcoholism	
Rheumatic Fever	

II. HOSPITALIZATIONS, SURGERIES, INJURIES

Please list all times you have been hospitalized, operated on, or seriously injured.

Year	Operation, Illness, Injury	Hospital and City
1990	Appendix removed	LA CA

III. ILLNESS AND MEDICAL PROBLEMS

Please mark with an (X) any of the following illnesses and medical problems you have or have had and indicate the year when each started. If you are not certain when an illness started, write down an approximate year.

Illness	(x)	(Year)	Illness	(x)	(Year)
Eye or eye lid infection			Hernia		
Glaucoma			Hemorrhoids		
Other eye problems			Kidney or bladder disease		
Ear trouble			Prostate problem (male only)		
Deafness or decreased hearing			Mental problems		
Thyroid trouble			Headaches		
Strep throat			Head injury		
Bronchitis			Stroke		
Emphysema			Convulsions, seizures		
Pneumonia			Arthritis		
Allergies, asthma or hay fever			Gout		
Tuberculosis			Cancer or tumor		
Other lung problems			Bleeding tendency		
High blood pressure			Diabetes		
Heart attack			Measles/Rubeola		
High cholesterol			German measles/Rubella		
Arteriosclerosis (Hardening of arteries)			Polio		
Heart murmur			Mumps		
Other heart condition			Scarlet fever		
Stomach/duodenal ulcer			Chicken pox		
Diverticulosis			Mononucleosis		
Colitis			Eczema		
Other bowel problems			Psoriasis		
Hepatitis			Venereal disease		
Liver trouble			Genital herpes		
Gallbladder trouble			HIV test		
			AIDS		

CONFIDENTIAL

Page 2

To Order Call:800-BIBBERO (800 242-2376) Or Fax: (800 242-9330)

STOCK NO. 19-742-4 8/95

Health history questionnaire—cont'd

Chapter 11 Quiz

Name: ____________________

1. List two activities that should take place before the patient arrives.

   a. ____________________

   b. ____________________

2. __________ spelling of patient names may help with pronunciation.

3. True or False: After pulling the charts for the day, they should be arranged alphabetically. __________

4. What are the disadvantages to offering coffee or water to patients while they are waiting?

   ____

   ____

5. A registration form helps collect current __________ information.

6. What are the effective ways to deal with a talkative patient who has been known to take up a lot of the doctor's time?

   ____

   ____

7. List three routine tasks that are done before closing the office.

   a. ____________________

   b. ____________________

   c. ____________________

8. Describe how to ask for payment before the patient leaves the office.

   ____

   ____

9. What instructions do you give a patient about disrobing in the exam room?

   ____

   ____

10. List two of the essentials of an adequate waiting area.

    a. ____________________

    b. ____________________

Chapter 12 Quiz

Name: ______________________________

1. A durable formal paper used for office documents is called bond.

2. COD stands for cash on delivirg.

3. Domestic mail is sent within the US borders.

4. Define portfolio.
pictures drawing documents in book or folder form.

5. A ream of paper usually contains 500 sheets.

6. A watermark is a marking in a paper that is visible when held up to the light.

7. The process of making notes of explanation is annotating.

8. The second page of a letter is the continuation page.

CHAPTER 13

Medical Records Management

Part I. Vocabulary

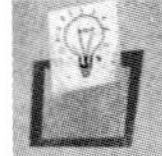

Directions: Insert the correct vocabulary word.

1. ________________ Systems made up of combinations of letters and numbers.
2. ________________ A formal examination of an organization's or individual's accounts or financial situation; a methodical examination and review.
3. ________________ To make greater, more numerous, larger, or more intense.
4. ________________ A heading, title, or subtitle under which records are filed.
5. ________________ Of, relating to, or arranged in or according to the order of time.
6. ________________ The act or manner of uttering words to be transcribed.
7. ________________ ________________ ________________ A filing system in which materials can be located without consulting an intermediary source of reference.
8. ________________ ________________ ________________ A filing system in which an intermediary source of reference, such as a card file, must be consulted to locate specific files.
9. ________________ A film bearing a photographic record on a reduced scale of printed or other graphic matter.
10. ________________ Information that is gathered by watching or observing a patient.
11. ________________ A method of filing whereby one report is laid on top of the older report, resembling the shingles of a roof.
12. ________________ Information that is gained by questioning the patient or taken from a form.
13. ________________ A chronological file used as a reminder that something must be taken care of on a certain date.
14. ________________ To make a written copy of, either in longhand or by machine.

Part II.

A. **Directions:** Indicate where you would look for information on the following patients.

1. Veronica Marcengill ____________________
2. Jennings Carter ____________________
3. Madison Jennings ____________________
4. Mary Lismore-Golden ____________________

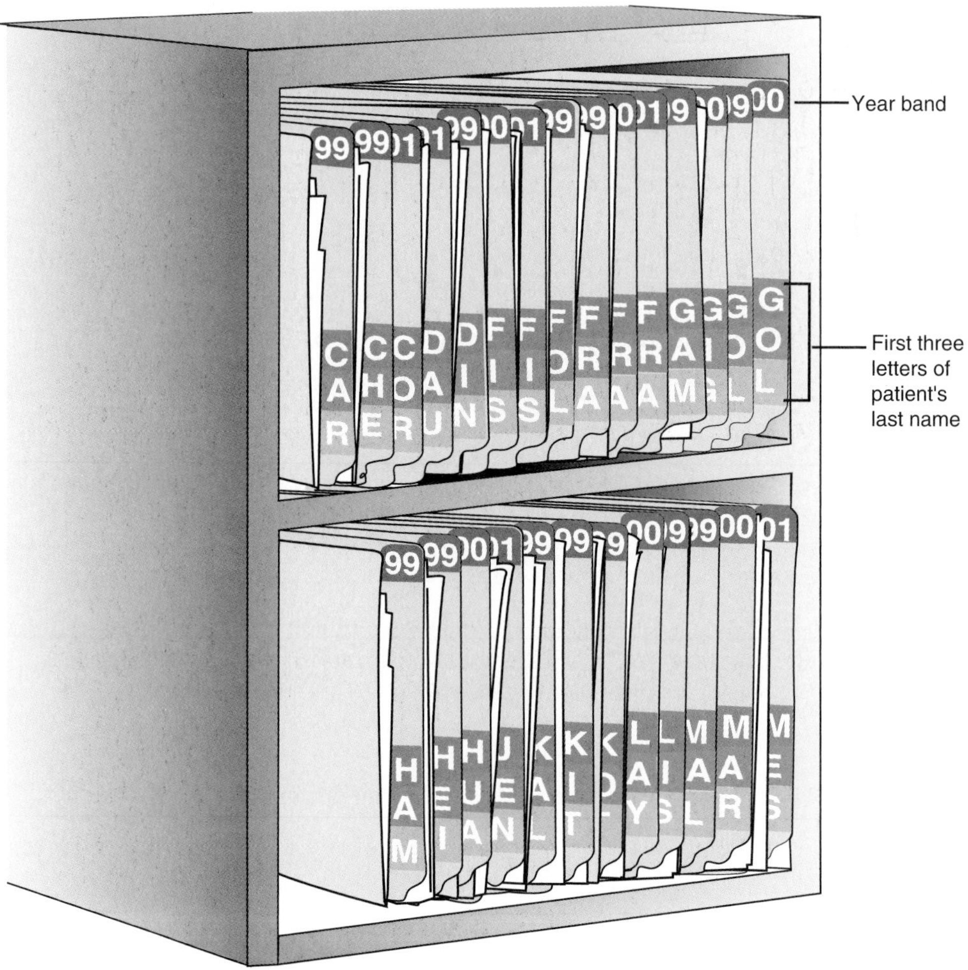

B. Indicate where you would file the records for the following patients.

1. Mary Smith ______________________________

2. Mike Smith ______________________________

3. Ann Davis-Adams ______________________________

4. Joe Brown, Jr. ______________________________

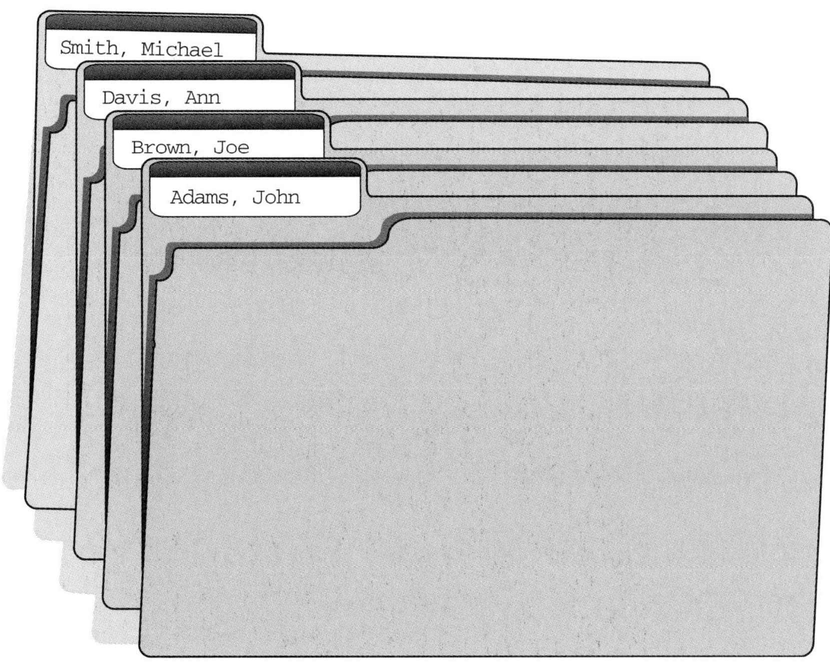

File folder labeling showing top tabs.

Part III. ______________________________

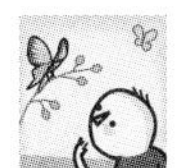

A. **Directions:** Examine the file folder on p. 88. What information is available on the folder? What is the major advantage of this filing system?

____

____

____

____

____

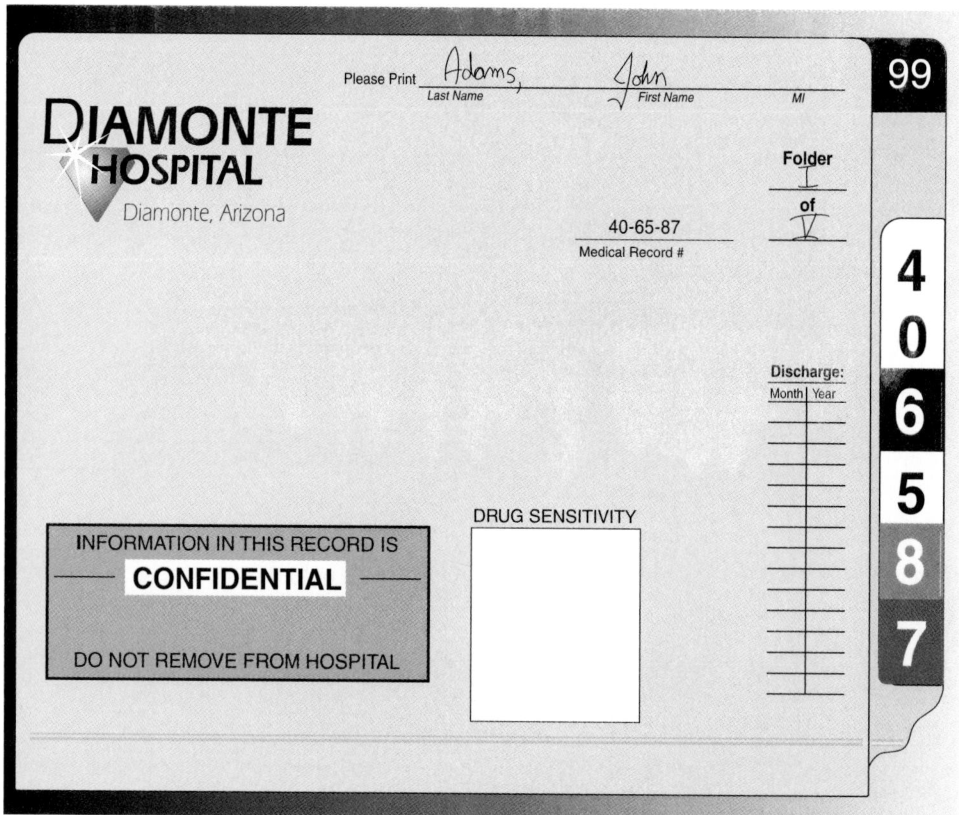

B. **Directions:** Label each type of filing system. What are some of the advantages and disadvantages?

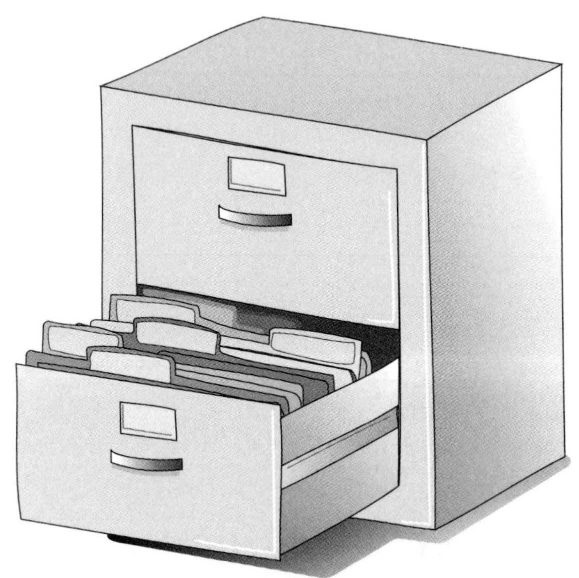

Type of system: ______________________________.

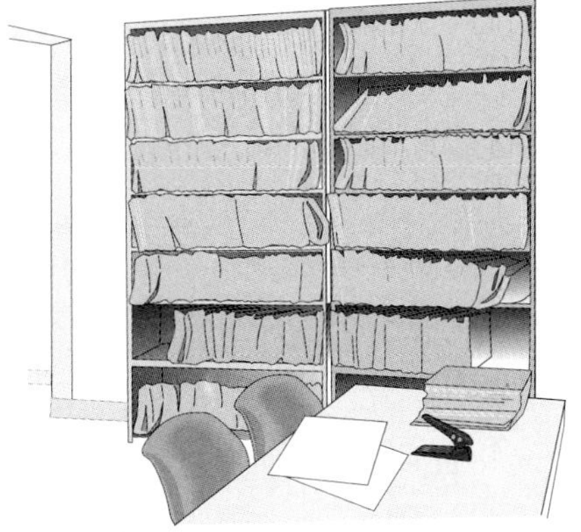

Type of system: ____.

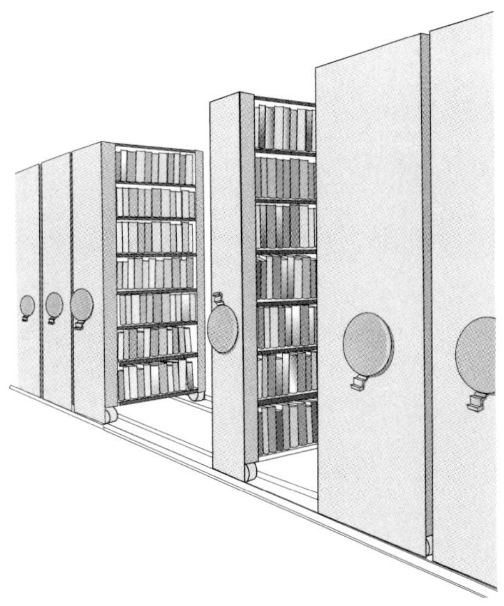

Type of system: ____.

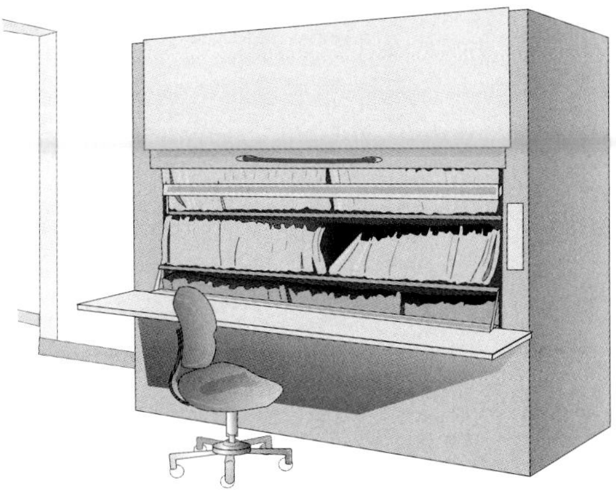

Type of system: ____.

Part IV. ______________________________

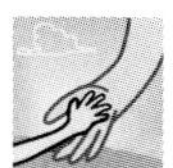

A. **Directions:** Research various information storage systems. Describe the information storage systems pictured below.

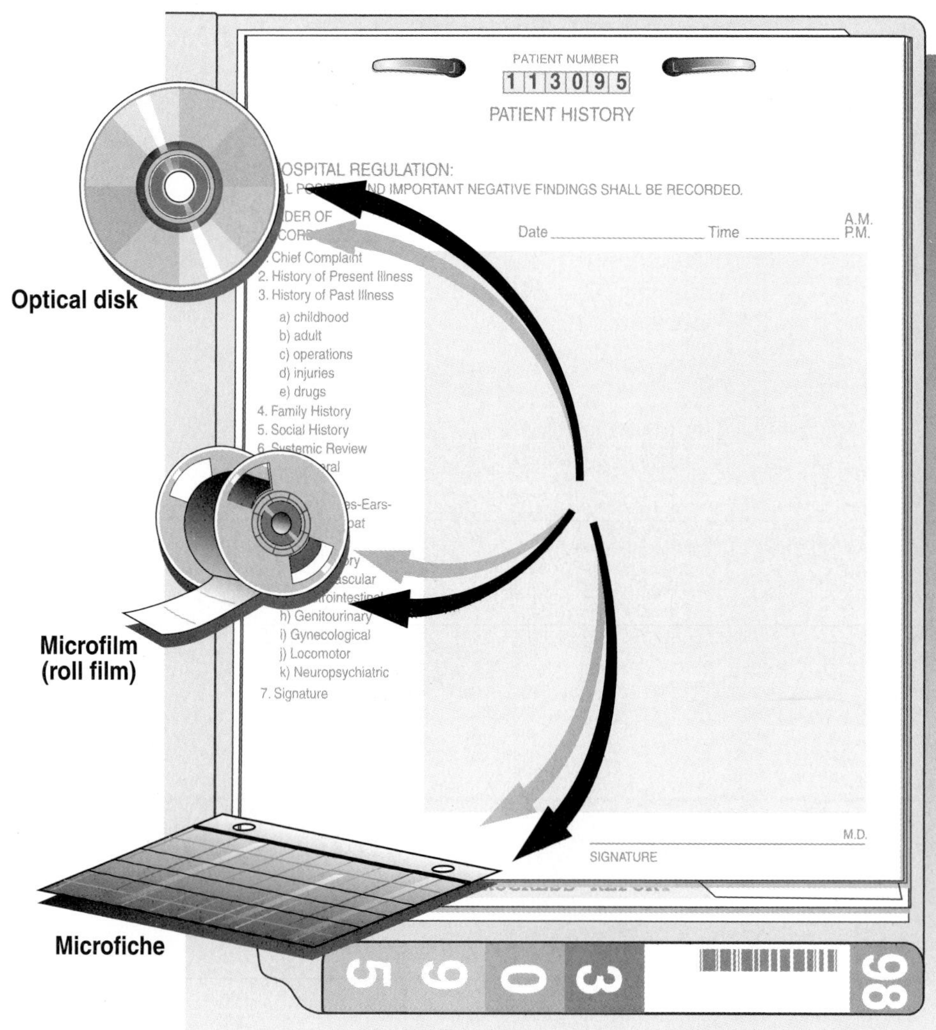

Disk: ______________________________

____

____

Microfilm: ______________________________

____

____

Microfiche: ______________________________

____

____

B. Identify the item in the picture below. What are the advantages of using this item?

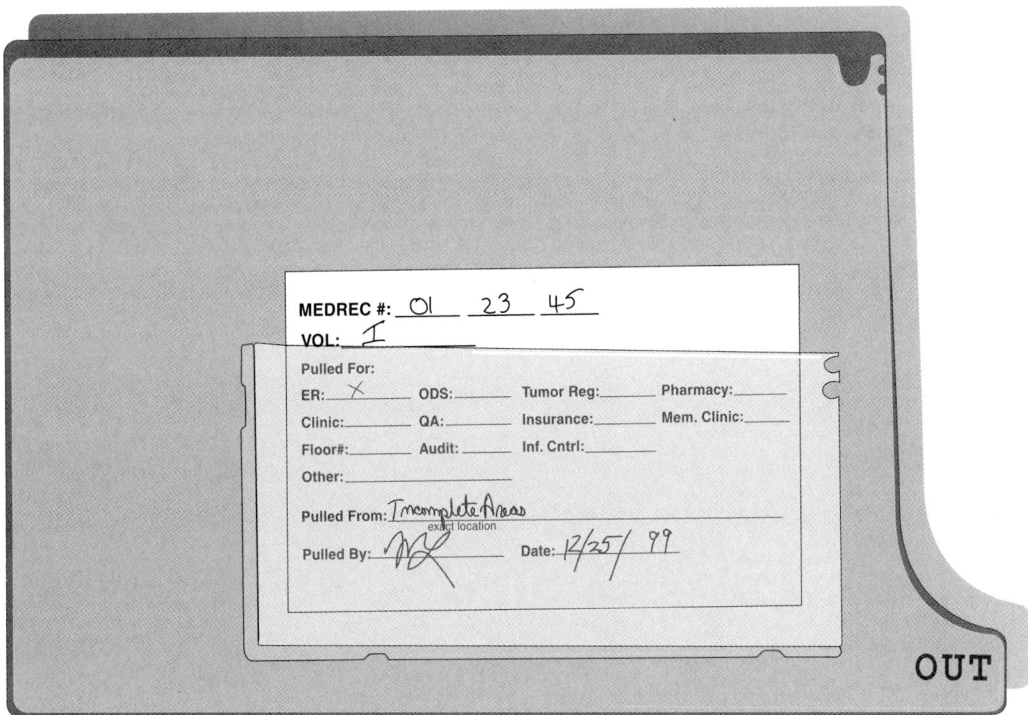

Chapter 13 Quiz

Name: ______________________________

1. List three classifications of files.

   a. ______________________

   b. ______________________

   c. ______________________

2. What information should be included on an outguide or OUTfolder?

   ____

   ____

3. What is the disadvantage of shelf filing systems?

   ____

   ____

4. True or False: Hyphenated elements of a name are treated as two separate units.

   ____

5. True or False: Numeric filing systems can be expanded without relocating all of the other files. ______________

6. Who owns a patient's medical record?

   ____

   ____

7. The process of recording something for transcription is called ____________ .

8. True or False: Wall files offer less privacy and security than other systems.

   ____

9. POMR stands for ________ ________ ________ ________ .

10. The process of writing or typing dictated material is called

    ______________________ .

Chapter 14 Quiz

Name: ____

1. A statement that shows finance charges is a ____________________.

2. What is a skip?

   ____

3. Name an advantage of small claims court.

   ____

   ____

4. True or False: Collection agencies can charge 40-60%. ____________

5. The total of all account balances that are due to the physician is called

   ____

   ____________________.

6. The pegboard is also called a

   ________ ________ ________.

7. What kind of balance occurs when an account is overpaid?

   ____

   ____

8. What is the term for the person who is responsible for a bill?

   ____

9. What is the name of the form that is attached to a chart and is used to help with charges?

   ____

10. UCR stands for

   ________ ________ ________.

CHAPTER 15

Basics of Diagnostic Coding

Part I.

Symbols, abbreviations, punctuation, and notations appear in the listings to serve as instructional notes. Understanding their meaning and using them for guidance are crucial to accurate coding.

Directions: Fill in the blanks with the appropriate vocabulary terms.

1. □ The ________________ symbol precedes a disease code to indicate that the content of a four-digit category has been moved or modified.
2. § This ________________ ________________ symbol is only used in the Tabular List of Diseases.
3. ● The ________________ symbol indicates a new entry.
4. ▲ The ________________ indicates a revision in the Tabular List of Diseases and a code change in the alphabetical index.
5. ▶◀ These symbols mark both the ________________ and ________________ of new or revised text.
6. ♀ ________________ diagnosis only.
7. ♂ ________________ diagnosis only.
8. √4th Code requires a ________________ digit.
9. √5th Code requires a ________________ digit.
10. [ ] ________________ are used to enclose synonyms, alternative wordings, or explanatory phrases.
11. ( ) ________________ are used to enclose supplementary words, which may be present or absent in the statement of a disease or procedure without affecting the code number to which it is assigned.
12. : A ________________ is used in the Tabular List of Diseases after an incomplete term that needs one or more of the modifiers that follow it to make the assignable to a given category.
13. { } ________________ enclose a series of terms, each of which is modified by the statement appearing to the right of the brace.

Part II.

Directions: Using this checklist, code the diagnoses listed below.

- Identify the key terms in the diagnostic statement, determining the main reason for the encounter.
- Locate the diagnosis in the alphabetic index (volume II).
- Read and understand any footnotes, symbols, or instructions following any cross-references.
- Locate the diagnosis in the Tabular List of Diseases.
- Read and understand the inclusions and exclusions.
- Make sure you include fourth and fifth digits when available, assigning to the highest level of specificity.
- Assign the code, until all diagnosis elements are identified.
- After assigning the code, double-check to ensure accurate transfer from the book to the patient form and subsequent data entry.
- Use the same process for secondary diagnoses and other conditions addressed during the encounter.

Diagnosis	International Classification of Diseases, Ninth Revision *(ICD-9)* Code
1. Polycystic kidney	
2. Amenorrhea	
3. Measles	
4. Hematuria	
5. Catatonic schizophrenia, chronic	
6. Cancer of the duodenum (neoplasm)	
7. Nodular tuberculosis (lung)	
8. High blood pressure	
9. Left-sided congestive heart failure	
10. Croup	
11. Ear wax	
12. Exophthalmos R/T thyroid	
13. Gout	
14. Active rickets	
15. Cat scratch fever	
16. Benign prostatic hypertrophy (enlarged prostate)	
17. Encephalitis from West Nile virus	
18. Thrush	
19. Parkinson's disease	

Diagnosis	International Classification of Diseases, Ninth Revision *(ICD-9)* Code
20. Senile cataract	
21. Huntington's chorea	
22. Mitral valve prolapse	
23. Transient ischemic attack	
24. Asthma	
25. Cushing's syndrome	

Diagnosis	V-Code
1. Ear piercing	
2. Gynecologic exam	
3. Annual physical	
4. Venereal disease exposure	
5. History of mental illness	

Situation	E-Code
1. Bathtub drowning	
2. Rattlesnake bite	
3. Sunstroke	
4. Pedestrian hit by a train	
5. Parachute failure	

Part III.

A. **Directions:** Fill in the blanks.

1. Volume I contains ________________ appendices and ________________ chapters.
2. ________________ is referred to as the *Tabular List of Diseases*.
3. Volume II contains an ________________ index of disease and injury.

B. **Directions:** Complete Box 21 of the Health Care Financing Administration (HCFA) 1500 form by writing in the *International Classification of Diseases, Ninth Revision* (*ICD-9*) codes that you found for Part II.

1. Gout and hypertension (code as primary)

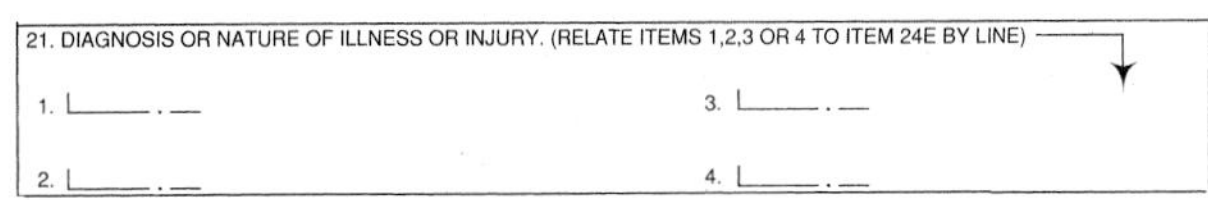
21. DIAGNOSIS OR NATURE OF ILLNESS OR INJURY. (RELATE ITEMS 1,2,3 OR 4 TO ITEM 24E BY LINE)

1. ____ . __ 3. ____ . __

2. ____ . __ 4. ____ . __

2. Croup and thrush

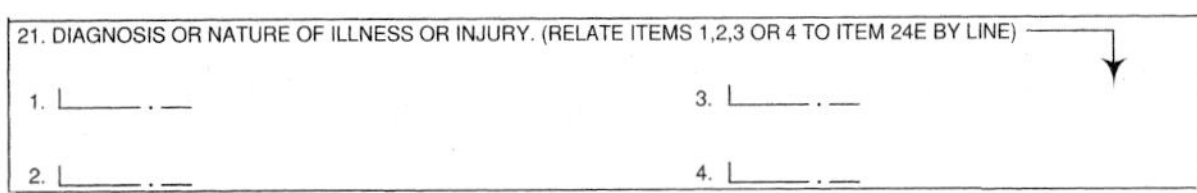
21. DIAGNOSIS OR NATURE OF ILLNESS OR INJURY. (RELATE ITEMS 1,2,3 OR 4 TO ITEM 24E BY LINE)

1. ____ . __ 3. ____ . __

2. ____ . __ 4. ____ . __

3. Hematuria and benign prostatic hypertrophy (code as primary)

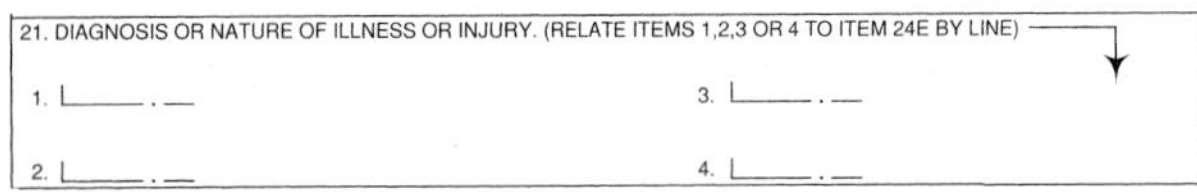
21. DIAGNOSIS OR NATURE OF ILLNESS OR INJURY. (RELATE ITEMS 1,2,3 OR 4 TO ITEM 24E BY LINE)

1. ____ . __ 3. ____ . __

2. ____ . __ 4. ____ . __

4. Left-sided congestive heart failure and gout

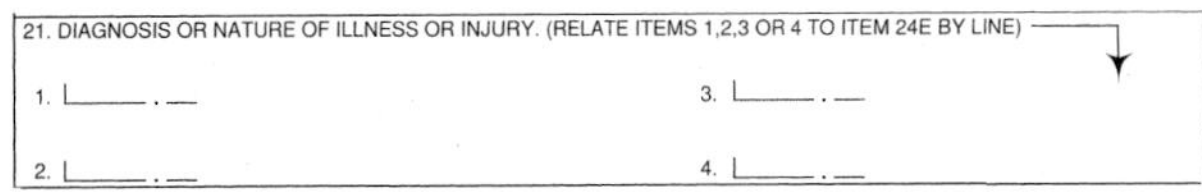
21. DIAGNOSIS OR NATURE OF ILLNESS OR INJURY. (RELATE ITEMS 1,2,3 OR 4 TO ITEM 24E BY LINE)

1. ____ . __ 3. ____ . __

2. ____ . __ 4. ____ . __

Part IV.

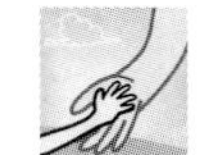

A. Why would an *ICD-9* coding book be a good reference tool for a medical transcriptionist?

____

____

____

____

B. Indicate which statements are true (T) and which statements are false (F).

1. _____ Documentation regarding preexisting condition is required.
2. _____ Conditions described as "rule out," "suspected," "probable," or "questionable" should be coded.
3. _____ It is okay to substitute another *ICD-9* code if a patient requests that a diagnosis other than the correct or appropriate diagnosis be used for the visit because that patient's insurance company will not reimburse for the actual diagnosis.
4. _____ You have a legal and ethical responsibility to code the diagnosis correctly.
5. _____ If no definitive diagnosis is made, the symptoms should be coded.

Chapter 15 Quiz

Name: ____

1. True or False: The tabular list contains the codes, categories, and subcategories.

   ____

2. True or False: Volume 2 serves as an index. ______________________

3. V-codes are used for

   ____

   ____

4. E-codes are used for

   ____

   ____

5. NOS is used for ______________ diagnoses.

6. A condition that was present before a person was included is called

   ______________________________.

7. ______________ are conditions that occur together and lengthen a hospital stay.

8. A condition that arises during a hospital stay is called a

   ______________________________.

9. Services that support a patient diagnosis such as labs and x-rays are

   ______________ ______________

   ______________________________.

10. A condition that is determined to be responsible for an admission to the hospital is called

    ______________ ______________.

CHAPTER 16

Basics of Procedural Coding

Part I. Vocabulary

Directions: Fill in the blanks with the appropriate vocabulary terms.

A. *Current Procedural Terminology (CPT)* was first published in ________________ by the American Medical Association (AMA). It was based on the California Relative Value Study, developed by the California Medical Society. Its primary purpose was to simplify the reporting of ________________ and/or ________________ provided by physicians.

B. 1992 marked the most significant change to *CPT,* with the replacement of the office and hospital visit codes with the ________________ (E&M) codes, identifying key elements to be documented in the medical record.

C. *CPT* has been revised three times, and the edition in current use is ________________.

D. *CPT* is updated every ________________ by the AMA and published for the next calendar year.

E. ________________ codes describe procedures or services that are grouped together and paid as one. An example would be code 90700 for a Diphtheria, Tetanus, and Pertussis vaccine for intramuscular use.

F. ________________ codes means reporting the components of a procedure separately. In the example above (code 90700), if you report the three vaccines separately, it gives the impression that three injections, and not one, were given.

G. ________________ is a deliberate increase in a *CPT* code to receive higher reimbursements. This is a target of Centers for Medicare & Medicaid Services (CMS) investigations and should never be done.

H. ________________ is usually done by insurance companies for several reasons, either when one coding system is converted to another or if, on review, the examiner believes the documentation does not match the code description.

Part II.

Directions: Use these steps in *CPT* coding to find the following codes.

- Know your *CPT* code book: changes are made each year, so even if you have been coding for years, you need to read the introduction, guidelines, and notes.
- Review all services and procedures performed on the day of the encounter; include all medications administered and trays and equipment used.
- Find the procedures and/or services in the index in the back of the *CPT* book. This will direct you to a code (not a page number). The code you are looking for may be listed as a procedure, body system, service, or abbreviation (which will usually refer you to the full spelling).

- Read the description in the code and also any related descriptions that follow a semicolon; this will lead you to the most accurate code.
- If the service is an Evaluation and Management code do the following:

  Determine whether the person is a new or established patient.

  Determine whether this is a consultation.

  Indicate where the service was performed.

  Review the documentation to determine the level of service.

  Check to see whether there is a reason to use a modifier.

  Assign the five-digit *CPT* code.

Procedure	*CPT* Code
1. Liver biopsy, needle	
2. Cholecystectomy	
3. Newborn circumcision	
4. Gastric motility study	
5. Right heart catheterization	
6. Intradermal allergy testing	
7. Removal of foreign body from nose	
8. X-ray examination of ankle, three views	
9. Computed axial tomography (CAT) scan of arm with contrast	
10. Partial thromboplastin time (PTT)	

Find the Appropriate Modifier	Modifier
1. Bilateral	
2. Two surgeons	
3. Repeat procedure same surgeon	
4. Multiple procedures	

Part III. ____________________

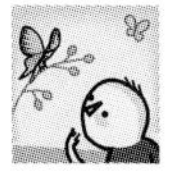

A. Symbols appear in the listings to serve as instructional notes. Understanding their meaning and using them for guidance are crucial to accurate coding.

Directions: Describe each symbol.

1. ● ______________ procedure

2. ▲ code ______________

3. + *CPT* ________________ codes

4. Ø exempt from the use of ________________ –51

5. ▶◀ revised ________________, cross-________________ and explanations

6. → with a circle around it, which refers to *CPT* ________________

7. * ________________ procedure only

B. **Directions:** Look at a *CPT* book and list the sections.

1. ________________
2. ________________
3. ________________
4. ________________
5. ________________

Part IV. ________________

A. What three things must you know before assigning an E&M code?

1. ________________
2. ________________
3. ________________

B. Name the four levels of histories.

1. ________________
2. ________________
3. ________________
4. ________________

C. List the four levels of decision making.

1. ________________
2. ________________
3. ________________
4. ________________

D. Insert the appropriate E&M code in Box 24 of the Health Care Financing Administration (HCFA) 1500 form and relate it to the matching diagnosis in Box 21. Indicate the relationship in column E of Box 24.

1. New patient, comprehensive exam and history, 45 minutes, *International Classification of Diseases, Ninth Revision* (*ICD-9*) code for physical exam V70.0 and use 11 (doctor's office) for place of service in column B.

21. DIAGNOSIS OR NATURE OF ILLNESS OR INJURY. (RELATE ITEMS 1,2,3 OR 4 TO ITEM 24E BY LINE)

1. ___ . __   3. ___ . __

2. ___ . __   4. ___ . __

24.	A DATE(S) OF SERVICE From MM DD YY	To MM DD YY	B Place of Service	C Type of Service	D PROCEDURES, SERVICES, OR SUPPLIES (Explain Unusual Circumstances) CPT/HCPCS	MODIFIER	E DIAGNOSIS CODE	F $ CHARGES	G DAYS OR UNITS	H EPSDT Family Plan	I EMG	J COB	K RESERVED FOR LOCAL USE
1													
2													
3													
4													
5													
6													

2. Established patient, problem-focused exam and history, 10 minutes, *ICD-9* code for anemia is 281.9 and use 11 (doctor's office) for place of service in column B.

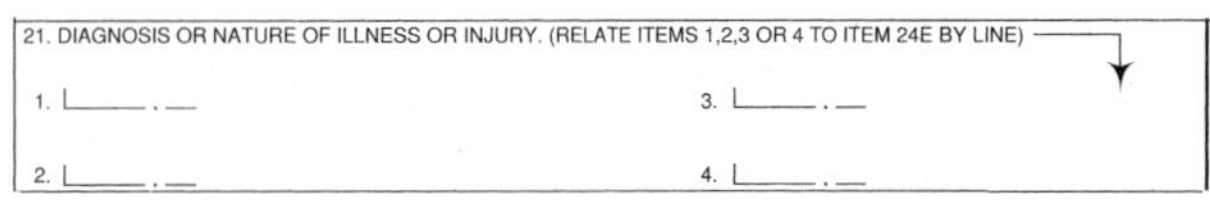
21. DIAGNOSIS OR NATURE OF ILLNESS OR INJURY. (RELATE ITEMS 1,2,3 OR 4 TO ITEM 24E BY LINE)

1. ____ . __ 3. ____ . __

2. ____ . __ 4. ____ . __

24.	A DATE(S) OF SERVICE From MM DD YY	To MM DD YY	B Place of Service	C Type of Service	D PROCEDURES, SERVICES, OR SUPPLIES (Explain Unusual Circumstances) CPT/HCPCS	MODIFIER	E DIAGNOSIS CODE	F $ CHARGES	G DAYS OR UNITS	H EPSDT Family Plan	I EMG	J COB	K RESERVED FOR LOCAL USE
1													
2													
3													
4													
5													
6													

3. Established patient, detailed exam and history, 25 minutes, *ICD-9* code for cervical cancer is 180.9. She also has anxiety, which is a secondary diagnosis of 308.3. A Papanicolaou smear *CPT* 88141 is performed. Use 11 (doctor's office) for place of service in column B.

21. DIAGNOSIS OR NATURE OF ILLNESS OR INJURY. (RELATE ITEMS 1,2,3 OR 4 TO ITEM 24E BY LINE)

1. ____ . __ 3. ____ . __

2. ____ . __ 4. ____ . __

24.	A DATE(S) OF SERVICE From MM DD YY	To MM DD YY	B Place of Service	C Type of Service	D PROCEDURES, SERVICES, OR SUPPLIES (Explain Unusual Circumstances) CPT/HCPCS	MODIFIER	E DIAGNOSIS CODE	F $ CHARGES	G DAYS OR UNITS	H EPSDT Family Plan	I EMG	J COB	K RESERVED FOR LOCAL USE
1													
2													
3													
4													
5													
6													

Chapter 16 Quiz

Name: ______________________________

1. True or False: The E&M code can be used for the doctor's exam.

   ____

2. The place of service code for an office is

   ______________________________ .

3. The levels of medical decision making are:

   ____

   ____

   ____

4. The types of histories are:

   ____

   ____

   ____

5. The place of service code for inpatient hospital is ______________________ .

6. CPT stands for ______________________

   ______________ ______________ .

7. Procedures and services grouped together and paid as one are called

   ______________________________ .

8. An addition to a CPT code is a

   ______________________________ .

9. The relative incidence of a disease is called

   ______________________________ .

10. The incidence of death from a disease is

    ______________________________ .

CHAPTER 17

The Health Insurance Claim Form

Part I.

List some of the advantages and disadvantages of paper claims.

1. ________________________________
2. ________________________________
3. ________________________________
4. ________________________________

List some of the advantages and disadvantages of electronic claims.

1. ________________________________
2. ________________________________
3. ________________________________
4. ________________________________

Part II.

A. **Directions:** Use the information included in this chapter to complete a registration form for a patient who was referred by Dr. Mills.

REGISTRATION
(PLEASE PRINT)

Home Phone: ________________ Today's Date: ____________

PATIENT INFORMATION

Name ________________________________ Soc. Sec.# ____________
Last Name First Name Initial

Address ________________________________

City ____________________ State ____________ Zip ____________

Single ___ Married ___ Widowed ___ Separated ___ Divorced ___ Sex M___ F___ Age ___ Birthdate ____________

Patient Employed by ________________________ Occupation ____________

Business Address ________________________ Business Phone ____________

By whom were you referred? ________________________________

In case of emergency who should be notified? ________________________ Phone ____________
Last Name Relationship to Patient

PRIMARY INSURANCE

Person Responsible for Account ________________________________
Last Name First Name Initial

Relation to Patient ____________ Birthdate ____________ Soc. Sec.# ____________

Address (if different from patient's) ________________________ Phone ____________

City ____________________ State ____________ Zip ____________

Person Responsible Employed by ________________________ Occupation ____________

Business Address ________________________ Business Phone ____________

Insurance Company ________________________________

Contract # ____________ Group # ____________ Subscriber # ____________

Name of other dependents covered under this plan ________________________

ADDITIONAL INSURANCE

Is patient covered by additional insurance? ___Yes ___ No

Subscriber Name ____________ Relationship to Patient ____________ Birthdate ____________

Address (if different from patient's) ________________________ Phone ____________

City ____________________ State ____________ Zip ____________

Subscriber Employed by ________________________ Business Phone ____________

Insurance Company ________________________________

Contract # ____________ Group # ____________ Subscriber # ____________

Name of other dependents covered under this plan ________________________

ASSIGNMENT AND RELEASE

I, the undersigned, certify that I (or my dependent) have insurance coverage with ________________________
Name of Insurance Company(ies)

and assign directly to Dr. ____________ insurance benefits, if any, otherwise payable to me for services rendered. I understand that I am financially responsible for all charges whether or not paid by insurance. I hereby authorize the doctor to release all information necessary to secure the payment of benefits. I authorize the use of this signature on all insurance submissions.

________________ ________________ ________________
Responsible Party Signature Relationship Date

ORDER# 58-8426 • © 1996 BIBBERO SYSTEMS, INC. • PETALUMA, CALIFORNIA • TO REORDER CALL TOLL FREE: (800) 242-9330

Sample registration form.

B. **Directions:** Complete as many boxes as you can by using the following information. Indicate who may sign the various signature boxes.

John M. Smith, Father, DOB 10-25-67 ID#123456789 Mary L. Smith, Mother, DOB 9-29-69 ID#987654321 Levi Smith, Patient, DOB 9-11-96, male	Blackburn Realty (Acme Insurance Group #12345) Diamonte Hospital (BCBS Insurance Group #5432) Child (student) Blackburn Middle School Child is insured by both parents. Mom's insurance is primary because of her birth month.
Date of Illness 4-15-20XX Similar illness last month 3-12-20XX Diagnosis Croup 464.4 Office Visit Established Patient, 15 min 99213, $86 Referred by Dr. Fred Mills ID#123-6543-8761	Patient Address: 408 West View Road Blackburn, IL 123456 (123) 555-5432

1. MEDICARE (Medicare #) ☐ MEDICAID (Medicaid #) ☐ CHAMPUS (Sponsor's SSN) ☐ CHAMPVA (VA File #) ☐ GROUP HEALTH PLAN (SSN or ID) ☐ FECA BLK LUNG (SSN) ☐ OTHER (ID) ☐

1a. INSURED'S I.D. NUMBER (FOR PROGRAM IN ITEM 1)

2. PATIENT'S NAME (Last Name, First Name, Middle Initial)

3. PATIENT'S BIRTH DATE MM | DD | YY   SEX M ☐ F ☐

4. INSURED'S NAME (Last Name, First Name, Middle Initial)

5. PATIENT'S ADDRESS (No., Street)
CITY | STATE
ZIP CODE | TELEPHONE (Include Area Code) ( )

6. PATIENT RELATIONSHIP TO INSURED
Self ☐ Spouse ☐ Child ☐ Other ☐

7. INSURED'S ADDRESS (No., Street)
CITY | STATE
ZIP CODE | TELEPHONE (INCLUDE AREA CODE) ( )

8. PATIENT STATUS
Single ☐ Married ☐ Other ☐
Employed ☐ Full-Time Student ☐ Part-Time Student ☐

9. OTHER INSURED'S NAME (Last Name, First Name, Middle Initial)

a. OTHER INSURED'S POLICY OR GROUP NUMBER

b. OTHER INSURED'S DATE OF BIRTH MM | DD | YY SEX M ☐ F ☐

c. EMPLOYER'S NAME OR SCHOOL NAME

d. INSURANCE PLAN NAME OR PROGRAM NAME

10. IS PATIENT'S CONDITION RELATED TO:

a. EMPLOYMENT? (CURRENT OR PREVIOUS)

☐ YES ☐ NO

b. AUTO ACCIDENT? PLACE (State)

☐ YES ☐ NO

c. OTHER ACCIDENT?

☐ YES ☐ NO

11. INSURED'S POLICY GROUP OR FECA NUMBER

a. INSURED'S DATE OF BIRTH MM | DD | YY SEX M ☐ F ☐

b. EMPLOYER'S NAME OR SCHOOL NAME

c. INSURANCE PLAN NAME OR PROGRAM NAME

d. IS THERE ANOTHER HEALTH BENEFIT PLAN?

☐ YES ☐ NO ***If yes***, return to and complete item 9 a-d.

READ BACK OF FORM BEFORE COMPLETING & SIGNING THIS FORM.

12. PATIENT'S OR AUTHORIZED PERSON'S SIGNATURE I authorize the release of any medical or other information necessary to process this claim. I also request payment of government benefits either to myself or to the party who accepts assignment below.

SIGNED ____________ DATE ____________

13. INSURED'S OR AUTHORIZED PERSON'S SIGNATURE I authorize payment of medical benefits to the undersigned physician or supplier for services described below.

SIGNED ____________

14. DATE OF CURRENT: MM | DD | YY ◀ ILLNESS (First symptom) OR INJURY (Accident) OR PREGNANCY(LMP)

15. IF PATIENT HAS HAD SAME OR SIMILAR ILLNESS. GIVE FIRST DATE MM | DD | YY

16. DATES PATIENT UNABLE TO WORK IN CURRENT OCCUPATION FROM MM | DD | YY TO MM | DD | YY

17. NAME OF REFERRING PHYSICIAN OR OTHER SOURCE

17a. I.D. NUMBER OF REFERRING PHYSICIAN

21. DIAGNOSIS OR NATURE OF ILLNESS OR INJURY. (RELATE ITEMS 1,2,3 OR 4 TO ITEM 24E BY LINE)

1. ___ . __

3. ___ . __

2. ___ . __

4. ___ . __

24. A DATE(S) OF SERVICE From MM	DD	YY	To MM	DD	YY	B Place of Service	C Type of Service	D PROCEDURES, SERVICES, OR SUPPLIES (Explain Unusual Circumstances) CPT/HCPCS	MODIFIER	E DIAGNOSIS CODE	F $ CHARGES	G DAYS OR UNITS	H EPSDT Family Plan	I EMG	J COB	K RESERVED FOR LOCAL USE
1																
2																
3																
4																
5																
6																

Part III.

Directions: Use the insurance log to answer the following questions.

1. For how many visits was Terry Holmes charged? ______
2. How much did the patient pay on the second visit? ______
3. How much did insurance pay for the first visit? ______
4. What was the patient's balance after insurance paid for the second visit? ______
5. How much did insurance pay for the last visit? ______
6. What does the patient need to be reimbursed? ______

General Physicians, Inc.
5515 Lake Dr.
Chicago, IL 00000

INSURANCE LOG

Patient's Name	Date of Service	Fee	Amt. Paid	Insurance Reimbursements Date	Amount	Amt. Due from Patient	Date	Amt. Reimbursed to Patient	Date	Current Balance
Terry Holmes	2/5/03	$85	0	3/15/03	$75	$10	3/15			
	2/17/03	$30	30	3/30/03	$25	$5	3/30			
	3/24/03	$65	40	4/15/03	$32			$22	5/25/03	0

Insurance log.

Part IV.

Complete a Health Care Financing Administration (HCFA) 1500 form below for yourself using your own address and insurance information. Use Diagnosis V70.0, E&M Code 99213, and $65 for charges.

PLEASE DO NOT STAPLE IN THIS AREA

CARRIER

PICA

HEALTH INSURANCE CLAIM FORM

PICA

1. MEDICARE (Medicare #) MEDICAID (Medicaid #) CHAMPUS (SponsorÕs SSN) CHAMPVA (VA File #) GROUP HEALTH PLAN (SSN or ID) FECA BLK LUNG (SN) OTHER (ID)

1a. INSURED'S I.D. NUMBER (FOR PROGRAM IN ITEM 1)

2. PATIENT'S NAME (Last Name, First Name, Middle Initial)

3. PATIENT'S BIRTH DATE MM DD YY SEX M F

4. INSURED'S NAME (Last Name, First Name, Middle Initial)

5. PATIENT'S ADDRESS (No., Street)

6. PATIENT RELATIONSHIP TO INSURED Self Spouse Child Other

7. INSURED'S ADDRESS (No., Street)

CITY STATE

8. PATIENT STATUS Single Married Other; Employed Full-Time Student Part-Time Student

CITY STATE

ZIP CODE TELEPHONE (Include Area Code) ( )

ZIP CODE TELEPHONE (INCLUDE AREA CODE) ( )

9. OTHER INSURED'S NAME (Last Name, First Name, Middle Initial)

10. IS PATIENT'S CONDITION RELATED TO:

11. INSURED'S POLICY GROUP OR FECA NUMBER

a. OTHER INSURED'S POLICY OR GROUP NUMBER

a. EMPLOYMENT? (CURRENT OR PREVIOUS) YES NO

a. INSURED'S DATE OF BIRTH MM DD YY SEX M F

b. OTHER INSURED'S DATE OF BIRTH MM DD YY SEX M F

b. AUTO ACCIDENT? PLACE (State) YES NO

b. EMPLOYER'S NAME OR SCHOOL NAME

c. EMPLOYER'S NAME OR SCHOOL NAME

c. OTHER ACCIDENT? YES NO

c. INSURANCE PLAN NAME OR PROGRAM NAME

d. INSURANCE PLAN NAME OR PROGRAM NAME

10d. RESERVED FOR LOCAL USE

d. IS THERE ANOTHER HEALTH BENEFIT PLAN? YES NO *If yes*, return to and complete item 9 a-d.

READ BACK OF FORM BEFORE COMPLETING & SIGNING THIS FORM.

12. PATIENT'S OR AUTHORIZED PERSON'S SIGNATURE I authorize the release of any medical or other information necessary to process this claim. I also request payment of government benefits either to myself or to the party who accepts assignment below.

SIGNED DATE

13. INSURED'S OR AUTHORIZED PERSON'S SIGNATURE I authorize payment of medical benefits to the undersigned physician or supplier for services described below.

SIGNED

PATIENT AND INSURED INFORMATION

14. DATE OF CURRENT: MM DD YY ILLNESS (First symptom) OR INJURY (Accident) OR PREGNANCY(LMP)

15. IF PATIENT HAS HAD SAME OR SIMILAR ILLNESS. GIVE FIRST DATE MM DD YY

16. DATES PATIENT UNABLE TO WORK IN CURRENT OCCUPATION MM DD YY FROM MM DD YY TO

17. NAME OF REFERRING PHYSICIAN OR OTHER SOURCE

17a. I.D. NUMBER OF REFERRING PHYSICIAN

18. HOSPITALIZATION DATES RELATED TO CURRENT SERVICES MM DD YY FROM MM DD YY TO

19. RESERVED FOR LOCAL USE

20. OUTSIDE LAB? YES NO $ CHARGES

21. DIAGNOSIS OR NATURE OF ILLNESS OR INJURY. (RELATE ITEMS 1,2,3 OR 4 TO ITEM 24E BY LINE)

1. ___ . __
2. ___ . __
3. ___ . __
4. ___ . __

22. MEDICAID RESUBMISSION CODE ORIGINAL REF. NO.

23. PRIOR AUTHORIZATION NUMBER

24. A DATE(S) OF SERVICE From MM DD YY To MM DD YY	B Place of Service	C Type of Service	D PROCEDURES, SERVICES, OR SUPPLIES (Explain Unusual Circumstances) CPT/HCPCS MODIFIER	E DIAGNOSIS CODE	F $ CHARGES	G DAYS OR UNITS	H EPSDT Family Plan	I EMG	J COB	K RESERVED FOR LOCAL USE
1										
2										
3										
4										
5										
6										

25. FEDERAL TAX I.D. NUMBER SSN EIN

26. PATIENT'S ACCOUNT NO.

27. ACCEPT ASSIGNMENT? (For govt. claims, see back) YES NO

28. TOTAL CHARGE $

29. AMOUNT PAID $

30. BALANCE DUE $

31. SIGNATURE OF PHYSICIAN OR SUPPLIER INCLUDING DEGREES OR CREDENTIALS (I certify that the statements on the reverse apply to this bill and are made a part thereof.)

SIGNED DATE

32. NAME AND ADDRESS OF FACILITY WHERE SERVICES WERE RENDERED (If other than home or office)

33. PHYSICIAN'S, SUPPLIER'S BILLING NAME, ADDRESS, ZIP CODE & PHONE #

PIN# GRP#

PHYSICIAN OR SUPPLIER INFORMATION

(APPROVED BY AMA COUNCIL ON MEDICAL SERVICE 8/88) **PLEASE PRINT OR TYPE** APPROVED OMB-0938-0008 FORM CMS-1500 (12-90), FORM RRB-1500, APPROVED OMB-1215-0055 FORM OWCP-1500, APPROVED OMB-0720-0001 (CHAMPUS)

Chapter 17 Quiz

Name: ______________________________

1. True or False: ICD-9 codes are not needed for the CMS 1500.

   ____

2. OCR stands for ______________ ______________ recognition.

3. A claim filed without any omissions or errors is called a __________ claim.

4. The point of service code for a doctor's office is ______________ .

5. The point of service code for inpatient hospitalization is ____________ .

6. The HCFA 1500 form is now called a ______________________ .

7. Giving permission for the doctor's office to receive payment from an insurance company is called ______________________ __________ __________ .

8. The ____________ is entitled to receive benefits from an insurance policy.

9. The company that assumes the risk of an insurance policy is the ______________________ .

10. PIN stands for ____________ ____________ number.

CHAPTER 18

Third-Party Reimbursement

Part I.

Directions: Define the following insurance terms in your own words.

1. allowed charge

2. authorization

3. benefits

4. birthday rule

5. coordination of benefits

6. copayment

7. deductible

8. government plan

9. group policy

10. health insurance

11. HMO

12. indemnity plan

13. individual policy

14. managed care

15. medical savings account

16. medically indigent

17. medically necessary

18. participating provider

19. policyholder

20. primary diagnosis

21. principal diagnosis

22. premium

23. RBRVS

24. rider

25. self-insured plans

26. service benefit plan

27. workers' compensation

28. utilization review

Part II.

A. Name five different types of health insurance plans.

1.
2.
3.
4.
5.

B. Name seven different types of insurance benefits.

1. ______
2. ______
3. ______
4. ______
5. ______
6. ______
7. ______

Part III.

A. List the advantages of managed care.

1. ______
2. ______
3. ______
4. ______
5. ______

B. List the disadvantages of managed care.

1. ______
2. ______
3. ______
4. ______
5. ______

Part IV.

Discussion Questions

Directions: Answer the following questions. Be prepared to discuss your answers with your classmates.

1. What is the difference between Medicare and Medicaid?

2. How do CHAMPUS, CHAMPVA, and TRICARE differ?

3. What is the difference between Medicare Part A and Medicare Part B?

4. What is the difference between an HMO and a PPO?

5. What is workers' compensation?

Chapter 18 Quiz

Name: ____

1. True or False: Coordination of benefits is when two insurance policies pay for the applicable portions of the same service.

   ____

2. A ____________ ____________ account allows for tax deferred contributions to an account that helps pay medical expenses.

3. Major medical covers ____________ illnesses.

4. RBRVS stands for ________ ________ ________ scale.

5. True or False: UCR stands for Usual, Customary, and Reasonable.

   ____

6. A program where military personnel and dependents may receive health care benefits is called

   ______________________________ .

7. The amount that a person has to pay out of pocket before insured benefits begin paying is called the

   ______________________________ .

8. The amount an insured person pays at the time of service is called the

   ______________________________ .

9. If a person has to pay 20% of all medical expenses, this is referred to as

   ______________________________ .

10. Insurance offered by an employer is an example of a ____________________ policy.

Chapter 19 Quiz

Name: ____

1. True or False: The ABA number is on the bottom of a check.

   ____

2. Always write the check stub

   ______________________________ .

3. A ______________ check has an itemized stub.

4. Why would you stop payment of a check?

   ____

   ____

5. Check washing is a type of

   ______________________________ .

6. The person presenting a check for payment is the ______________ .

7. The person who writes a check is the

   ______________________________ .

8. The person named on a check as the recipient of the amount shown is the

   ______________________________ .

9. The funds paid out are

   ______________________________ .

10. M-banking is banking by

    ______________________________ .

CHAPTER 20

Medical Practice Management

Part I. Vocabulary

Directions: Insert the correct vocabulary term.

1. The co-workers at Diamond Family Care are a ______________ group.
2. The bookkeeper who mishandled practice funds was found guilty of ______________.
3. One of the ______________ is a fifty-dollar bonus for perfect attendance each month.
4. Rumors abound when staff ______________ is low.
5. Refusal to perform a routine duty for the office manager might be perceived as ______________.
6. The office manager issues verbal ______________ to help correct deficiencies.

Part II.

A. List six tasks performed by the medical office manager

1. ______________
2. ______________
3. ______________
4. ______________
5. ______________
6. ______________

B. Examine the notice of practice closure below. Record your thoughts about the ad and discuss with your classmates.

____

____

____

____

ince April was $6543 that the Spro anufacturing Company spent in e for Rep. Alphonse Traubin, D-NH. if Thacburn, and his wife Shakira, comlass to Vancouver, British Co-BIA for a speech at a two day con-ence. Traubin spokesman, Kevin th, also traveled to the conference an additional $1643 in travel, lodg-and meals.

Smith said that because Traubin he conference for the entire time, the expenses are legally buisness

ut they aren't allowed to pay for the ips. Atttendence at events is not mandatory. Some staffers submit tdated forms that don't indicate, as e new ones require, whether they ok their spouses or children along

hat all legal channels will be pro-ly contacted.

When the Nuclear Energy Inst-te took Galveston and the other gressional staffers to France, in

see BUSINESS, B-13

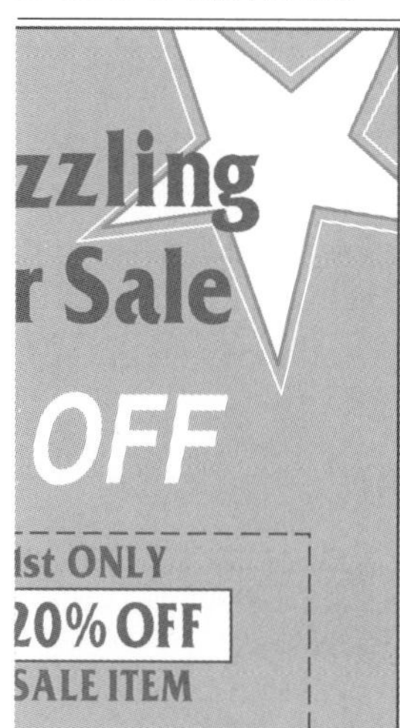

Dr. Fred Davenport

announces the transfer of his practice, Diamonte Cardiology, to the Cardiology Clinic of Dobbins, Arizona.

Patients of Dr. Davenport's have had their records transferred to the offices ot the Cardiology Clinic of Dobbins, Arizona.

Dr. Davenport thanks the community and patients who have entrusted their care to him over the years. Patients are urged to continue their care at the Cardiology Clinic of Dobbins, Arizona.

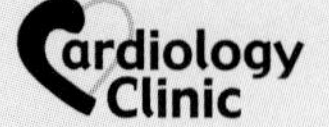

of Dobbins, Arizona
(998) 775-2323

Out-of-town referrals and consultations accepted

Answering Service and 24-Hour #
(998) 775-2323

BLUE CROSS • PRIVATE INSURANCE • MEDICARE (PARTICIPATING) • HMO and PPO PLANS ACCEPTED

Newspaper advertisement of facility closure.

C. List five essential elements of a team.

1. ____
2. ____
3. ____
4. ____
5. ____

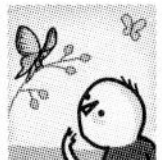

Part III.

AGENDA FOR HIM COMMITTEE

Health Information Management Committee
Meeting: October 19, 2000

Agenda

I. Call to order
II. Review of minutes
III. Old business
IV. Record review
V. New business
VI. Reports
  Delinquent record count
  Quality audit of HIM functions
VII. Adjourn

Next Meeting: November 16, 2000

Agenda for HIM committee.

Examine the agenda for the Health Information Management Committee and answer the following questions.

1. When would be an appropriate time to record attendance? ______
2. When would be an appropriate time to present a pilot staffing plan? ______
3. When would be the best time to discuss unresolved business? ______
4. What are the advantages of having a written agenda? ______

______

______

Part IV. ______

A. **Directions:** Examine the list of motivators below. Circle five motivators that are helping you to reach your educational goals.

a challenge	fulfillment
money	integrity
praise	honor
satisfaction	reputation
freedom	responsibility
fear	prestige
family	needs
insecurity	love
competition	

B. **Directions:** Examine the organizational chart for a fictitious doctor's office and answer the following questions.

1. The office manager is directly supervised by whom? ______
2. The office manager has the sole responsibility for which three groups? ______
3. Why do you think that nurses and medical assistants are also supervised by the physician? ______
4. In this organization, do licensed practical nurses (LPNs) and licensed visiting nurses (LVNs) supervise medical assistants? ______

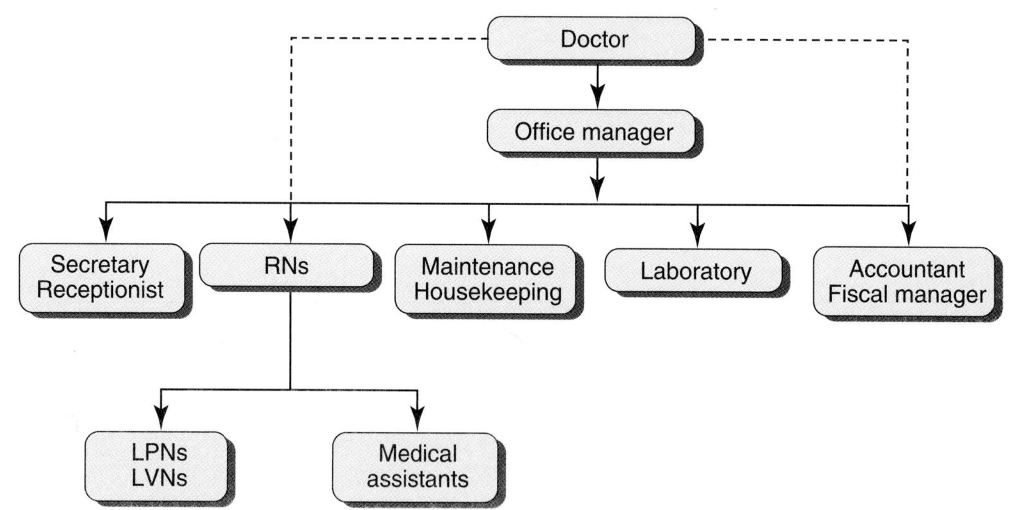

Sample of employees in a physician's office.

C. List the three types of leaders. Provide the name of a teacher, coach, or employer who fits the description of each of these types of leaders.

1. ______________________________

2. ______________________________

3. ______________________________

Chapter 20 Quiz

Name: ____

1. Name three types of leaders.
   a. ______________________
   b. ______________________
   c. ______________________

2. Name three types of managers.
   a. ______________________
   b. ______________________
   c. ______________________

3. True or False: Peer pressure is an example of internal motivation.

   ____

4. ______________________ evaluations involve other staff in the process.

5. True or False: It is illegal to ask about race or religion during an interview.

   ____

6. The ______________ is the order of a meeting.

7. ______________ is stealing from an employer.

8. Disobedience of authority is

   ______________________ .

9. A ______________ is criticism of fault or formal reproof.

10. A series of executive positions in order of authority is a ______________

    ______________ ______________ .

CHAPTER 21

Medical Practice Marketing and Customer Service

Part I. Vocabulary

Directions: Insert the appropriate vocabulary word for each definition.

1. ________________ Something toward which effort is directed; an aim, goal, or end of action.
2. ________________ The process of using marketing and education strategies to reach and involve diverse audiences through the use of key messages and effective programs.
3. ________________ The process or technique of promoting, selling, and distributing a product or service.
4. ________________ The surgical or dental specialty concerned with the design, construction, and fitting of prostheses, which are artificial devices that replace missing parts of the body.
5. ________________ Capable of being appraised at an actual or approximate value; capable of being precisely identified or realized by the mind.
6. ________________ A specific group of individuals to whom the marketing plan is directed.

Part II.

A. List the four P's of marketing.

1. ________________
2. ________________
3. ________________
4. ________________

B. Describe the steps in developing a marketing plan.

1. ________________
2. ________________
3. ________________
4. ________________
5. ________________

C. Give examples of community involvement that may promote a medical practice.

1. ______________________________

2. ______________________________

3. ______________________________

D. Differentiate between advertising and public relations.

____

____

____

____

____

E. List the eight deadly sins of customer service.

1. ______________________________

2. ______________________________

3. ______________________________

4. ______________________________

5. ______________________________

6. ______________________________

7. ______________________________

8. ______________________________

F. List the four basic steps for building a website.

1. ______________________________

2. ______________________________

3. ______________________________

4. ______________________________

Part III.

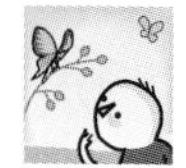

Directions: Visit www.aama-ntl.org and find websites for American Association of Medical Assistants affiliates in different states. Evaluate each website according to the following criteria.

Website	Overall Appeal	Content	Navigation	Font	Consistency

Part IV.

The patient is the most important customer in the medical practice. Name other customers in a medical practice.

1. ______

2. ______

3. ______

4. ______

Chapter 21 Quiz

Name: ____

1. Name the 4 P's of marketing.

   a. ______________________

   b. ______________________

   c. ______________________

   d. ______________________

2. List several free marketing resources.

   ____

   ____

3. What is a hyperlink?

   ____

   ____

4. What is the final stage of implementing a marketing plan?

   ____

   ____

5. True or False: Staff are internal customers.

   ____

6. Define marketing.

   ____

   ____

7. What is the first step of marketing?

   ____

   ____

8. A URL is a __________ __________ .

9. A group of individuals to whom marketing is focused is called the

   ____

   ______________________ .

10. An ISP is an ______________________

    ____

    ______________________ .

CHAPTER 22

Health Information Management

Part I. Vocabulary

Directions: Match the following terms and definitions.

1. _____ Proof of; with regard to medical records, it applies to a signature, initials, or computer keystroke by the maker of the record that verifies that the record is correct.
2. _____ To manage to get around, especially by ingenuity or stratagem.
3. _____ Something, as a symptom or condition, that makes a particular treatment or procedure inadvisable.
4. _____ Containing or made up of fundamentally different and often incongruous elements; markedly distinct in quality or character.
5. _____ To convert from one system of communication to another; encode.
6. _____ Containing or characterized by error or assumption.
7. _____ Originating or taking place in a hospital.
8. _____ Activities designed to increase the quality of a product or service through process or system changes that increase efficiency or effectiveness.
9. _____ An unexpected occurrence involving death or serious physical or psychological injury, or the risk thereof.
10. _____ Established by authority, custom, or general consent as a model or example; something set up and established by authority as a rule for the measure of quantity, weight, extent, value, or quality.
11. _____ To change the relative place or normal order of; to alter the sequence.

A. disparities
B. authenticated
C. erroneous
D. transposed
E. standards
F. circumvent
G. encrypted
H. quality assurance
I. sentinel events
J. nosocomial
K. contraindications

Part II.

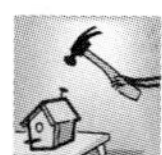

Phone-etics Game

Directions: Use the telephone keypad below to spell out the missing words.

A. The health information profession is supported by a national organization called the 2-4-4-6-2.

B. The 4-4-7-2-2 Act of 1996 was developed in part to help ensure the confidentiality of medical records.

C. 5-2-2-4-6 is a nonprofit organization that assists healthcare facilities by providing accreditation services.

1	ABC 2	DEF 3
GHI 4	JKL 5	MNO 6
PRS 7	TUV 8	WXY 9
*	0	#

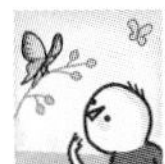

Part III.

A medical assistant gives an injection of penicillin to a patient who reported an allergy to amoxicillin. The patient complains of itching and experiences shortness of breath and wheezing while sitting in the treatment room. The patient collapses to the floor and stops breathing. Cardiopulmonary resuscitation (CPR) is initiated, and an ambulance is called. The patient is transported on life support to the local emergency department. The patient dies 12 hours later. Complete an incident report for this sentinel event.

Incident Report

Do Not File in Medical Records

Confidential and privileged health care quality improvement information prepared in anticipation of litigation

Name: ______________ Employee ☐ Patient ☐ Visitor ☐

Attending physician: ______________
MR # ______________ SS # ______________
D.O.B. __/__/__ Sex: M[ ] F[ ]
Admission date: __/__/__
Primary diagnosis: ______________

Facility name: ______________
Site (if applicable) ______________
City ______________
Facility ID# ______________
State ______________
Phone # ______________

SECTION I: General Information

General Identification (circle one)
001 Inpatient
002 Outpatient
003 Nonpatient
004 Equipment only

Location (circle one):
005 Bathroom/toilet
006 Beauty shop
007 Cafeteria/dining room
008 Corridor/hall
009 During transport
010 Emergency department
011 Exterior grounds
012 ICU/SCU/CCU
013 Labor/delivery/birthing
014 Nursery
015 Outpatient clinic
016 Patient room
017 Radiology
018 Recovery room
019 Recreation area
020 Rehab
021 Shower room
022 Surgical suite
023 Treatment/exam room

Treatment Rendered (circle one):
024 Emergency room
025 First aid
026 None
026 Transfer to other facility
027 X-ray

SECTION II: Nature of Incident **(Circle all that apply):**
001 Adverse outcome after surgery or anesthetic
002 Anaphylactic shock
003 Anoxic event
004 Apgar score of 5 or less
005 Aspiration
006 Assault or altercation/combative event
007 Blood or IV variance
008 Blood/body fluid exposure
009 Code/arrest
010 Damage/loss of organ
011 Death
012 Dental-related complication
013 Dissatisfaction/noncompliance*
014 Equipment operation*
015 Fall with injury*
016 Fall without injury*
017 Handling of and/or exposure to hazardous waste
018 Informed consent issue
019 Injury to other
020 Injury to self
021 Loss of limb
022 Loss of vision
023 Medication variance*
024 Needle puncture/sharp injury
025 Paralysis
026 Patient-to-patient altercation
027 Perinatal complication*
028 Poisoning
029 Suspected nonstaff-to-patient abuse
030 Suspected staff-to-patient abuse
031 Thermal burn
032 Treatment/procedure issue
033 Ulcer: nosocomial stage III/IV

* *Complete appropriate area in Section III*

SECTION III: Type of Incident

If death, circle all that apply:
001 After medical equipment failure
002 After power equipment failure or damage
003 During surgery or postanesthesia
004 Within 24 hours of admission to facility
005 Within 1 week of fall in facility
006 Within 24 hours of medication error

Blood/IV Variance Issues (circle all that apply):
007 Additive
008 Administration consent
009 Contraindications/allergies
010 Equipment malfunction
011 Infusion rate
012 Labeling issue
013 Reaction
014 Solution/blood type
015 Transcription
016 Patient identification
017 Allergic/adverse reaction
018 Infiltration
019 Phlebitis

Dissatisfaction/Noncompliance (circle all that apply):
020 AMA
021 Elopement
022 Irate or angry (either family or patient)
023 Left without service
024 Noncompliant patient
025 Refused prescribed treatment

Falls (circle all that apply):*
001 Assisted fall
002 Found on floor
003 From bed
004 From chair
005 From commode/toilet
006 From exam table
007 From stretcher
008 From wheelchair
009 Patient states—unwitnessed
010 Unassisted fall
011 While ambulating
012 Witnessed fall

* *For any marks in this field, Section V must be completed*

Medication Variance Issues (circle all that apply):
013 Contraindication/allergies
014 Delay in dispensing
015 Incorrect dose
016 Expired drug
017 Medication identification
018 Narcotic log variance
019 Not ordered
020 Ordered, not given
021 Patient identification
022 Reaction
023 Route
024 Rx incorrectly dispensed
025 Time of dose
026 Transcription

Incident report.

Part IV.

Evaluate the confidentiality statement for Diamonte Hospital. Reword the statement to make it appropriate for a medical practice setting. Indicate your proposed changes on the confidentiality statement.

DIAMONTE HOSPITAL

Diamonte, Arizona 89104 ▪ TEL. 602-484-9991

CONFIDENTIALITY STATEMENT

I, ______________________________, understand that in the course of my activities/business at or for Diamonte Hospital, I am required to have access to and am involved in the viewing, reviewing, and/or processing of patient care data and/or health information.

I understand that I am obligated by State Law, Federal Law, and Diamonte Hospital to maintain the confidentiality of these data and information at all times.

I understand that a violation of these confidentiality considerations may result in punitive legal action against me.

I certify by my signature below that this Confidentiality Statement has been explained to me, and I agree to the principles contained herein as a condition of my activity/business at or for Diamonte Hospital.

____
Signature/date

____
Witness/date

Confidentiality statement.

Chapter 22 Quiz

Name: ____

1. Coded data is called ________________ .

2. TQM stands for____________________

________________ ________________ .

3. What is JCAHO?

____

____

4. What is the NCHS?

____

____

5. What is a sentinel event?

____

____

6. What does HIPAA stand for?

____

____

7. What is the professional organization for health information professionals?

____

____

8. What does reliability of data mean?

____

____

9. How do third party payers use the medical record?

____

____

10. Signature of the maker that indicates that a record is accurate is called

________________________________ .

Chapter 23 Quiz

Name: ____________________

1. A bill inside a package is an ________ .

2. An itemized list of a package's contents is a __________________ slip.

3. How many years should you keep payroll records?

   ____

   ____

4. What is a W-4 form?

   ____

   ____

5. What is FUTA?

   ____

   ____

6. What is bookkeeping?

   ____

   ____

7. Name two bases of accounting?

   a. ____________________

   b. ____________________

8. What is a disbursement?

   ____

   ____

9. What type of fund is used for minor expenses?

   ____

   ____

10. Name two types of bookkeeping systems.

    a. ____________________

    b. ____________________

CHAPTER 24

Infection Control

Part I. Vocabulary

Directions: Define the following terms in your own words.

1. anaphylaxis

2. antibody

3. antigen

4. antiseptic

5. autoimmune

6. contaminated

7. germicides

8. pathogenic

9. permeable

____

____

10. relapse

____

____

11. remission

____

____

12. vector

____

____

Part II. Chain of Infection

Directions: Label the diagram below with the following terms.

A. Reservoir host

B. Entry (any body opening)

C. Transmission mode (air, food, hand, insects, body fluid)

D. Exit mode (mouth, skin, rectum, body fluid)

E. Susceptible host

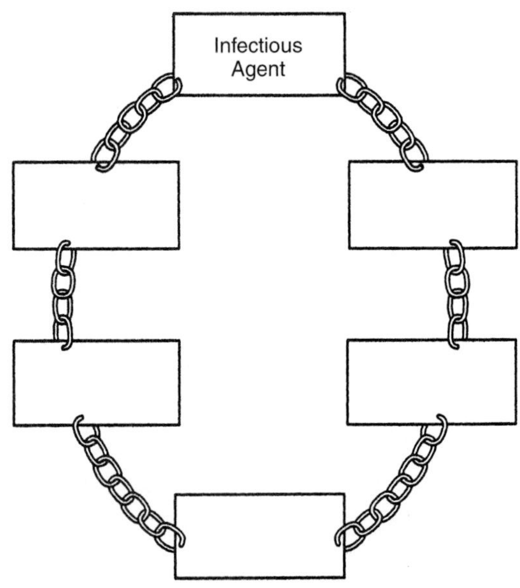

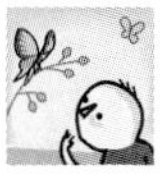

Part III. Inflammation

A. Describe the first four stages of inflammation in response to pathogenic invasion.

1. ______

2. ______

3. ______

4. ______

B. Describe the conditions that may result if the pathogen continues to invade the entire body.

1. Pus formation

2. Enlarged lymph nodes

3. Septicemia

C. List four types of infection and describe them.

1. ______
2. ______
3. ______
4. ______

Part IV. Pathogens and Barriers

A. List five groups of infectious organisms.

1. __________
2. __________
3. __________
4. __________
5. __________

B. Complete the table with information about various viruses.

Disease	Organism	Description	Transmission	Symptoms	Specimens	Tests
HIV-positive acquired	HIV	DNA retrovirus				
Immuno-deficiency syndrome (AIDS)						
Hepatitis A	HAV	RNA virus				
Hepatitis B	HBV	DNA virus				
Hepatitis delta	HDV	RNA virus				
Hepatitis C	HCV	RNA flavivirus				
Herpes simplex	HSV	Exhibits latency				
Chicken pox or shingles	Varicella zoster virus (VZV)	Exhibits latency, may cause shingles (herpes zoster) in patients who have had chicken pox				

C. List three types of bacteria and describe their shapes.

1. __________
2. __________
3. __________

D. List several barriers or types of personal protective equipment that are commonly used in physicians' offices.

1. ___
2. ___
3. ___
4. ___
5. ___
6. ___

E. Hypersensitivity to latex products may include the following symptoms:

1. ___
2. ___
3. ___
4. ___
5. ___
6. ___

Part V. Exposure Control

Employers with workers who are at risk for occupational exposure to blood or other infectious materials must implement an Occupational Safety and Health Administration (OSHA) Exposure Control Plan that details employee protection procedures. List seven items that should be included in the plan.

1. ___
2. ___
3. ___
4. ___
5. ___
6. ___
7. ___

Part VI. Asepsis

Directions: Define the following terms.

1. Disinfection

___

___

2. Medical asepsis

3. Surgical asepsis

4. Proper hand washing (two factors)

5. Sanitization

6. Sterilization

Part VII. Hand Washing

Directions: Review Procedure 24.1: Performing Medical Aseptic Hand Washing in your textbook. What did you learn? Practice proper hand washing for the next 24 hours. Note any new habits you have formed. Do you see any improvement? Have you noticed hand washing behaviors of others?

Chapter 24 Quiz

Name: ____________________

1. The relief of systems is called ____________.

2. Viruses form a substance called
   a. interferon
   b. spores

   ____

3. List three potentially infectious fluids.
   a. ____________________
   b. ____________________
   c. ____________________

4. CDC stands for ____________.

5. True or False: Cocci bacteria are rod-shaped.

   ____

6. Name a symptom or sign of latex allergy.

   ____

7. True or False: Hepatitis A can be food borne.

   ____

8. Instruments in surgery are ____________.

9. OSHA stands for ____________.

10. Rhinitis means ____________.

CHAPTER 25

Patient Assessment

Part I.

List five components of the medical history.

1. ______________________
2. ______________________
3. ______________________
4. ______________________
5. ______________________

Part II.

Describe things that influence someone's value system.

____

____

____

Do you think these things have influenced your values?

____

____

Part III.

List and describe three processes of active listening.

____

____

____

The receiver of a message attaches meaning to a message based on:

____

____

____

Part IV. ______

Directions: Complete the diagram below by including examples of nonverbal communication.

Area Observed	Observation
Breathing patterns	
Eye patterns	
Hands	
Arm placement	
Leg placement	

List four important rules to remember in preparing the appropriate environment for patient interaction.

1. ______
2. ______
3. ______
4. ______

Part V.

Directions: Label the following questions as either open-ended or closed-ended.

1. ______ How have you been getting along?
2. ______ Do you have a headache?
3. ______ Have you ever broken a bone?
4. ______ What brings you to the doctor?
5. ______ Are you feeling better?
6. ______ Do you have high blood pressure?
7. ______ Tell me about your back pain?
8. ______ When did the nausea start?
9. ______ Did your mother have a history of cancer?
10. ______ Do you smoke?

Part VI.

Consider the following interview barriers. Give an example of each.

1. Providing unwarranted assurance

2. Giving advice

3. Using professional terms

4. Leading questions

Part VII.

List some of the important guidelines to follow in obtaining the health history of a child.

1. ______
2. ______
3. ______
4. ______
5. ______

Part VIII.

Directions: Label the following as "Subjective" (symptom) or "Objective" (sign).

1. Pain ______
2. Nausea ______
3. Dizziness ______
4. Elevated blood pressure ______
5. Labored respirations ______
6. Headache ______

7. Temperature of skin ______________________________

8. Back pain ______________________________

9. Color of skin ______________________________

10. Abdominal pain ______________________________

Part IX. ______________________________

Directions: Review the correct method of charting in your textbook and answer the following questions.

1. What is the first step in charting? ______________________________

____

____

2. What color ink do you use? ______________________________

3. What appears on every entry? ______________________________

4. What three things do you include about symptoms?

____

____

5. How do you chart intensity of pain? ______________________________

____

____

6. How do you correct an error? ______________________________

____

____

7. How do you add additional information at a later time? ______________________________

____

____

8. Why are neatness and legibility important? ______________________________

____

____

Part X. Charting Methods

A. List four components of the POMR.

1. ______
2. ______
3. ______
4. ______

B. The first letter of each part of the progress note makes up the word *SOAPE*. Describe what each of these letters stands for.

S ______

O ______

A ______

P ______

E ______

C. What is an SOMR? ______

D. What are some of the sections in an SOMR?

1. ______
2. ______
3. ______
4. ______

E. What is a CMR? ______

Part XI. Workplace Applications

Directions: Document the following four scenarios by using the POMR method.

1. The patient c/o chest with pain of 4 on a 1-10 scale and sweating for 2 hours. He has been taking NTG for relief of symptoms. His VS are T-99, P-68, R-24. He also has an irregular pulse and left arm pain.

   S: ______

   O: ______

2. The patient c/o a sore throat with pain of 7 on a 1-10 scale and fever for 2 days. He has been taking OTCs and gargling with warm salt water for relief of symptoms. His VS are T-102.4, P-108, R-20. He also has an erythematous papular rash across his chest. He was exposed to strep last week.

   S: ____

   O: ____

   ____

   ____

3. The patient c/o a headache with pain of 8 on a 1-10 scale and nausea for 3 days. She has been taking Lortab 5 for relief of symptoms. Her VS are T-97.6, P-110, R-20. She also has dizziness and her eyes hurt. She is pale and her skin is damp.

   S: ____

   O: ____

   ____

   ____

4. The patient fell off a ladder 2 days ago and c/o low back pain of 5 on a 1-10 scale. He has been taking Advil for relief of symptoms. His VS are T-98.7, P-98, R-20. He also has an ecchymosis across his flank and c/o blood in his urine.

   S: ____

   O: ____

   ____

   ____

Chapter 25 Quiz

Name: ____________________

1. True or False: An example of pain quality is "stabbing."

   ____

2. True or False: An earache is a symptom.

   ____

3. True or False: SOAPE is part of a POMR.

   ____

4. True or False: Objective data are signs.

   ____

5. ____________ complaint is the reason for seeking medical care.

6. ____________ is a relationship of harmony between the patient and healthcare personnel.

7. Health insurance information is part of the

   ____________.

8. Smoking is part of the ____________ history.

9. Age of a parent at death is part of the

   ____________ history.

10. True or False: Open-ended questions often provide better data.

    ____

CHAPTER 26

Patient Education

Part I. Vocabulary

Directions: Fill in the blanks with the appropriate terms.

1. The holistic model suggests that patient education should take into consideration all aspects of patient life including patients' __________, __________, __________, __________, __________, and __________ needs.

Part II.

Directions: List six guidelines for patient education.

1. __________
2. __________
3. __________
4. __________
5. __________
6. __________

Part III.

Directions: List seven factors that influence learning.

1. __________
2. __________
3. __________
4. __________
5. __________
6. __________
7. __________

Part IV.

Directions: Identify eight approaches to language barriers.

1. ______________________________
2. ______________________________
3. ______________________________
4. ______________________________
5. ______________________________
6. ______________________________
7. ______________________________
8. ______________________________

Part V.

Directions: Fill in the blanks with the appropriate terms.

1. One of the most important aspects of patient teaching is to be ______________ and provide information about ______________ patients want to know ______________ patients want to know it.

Part VI.

Directions: List 10 barriers to patient learning.

1. ______________________________
2. ______________________________
3. ______________________________
4. ______________________________
5. ______________________________
6. ______________________________
7. ______________________________
8. ______________________________
9. ______________________________
10. ______________________________

Part VII.

Directions: Identify five guidelines for ordering educational materials.

1. ______________________________
2. ______________________________
3. ______________________________
4. ______________________________
5. ______________________________

Part VIII.

Directions: Complete the statement.

The role of the medical assistant educator includes:

1. ______________________________
2. ______________________________
3. ______________________________
4. ______________________________
5. ______________________________
6. ______________________________
7. ______________________________
8. ______________________________

Part IX.

Directions: Fill in the blanks with the appropriate terms.

Teaching methods that are effective include use of ______________ materials, videos, and approved ______________ sites to gather information; referral to community ______________ and experts; ______________ demonstration of medical skills; examination of patients' records of events; and involving ______________ in the education process.

Part X. Teaching Plan Checklist

Directions: Use the following checklist to design and present a patient education program for a patient during your externship, or role play with a fellow classmate.

1. Conduct patient assessment.
   - Consider pertinent patient factors.
   - Identify barriers to learning.
   - Prioritize patient information.
   - Determine immediate and long-term needs.
   - Decide on appropriate teaching materials and methods.

   Complete ______________

2. Prepare the teaching area and assemble necessary equipment and materials.
   - Use supplies and equipment the patient will use at home.
   - Provide positive feedback for correct display of skills.

   Complete ______________

3. Maintain adequate, not too fast, pace.

   Complete ______________

4. Repeatedly ask for patient feedback to confirm understanding.
   - Eliminate barriers to learning.
   - Address immediate learning needs.
   - Use repetition and rephrasing to promote understanding.

   Complete ______________

5. Summarize the material learned or the skill mastered at the end of each teaching interaction.

   Complete ______________

6. Outline a plan for the next meeting.

   Complete ______________

7. Evaluate the teaching plan.
   - Was there enough time to complete the lesson?
   - Was the patient physically and psychologically ready for the information?
   - Were the goals for the session reached?

   Complete ______________

8. Document the teaching intervention.
   - Material covered
   - Patient response or level of skill performance
   - Plans for next session
   - Community referrals

   Complete ______________

Chapter 26 Quiz

Name: ______________________________

1. Describe the holistic model of patient education.

 ____

 ____

2. List some areas in which patient education might focus.

 ____

 ____

3. True or False: The sixth to eighth grade level is recommended for brochures for the general public. ______________

4. List some examples of teaching materials.

 a. ______________________________

 b. ______________________________

 c. ______________________________

5. True or False: A quiet area is recommended for patient education.

 ____

6. Include ____________ and significant others in patient education.

7. True or False: Emotional state can affect patient learning.

 ____

8. Name two physical barriers to learning.

 a. ______________________________

 b. ______________________________

9. What is this first step in developing a teaching plan?

 ____

10. List ways to evaluate learning.

 ____

 ____

CHAPTER 27

Nutrition and Health Promotion

Part I. ___

A. **Directions:** Describe the dietary imbalances that contribute to each of these health problems.

1. Anemia ___
2. Cancer ___
3. Constipation ___
4. Diabetes ___
5. Hypercholesterolemia ___
6. Hypertension ___
7. Osteoporosis ___

B. **Directions:** Fill in the blanks with the appropriate terms.

1. Dietary fiber is commonly called ___.
2. ___ are chemical organic compounds composed of carbon, hydrogen, and oxygen and are primarily plant products in origin. They are divided into three groups based on the complexity of their molecules: simple sugars, complex carbohydrates (starch), and dietary fiber.
3. ___ is a storage form of fuel that is used to supplement carbohydrates as an available energy source.
4. Naturally occurring ___ are found in many fruits, vegetables, and certain seasonings.
5. ___ are composed of units known as amino acids, which are the materials that our bodies use to build and repair tissues.
6. Vitamins are divided into two groups: ___-soluble (A, D, E, and K) and ___-soluble (B complex and C).
7. ___ present in the largest amounts include sodium, potassium, calcium, chlorine, phosphorus, and magnesium.

Part II.

A. **Directions:** Examine the nomogram below and answer the following questions.

1. How much does this patient weigh in pounds? ______________

   In kilograms? ______________

2. What is the height in inches? ______________ In centimeters? ______________

3. What is the body surface area (BSA)? ______________

4. Use the nomogram to calculate your own BSA. ______________

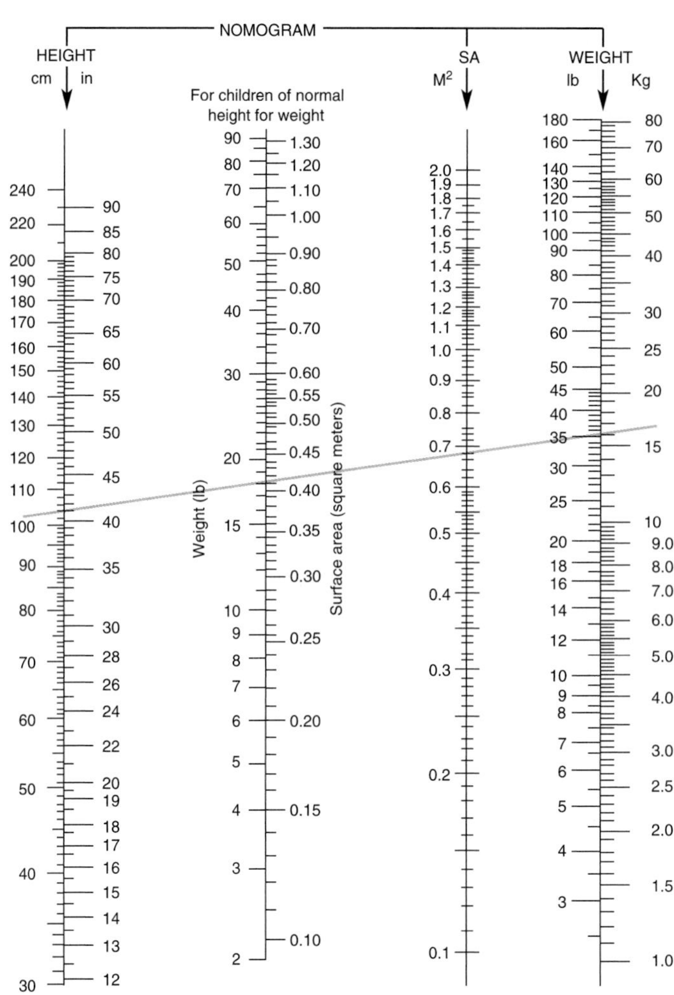

B. **Directions:** List four functions of water.

1. ______________
2. ______________
3. ______________
4. ______________

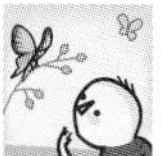

Part III.

A. **Directions:** Label each food group.

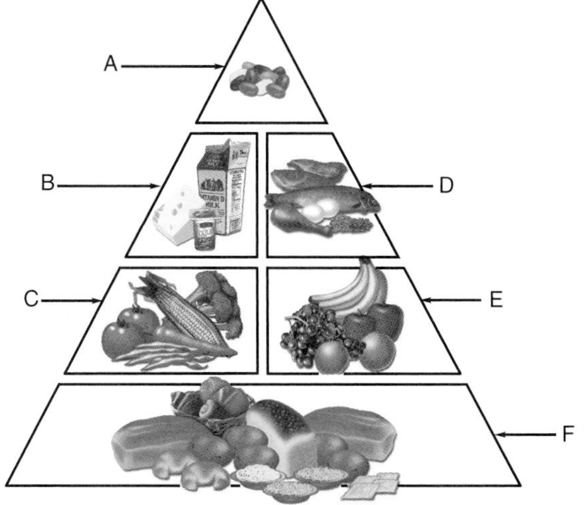

B. **Directions:** Examine the nutrition facts label below and answer the following questions.

1. What is the normal serving size?

 ____

2. How many calories are in one serving without milk? ______________

3. How many grams of fiber are present in one serving? ______________

4. This food is high in ______________ and ______________.

NUTRITION FACTS

Services size $1\frac{1}{4}$ cups (30 g)
Servicing per container about 16

Amount per serving		Cereal	Cereal with $\frac{1}{2}$ cup skim milk
Calories		110	190
Calories from fat		0	0
		% Daily value**	
Total fat 9 g*		0%	0%
Saturated fat 0 g		0%	1%
Cholesterol 0 mg		0%	1%
Sodium 270 mg		11%	14%
Total carbohydrate 26 g		9%	11%
Dietary fiber less than 1 g		0%	0%
Sugars 3 g			
Other carbohydrate 22 g			
Protein 2 g			
Vitamin A		0%	6%
Vitamin C		10%	10%
Calcium		0%	15%
Iron		50%	50%
Thiamin		25%	25%
Niacin		25%	25%
Vitamin B_6		25%	25%
Folate		25%	25%
Vitamin B_{12}		25%	30%

Amount per serving		Cereal	Cereal with $^1/_2$ cup skim milk
	Calories	**2000**	**2500**
Total fat	Less than	65 g	60 g
Saturated fat	Less than	20 g	25 g
Cholesterol	Less than	300 mg	300 mg
Sodium	Less than	2400 mg	2400 mg
Total carbohydrate		300 g	375 g
Dietary fiber		25 g	30 g
Calories per gram:			
Fat 9 –			
Carbohydrate 4 –			
Protein 4			
*Amount in cereal. One half cup skim milk an additional 40 calories. Less than 5 mg cholesterol, 65 mg sodium, 6 g total carbohydrate (6 g sugars) and 4 g protein. **Percent daily values are based on 2000 calorie diet. Your daily values may be higher may be higher or lower depending on your calorie needs.			

Part IV.

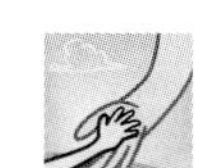

Directions: Record your dietary intake for the next 24 hours. Save nutrition labels from packages so that you can examine your caloric intake. Any surprises?

	Foods	Calories	Grams of Fat
Breakfast			
Snack Water			
Lunch			
Snack Water			
Dinner			
Snack Water			
Totals			

Chapter 27 Quiz

Name: ____

1. Name two types of protein.

   a. ______________________________

   b. ______________________________

2. Name two types of cholesterol.

   a. ______________________________

   b. ______________________________

3. What is the benefit of Omega 3 fatty acids?

   ____

   ____

4. Name two eating disorders.

   a. ______________________________

   b. ______________________________

5. What types of oil are monounsaturated?

   a. ______________________________

   b. ______________________________

6. Obesity is caused by excessive ______________ intake.

7. ______________ includes sugars and starches.

8. Fiber is also called ______________ .

9. Name two types of fat.

   a. ______________________________

   b. ______________________________

10. Antioxidants include Vitamins ______________ and ______________ .

CHAPTER 28

Vital Signs

Part I. Vocabulary

Directions: Define the following medical terms.

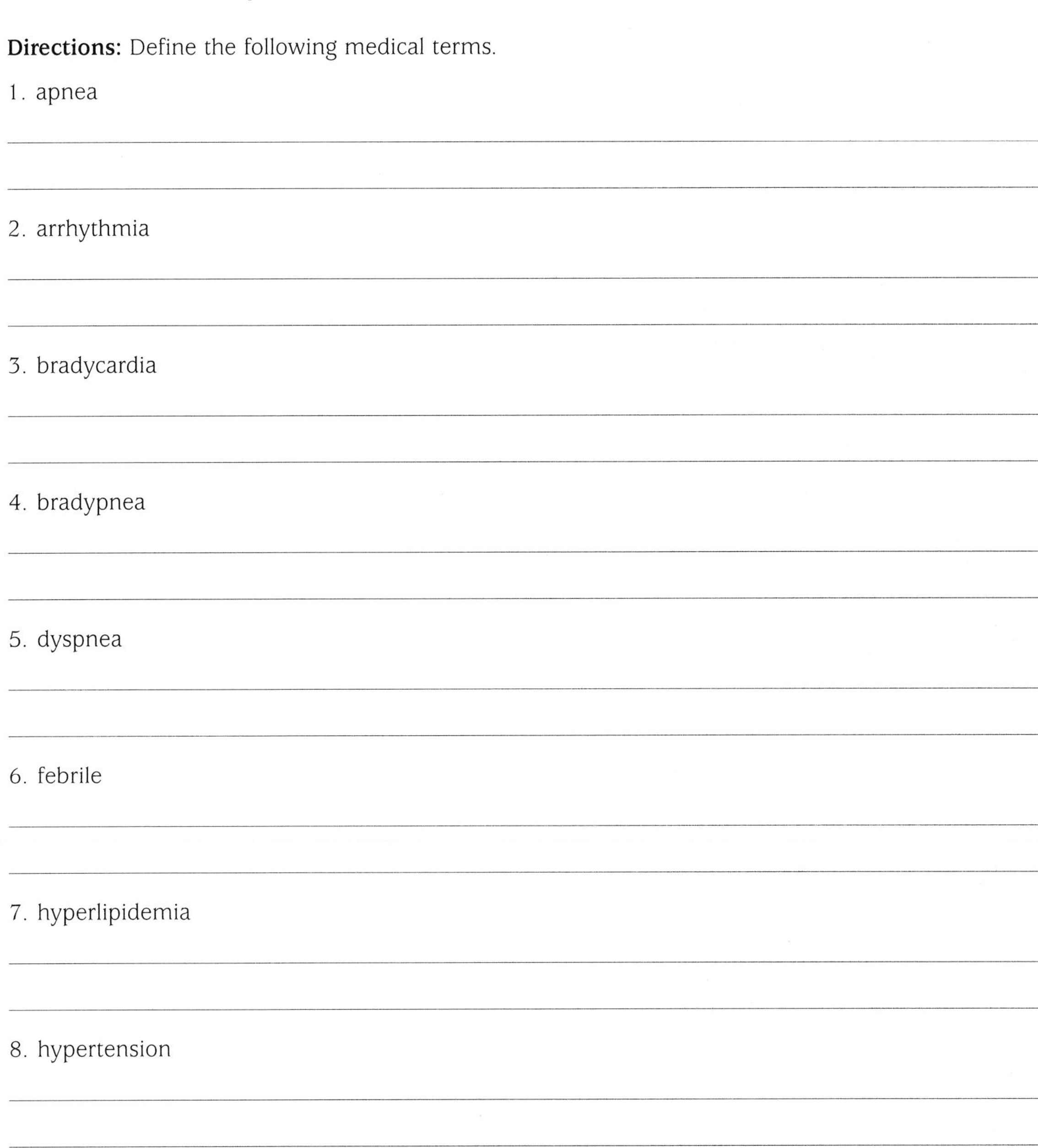

1. apnea

2. arrhythmia

3. bradycardia

4. bradypnea

5. dyspnea

6. febrile

7. hyperlipidemia

8. hypertension

9. hyperventilation

____

____

10. hypotension

____

____

11. orthopnea

____

____

12. rales

____

____

13. rhonchi

____

____

14. syncope

____

____

15. tachycardia

____

____

16. tachypnea

____

____

17. vertigo

____

____

Part II.

Directions: Complete the statement.

The cardinal four vital signs are:

1. ____
2. ____
3. ____
4. _______________________ _______________________

Part III.

Directions: Complete the statement.

Anthropometric measurements include:

1. ______________________________

2. ______________________________

3. ______________ ______________

4. ______________ and ______________ ______________

Part IV.

Directions: Indicate which statements are true (T) and which statements are false (F).

1. _____ A change in one or more of the patient's vital signs may indicate a change in general health.

2. _____ It sometimes is necessary to obtain some measurements a second time, after the patient is calmer or more comfortable.

3. _____ The body temperature is regulated by the hypothalamus.

4. _____ The body temperature ranges from being highest in the morning to lowest in the late afternoon.

Part V.

Directions: Complete the table of normal ranges for vital signs.

Age Group	Pulse	Respirations	Blood Pressure
Newborn			
Toddlers (1-3 yr)			
Preschool (4-6 yr)			
School Age (7-11 yr)			
Adolescent (12-16 yr)			
Adult			

Part VI. Temperatures

A. **Directions:** Use the correct terms to fill in the blanks.

1. A ______________ fever rises and falls only slightly during the 24-hour period. It remains above the patient's average normal range and is called *continuous* because that is exactly what the pattern shows.

2. A ______________ fever comes and goes, or it spikes and then returns into average range.

3. A ________________ fever has great fluctuation but never gets back into the average range. It is a constant fever with fluctuating levels and thus is remittent.
4. ________________ temperatures, when taken accurately, are approximately 1° F or 0.6° C higher than oral readings.
5. ________________ temperatures are approximately 1° F or 0.6° C lower than accurate oral readings.
6. ________________ readings are close to the core body temperature because the mucous membrane lining with which the thermometer comes in contact is not exposed to the air.
7. ________________ thermometers are battery-operated and are available in both Fahrenheit and Celsius scales. One type is a unit equipped with two probes: a ________________ one for oral use and a red one for ________________ use only.
8. The ________________ measurement system consists of a hand-held processor unit equipped with a probe that is covered with a disposable speculum that is placed at the opening of the ear canal. It should not be used for patients with ________________ ________________ or impacted ________________.
9. ________________ temperatures take the longest to register.
10. Water-soluble lubrication jelly is needed for obtaining ________________ temperatures. The patient should be placed in the ________________ position.

B. **Directions:** Document temperatures that are considered febrile.

1. Rectal or aural (ear) temperatures higher than ________________° F (38° C)
2. Oral temperatures higher than ________________° F (37.5° C)
3. Axillary temperatures higher than ________________° F (37° C)
4. Fever of unknown origin (FUO) is a fever higher than ________________° F (38.3° C) for ________________ ________________ in adults and ________________ in children without a known diagnosis.

C. Converting Temperatures

$$C = (F - 32) \times 5/9$$

$$F = \frac{9 \times C}{5} + 32$$

Directions: Using the above formulas, convert the following temperatures from one system to the other.

1. 98.6° F = ________________ C
2. 37° C = ________________ F
3. 97.6° F = ________________ C
4. 38° C = ________________ F
5. 99.4° F = ________________ C
6. 36° C = ________________ F
7. 104° F = ________________ C
8. 42° C = ________________ F
9. 101° F = ________________ C
10. 41° C = ________________ F
11. 102° F = ________________ C
12. 43° C = ________________ F

Part VII. Pulses

A. **Directions:** List eight pulse sites and label their correct locations on the figure below.

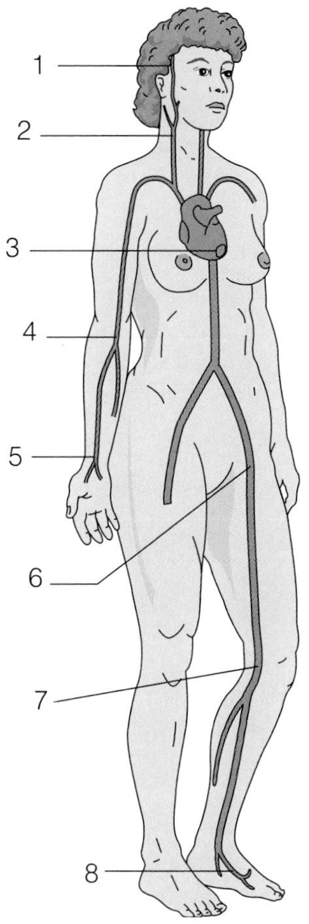

1. ______________________________
2. ______________________________
3. ______________________________
4. ______________________________
5. ______________________________
6. ______________________________
7. ______________________________
8. ______________ ______________

Part VIII. Respirations

Directions: Complete the sentences with the correct terms.

1. When Grace counts respirations, she understands that one respiration includes ____________________
2. Geri is documenting the three characteristics of respirations, which include ____________, ____________, and ____________.
3. Dianne counts eight respirations for 30 seconds and multiplies by ____________. She documents the rate as ____________ per minute.

Part IX. Blood Pressure

Directions: Complete the sentences with the correct terms.

1. Blood pressure is a reflection of the pressure of the blood against the walls of ____________.
2. The difference between the systolic and diastolic pressures is the ____________ ____________.
3. Blood pressure is recorded as a fraction, with the ____________ reading the numerator (top) and the ____________ reading the denominator (bottom).

Directions: Review the process of taking a blood pressure and complete the chart below.

The sphygmomanometer must be used with a stethoscope. The objective of the procedure is to use the inflatable cuff to obliterate (cause to disappear) circulation through an artery. The stethoscope is placed over the artery just below the cuff, and then the cuff is slowly deflated to allow the blood to flow again. As blood flow resumes, cardiac cycle sounds (Korotkoff sounds) are heard through the stethoscope, and gauge readings are taken when the first (systolic) and the last (diastolic) sounds are heard.

Phase I: This is the first sound heard as the cuff deflates. The blood is resurging into the patient's artery and can be heard quite clearly as a sharp, tapping sound. Note the gauge reading when this **first** sound is heard. **Record this as the systolic pressure.**

Phase V: All sounds disappear in this phase. Note the gauge reading when the **last** sound is heard. **Record this as the diastolic pressure.**

Phase I	Phase V	Document Blood Pressure
110	80	
204	114	
116	72	
98	56	
142	88	

Part X. Workplace Applications

Directions: Vital signs are documented with temperature (T) first, pulse (P) second, and respirations (R) last; the blood pressure is recorded after the TPR. Correctly document the following vital signs in the boxes provided. Date and sign each entry as you would on a patient record.

1. Oral temperature of 98.7, apical pulse of 60, respirations 22, and orthostatic blood pressure of 152/98 supine and 114/76 standing.

2. Tympanic temperature of 96.8, radial pulse of 86, respirations 18, and bilateral blood pressure of 132/76 in the left arm and 128/80 in the right arm.

3. Rectal temperature of 101.2, pulse of 100, respirations 20, and blood pressure 126/70.

4. Axillary temperature of 97.5, carotid pulse of 78, respirations 20, and palpated blood pressure of 120.

Chapter 28 Quiz

Name: ______________________________

1. The first tapping heard when taking a blood pressure is the ______________.

2. Respirations that are counted as 9 for 30 seconds are documented as ______________ per minute.

3. A ______________ blood pressure is done without a stethoscope.

4. Convert 146 pounds to kilograms.

   ____

5. Convert 73 kilograms to pounds.

   ____

6. True or False: Head circumference is an anthropometric measurement.

   ____

7. True or False: An apical pulse is taken with a stethoscope and counted for one full minute.

   ____

8. True or False: The dorsalis pedis is behind the knee.

   ____

9. The ______________ pulse is located on the side of the head.

10. True or False: The radial pulse is best found on the thumb side of the wrist, 1 inch above the base of the thumb.

    ____

CHAPTER 29

Assisting with the Primary Physical Examination

Part I. Vocabulary

Directions: Use the appropriate vocabulary word to complete each sentence.

1. The physician uses ______________ to assess the sinuses.
2. A patient undergoing dialysis may have ______________.
3. During jaundice, the ______________ of the eyes turn yellow.
4. A faulty heart valve creates a ______________.
5. A ______________ is a small lump, lesion, or swelling felt when the skin is palpated.
6. When the carotid arteries fill with plaque, a ______________ can be heard on the neck.

Part II.

A. Histology is the study of tissues. List four types of tissue in the human body.

1. ______________________________
2. ______________________________
3. ______________________________
4. ______________________________

B. What are the differences among tissue, organs, and body systems?

____

____

____

C. List the 11 systems of the body and name two organs in each system.

Body System	Organs

Part III.

The medical assistant's duties can be divided into three areas:

1. ______________________________

2. ______________________________

3. ______________________________

Part IV. Instruments and Equipment Needed for Physical Exam

Identify the instruments shown in the following figures.

1. ______________________________

2. ____

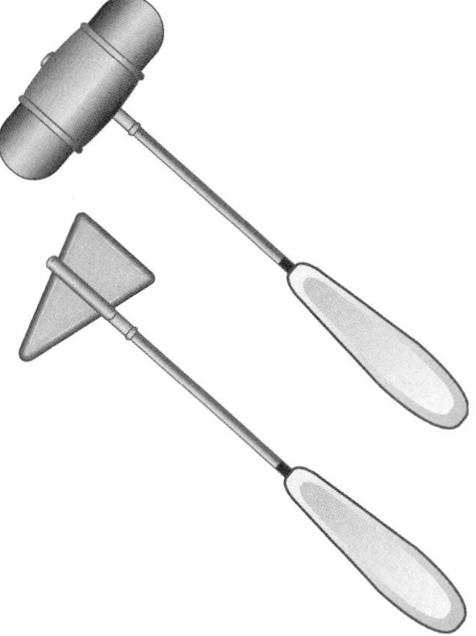

3. ____

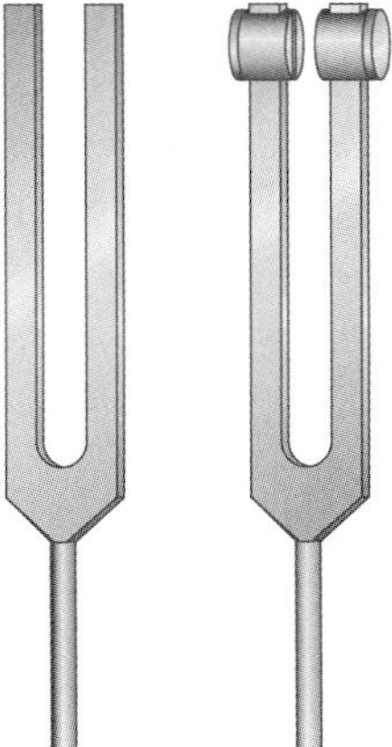

4. ____

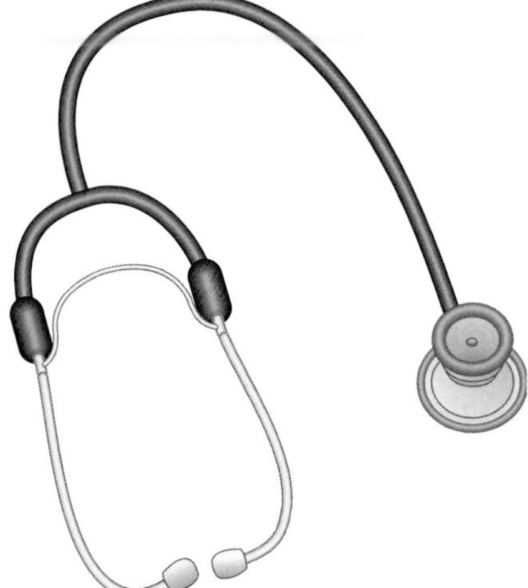

5. ______________________________

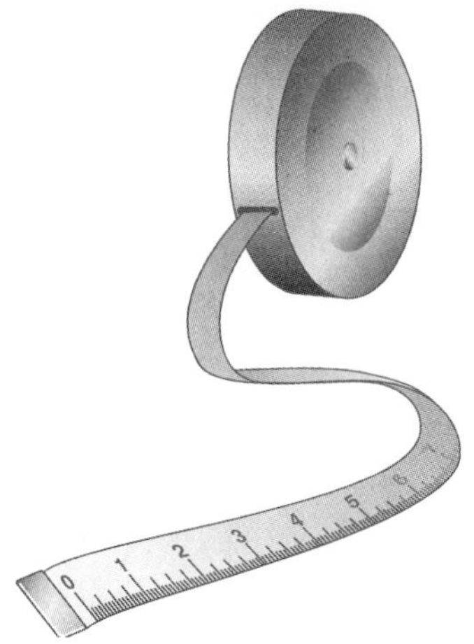

6. ______________________________

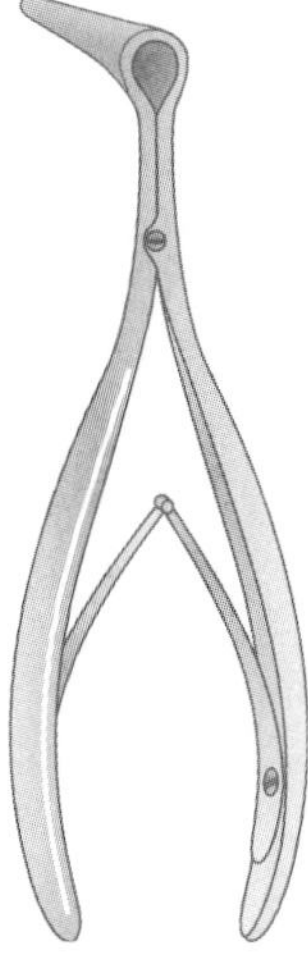

7. ______________________________

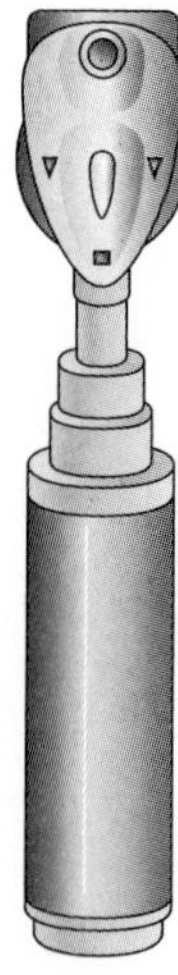

8. ______________________________

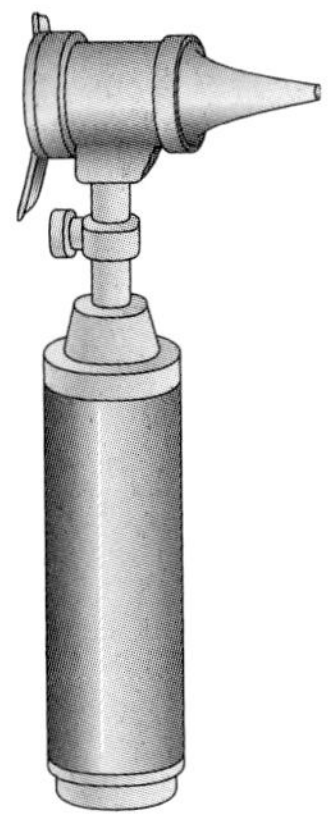

Part V.

Directions: Describe the following methods of assessment.

1. Inspection ______________________________
2. Palpation ______________________________
3. Percussion ______________________________
4. Auscultation ______________________________
5. Mensuration ______________________________
6. Manipulation ______________________________

Part VI. Positions for Examination

Directions: Label each position shown in the following figures.

1. ______________________________

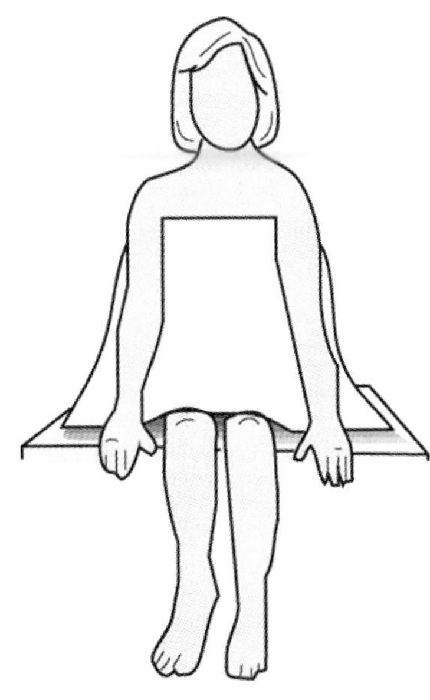

2. ______________________________

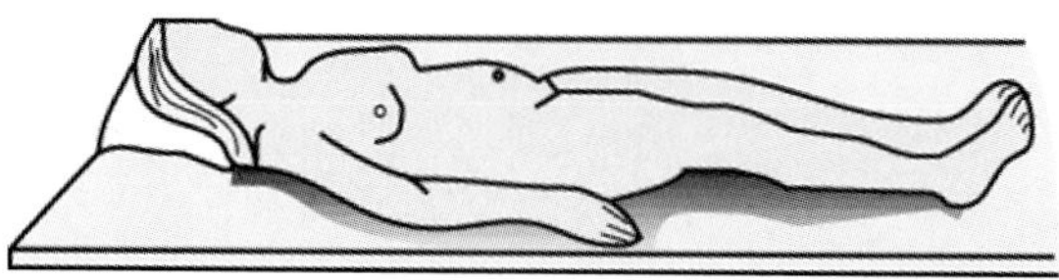

3. ______________________________

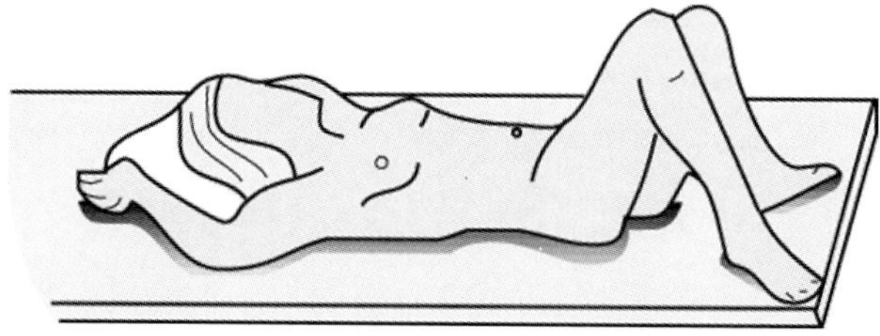

4. ______________________________

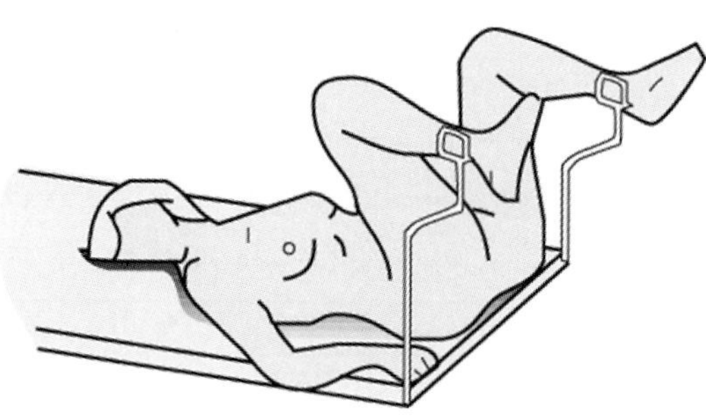

5. ______________________________

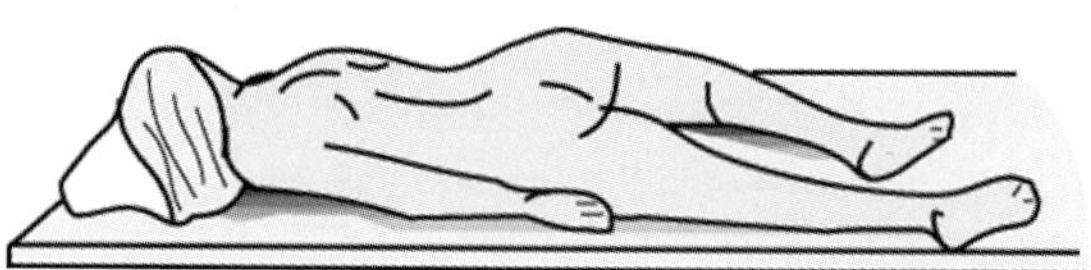

6. ______________________________

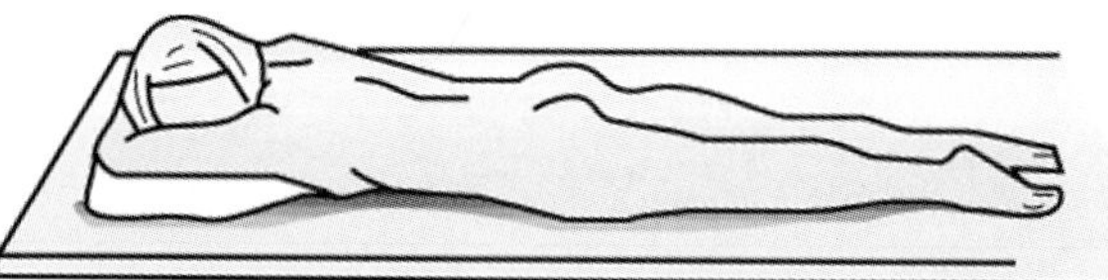

7. ______________________________

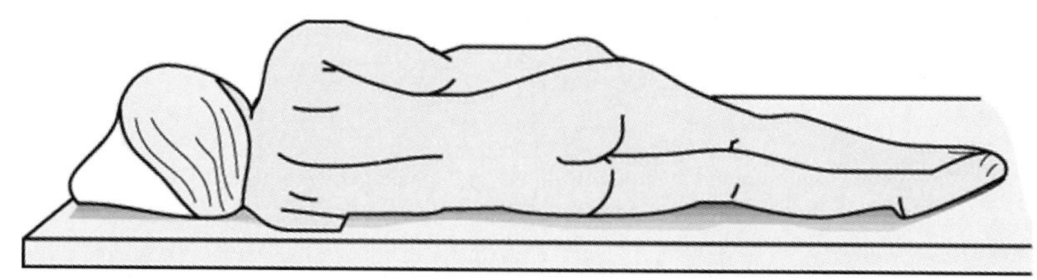

8. ____________________

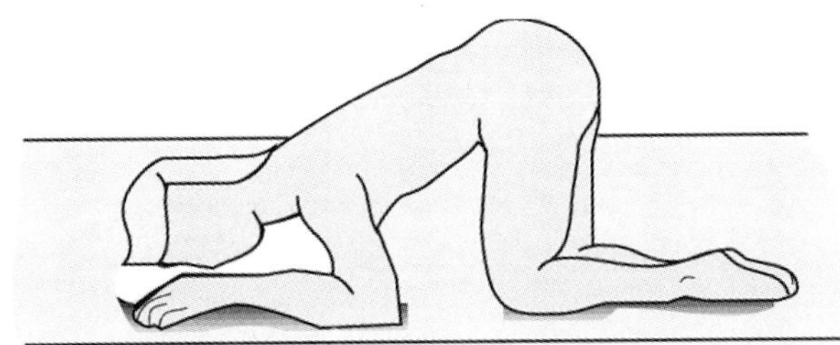

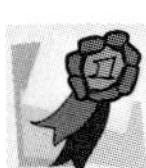

Part VII. Extra for Experts

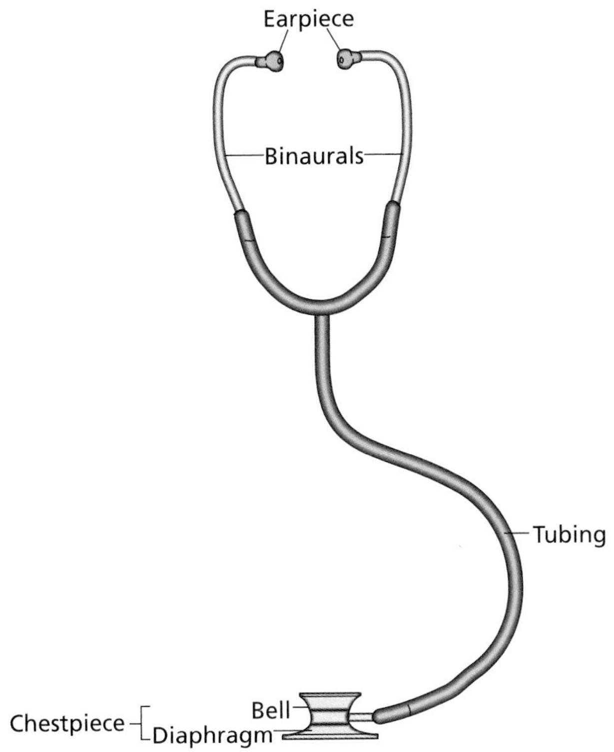

Directions: Examine the diagram of the stethoscope. Describe the function of the following.

1. Diaphragm ____________________

2. Bell ____________________

Chapter 29 Quiz

Name: ____

1. The kidneys are part of the

   ____________ system.

2. The otoscope is used to examine the

   ____________.

3. A tape measure is used for:

   a. palpation

   b. auscultation

   c. manipulation

   d. mensuration

   ____

4. The spinal cord is part of the

   ____________ system.

5. Ligaments are included in the

   ____________ system.

6. The liver is in the ____________ system.

7. Blood cells belong to the

   ____________ system.

8. Rectal medications are usually administered with the patient in the

   ____________ position.

9. True or False: The dorsal recumbent position includes having the patient's feet in stirrups.

   ____

10. True or False: Supine is flat on the back.

    ____

CHAPTER 30

Principles of Pharmacology

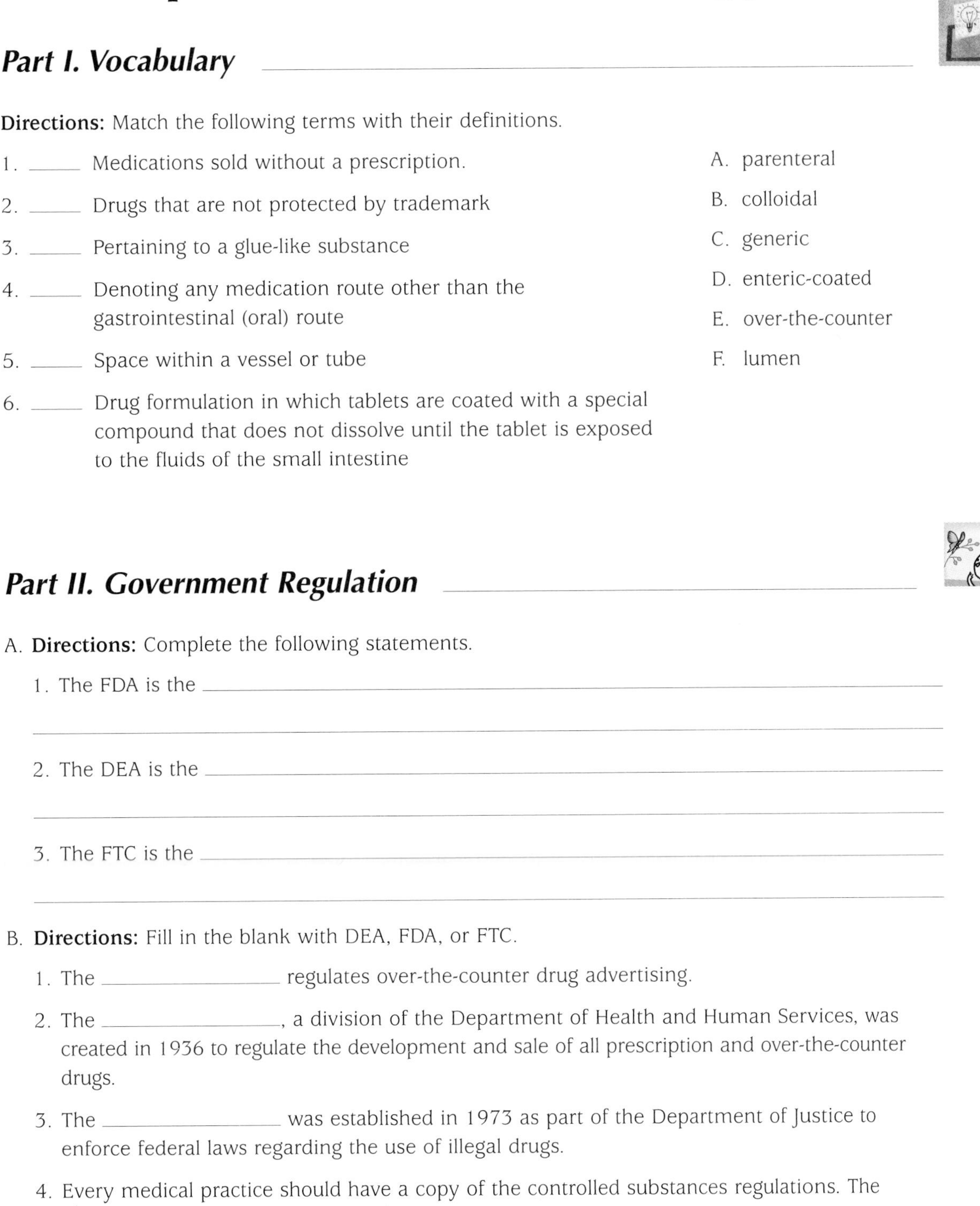

Part I. Vocabulary

Directions: Match the following terms with their definitions.

1. ______ Medications sold without a prescription.
2. ______ Drugs that are not protected by trademark
3. ______ Pertaining to a glue-like substance
4. ______ Denoting any medication route other than the gastrointestinal (oral) route
5. ______ Space within a vessel or tube
6. ______ Drug formulation in which tablets are coated with a special compound that does not dissolve until the tablet is exposed to the fluids of the small intestine

A. parenteral
B. colloidal
C. generic
D. enteric-coated
E. over-the-counter
F. lumen

Part II. Government Regulation

A. **Directions:** Complete the following statements.

1. The FDA is the ____

____

2. The DEA is the ____

____

3. The FTC is the ____

____

B. **Directions:** Fill in the blank with DEA, FDA, or FTC.

1. The ______________ regulates over-the-counter drug advertising.
2. The ______________, a division of the Department of Health and Human Services, was created in 1936 to regulate the development and sale of all prescription and over-the-counter drugs.
3. The ______________ was established in 1973 as part of the Department of Justice to enforce federal laws regarding the use of illegal drugs.
4. Every medical practice should have a copy of the controlled substances regulations. The medical assistant may secure this list from a regional office of the ______________.

5. Besides approving new drugs for the marketplace, the ________________ is also responsible for establishing standards for their purity and strength during the manufacturing process and for ensuring that generic brands are effective and safe.

6. Each physician who prescribes or who has controlled substances on site must register with the ________________ for a Controlled Substance Registration Certificate and will receive a specific registration number that must be included on all controlled substance prescriptions.

C. **Directions:** List six specific guidelines for prescription orders of controlled substances.

1. ________________
2. ________________
3. ________________
4. ________________
5. ________________
6. ________________

Part III. ________________

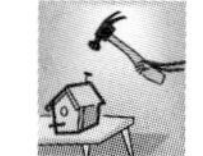

Directions: Use your text to complete the table of classification of controlled substances.

Schedule	Guidelines	List Three Drug Examples
I	________________ medical use ________________ potential for abuse Possession of these drugs is illegal.	
II	Accepted for medical use ________________ restrictions ________________ potential for abuse May cause severe psychological or physical dependence	
III	Accepted for medical use Potential for abuse less than I or II May cause ________________ physical dependence or high psychological dependence Includes combination drugs that contain limited amounts of narcotics or stimulants	
IV	Accepted for medical use ________________ potential for abuse May cause limited physical or psychological dependence in comparison with schedule III drugs Includes minor tranquilizers and hypnotics	
V	Accepted for medical use ________________ potential for abuse May cause limited physical or psychological dependence in comparison with schedule IV drugs Includes drug mixtures containing limited amounts of narcotics	

Part IV. Conflict Resolution

Directions: Indicate which statements are true (T) and which statements are false (F).

1. ______ The chemical name represents the drug's exact formula.
2. ______ The generic drug name is assigned by the manufacturer and is protected by copyright.
3. ______ Brand names are capitalized.
4. ______ The *PDR* is the most commonly used drug reference book.
5. ______ A prescription is an order written by the physician for the compounding or dispensing and administration of drugs to a particular patient.

Directions: Fill in the blanks by choosing the correct terms from the list below.

1. ______ drugs are used to treat the disorder and cure it; antibiotics cure bacterial infections.
2. ______ drugs do not cure but provide relief from pain or symptoms related to the disorder; an example is the use of an antihistamine for allergic symptoms.
3. ______ drugs prevent the occurrence of a condition; vaccines prevent the occurrence of specific infectious diseases.
4. ______ drugs help determine the cause of a particular health problem; an example is injection of antigen serum for allergy testing.
5. ______ drugs provide patients with substances needed to maintain health; examples are estrogen replacement therapy for menopausal women and administration of insulin to patients with diabetes.

A. Prophylactic
B. Therapeutic
C. Replacement
D. Palliative
E. Diagnostic

Part V. Pharmacokinetic Terms

Directions: Complete each sentence

Excretion

Distribution

Metabolism

Absorption

1. How a drug is absorbed into the body's circulating fluids, which depends on the route by which it is administered, is called ________________.
2. How a drug is transported from the site of administration to the various points in the body is called ________________.
3. How a drug is inactivated, including the time it takes for the drug to be detoxified and broken down into by-products, is called ________________.
4. The route by which a drug is excreted, or eliminated, from the body and the amount of time such a process requires is called ________________.

Part VI. Workplace Applications

Routes of Absorption

Oral route

Topical absorption

Mucous membrane absorption

Parenteral route

Step One: Think of an example of each of the listed routes of absorption. Record your ideas.

Step Two: Pair up with a classmate and discuss your examples.

Step Three: Share your ideas with your classmates. Make notes of any examples that you did not think of before.

List six of the factors that can affect drug action.

1. __________
2. __________
3. __________
4. __________
5. __________
6. __________

Part VII. Extra for Experts

Directions: Complete the table below by describing the action of each type of drug and giving an example of each type.

Type of Drug	Action and Example
Analgesic	
Anesthetic	
Antibiotic	
Antidepressant	
Antihistamine	
Antihypertensive	
Anti-inflammatory	
Antineoplastic	
Antitussive	

Part VIII. Self-Awareness

My biggest concern about giving medications is ______________________________

____

____

____

I look forward to ______________________________

____

____

____

I dread ______________________________

____

____

____

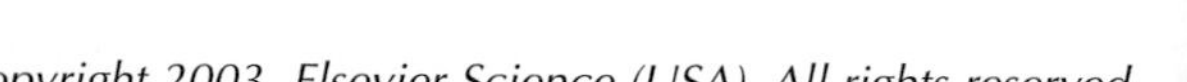

Chapter 30 Quiz

Name: ____________________

1. List three factors that affect drug action.

   a. ____________________

   b. ____________________

   c. ____________________

2. A ____________ increases peristaltic activity of the large intestine.

3. True or False: Pharmacology is the broad science that deals with the origin, nature, chemistry, effects, and uses of drugs.

   ____

4. True or False: Pharmaceutical companies developing new medications must first gain DEA approval before the drugs can be sold to consumers.

   ____

5. True or False: A diuretic increases urinary output and decreases blood pressure.

   ____

6. True or False: Schedule II drugs are closely monitored and controlled.

   ____

7. List three types of drug names.

   a. ____________________

   b. ____________________

   c. ____________________

8. PDR stands for ____________

   ____________ ____________.

CHAPTER 31

Pharmacology Math

Part I. Drug Labels

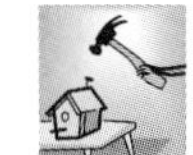

Directions: Visit a local pharmacy or grocery store that has a variety of over-the-counter (OTC) medications. Locate containers of aspirin, Tylenol, and Advil in both tablet and liquid forms for children. Complete the following table.

Drug Brand Name	Generic Name	Strength (weight in mg)	Dosage (per tablet or teaspoon)
Aspirin			
Baby aspirin tablets			
Tylenol tablets			
Tylenol liquid			
Advil or Motrin			
Advil liquid			

Part II. Metric System

Consider the following fundamental units of the metric system:

Mass or weight: gram (g) *always lowercase*

Volume: liter (L) *always capitalized*

Length: meter (m) *always lowercase*

Consider the following equivalents:

Mass and weight	*Volume*
1 kg = 1000 g	1 kl = 1000 liters
1 g = 1000 mg	1 L = 1000 ml (or cc)
1 mg = 1000 ìg	1 ml (or 1 cc) = 1000 ìl
1 dg = 0.1 g or 1/10 g	1 dl = 0.1 L or 1/10 L
1 cg = 0.01 g or 1/100 g	1 cl = 0.01 L or 1/100 L
1 mg = 0.001 g or 1/1000 g	1 ml (or 1 cc) = 0.001 L or 1/1000 L

A. **Directions:** Write the prefix for the following (remember to write them in lowercase).

1. ________________ one hundredth of a unit
2. ________________ one tenth of a unit
3. ________________ one thousandth of a unit
4. ________________ one millionth of a unit
5. ________________ ten units
6. ________________ one hundred units
7. ________________ one thousand units

B. **Directions:** Convert the following by moving the decimals or by multiplication or division.

Show your work here.

1. 1.5 L = ________________ ml
2. 500 mg = ________________ g
3. 3 g = ________________ mg
4. 2000 mg = ________________ g
5. 2.5 g = ________________ mg
6. 0.5 g = ________________ mg
7. 500 ml = ________________ L
8. 0.75 g = ________________ mg
9. 1 kg = ________________ g
10. 1000 mg = ________________ g

Part III. Apothecary System and Household Measurements

A. **Directions:** Insert roman numerals for use with the apothecary system.

Arabic	Roman	Arabic	Roman
1	I	15	
2		20	
3		30	
4		40	
5	V	50	L
6		60	
7		70	
8		80	
9		90	XC
10	X	100	C

Directions: Supply the abbreviations or symbols for these metric, apothecary system, and common household units.

1. ounce symbol __________
2. teaspoon __________
3. milligram __________
4. grain __________
5. pint __________
6. dram symbol __________
7. tablespoon __________

Directions: Use the conversions to complete the questions below.

1 cup = 8 oz
1 oz = 2 tablespoons
1 tablespoon = 3 teaspoons
1 teaspoon = 60 drops

1 teaspoon = 5 ml (cc)
1 tablespoon = 15 ml (cc)
1 fluid ounce = 30 ml (cc)
1 grain = 60 mg

1. A standard teaspoon equals 5 ml. If a liquid drug has 100 mg per teaspoon, how many milligrams are in each milliliter? __________

   How did you determine your answer?

   ____

   ____

2. You are asked to give 2 teaspoons of cough medicine to a child. How many milliliters will you give? ____________

3. How many teaspoons are in one ounce? ____________

4. Now that you know that 5 ml is the same as one teaspoon, how many milliliters are in one ounce? ____________

Part IV. Conversions Between Systems of Measurement

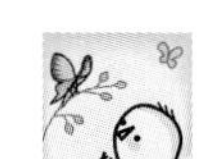

Conversions between units of measurements can also be done by using the following formula:

$$\text{Have} \times \frac{\text{Wanted}}{\text{Have (conversion)}} = \text{Unit Wanted in New System}$$

Using the 15 gr/g conversion, convert 30 grains to milligrams:

$$30 \text{ gr} \times \frac{1.0 \text{ g}}{15 \text{ gr}} = \text{Unit Wanted}$$

Cross-multiply the problem and the gr unit cancels out to give:

$$\text{Have} \times \frac{\text{Wanted}}{\text{Have (conversion)}} = \text{Unit Wanted in New System}$$

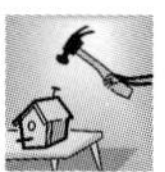

Directions: Convert pounds to kilograms. The conversion factor is 2.5 lb/kg.

Show your work here.

1. 150 lb = ____________ kg
2. 78 lb = ____________ kg
3. 22 lb = ____________ kg
4. 210 lb = ____________ kg
5. 64 lb = ____________ kg
6. 198 lb = ____________ kg
7. 112 lb = ____________ kg
8. 163 lb = ____________ kg
9. 13 lb = ____________ kg
10. 4.4 lb = ____________ kg

Directions: Convert inches to centimeters. There are 2.2 cm per inch.

Show your work here.

1. 62 inches = ____________ cm
2. 34 inches = ____________ cm
3. 97 inches = ____________ cm
4. 5′0″ = ____________ inches = ____________ cm
5. 6′2″ = ____________ inches = ____________ cm

Part V. Decimals and Percents

The act of dividing a fraction results in a decimal number. Decimal numbers can then be converted to percentages by moving the decimal two spaces to the right:

0.25 = 25.0%, commonly written 25%

Directions: Convert these decimals to percentages.

Show your work here.

1. 0.75 = ____________ %
2. 0.33 = ____________ %
3. 0.25 = ____________ %
4. 1.0 = ____________ %
5. 0.50 = ____________ %

Part VI. Ratio and Proportion

A proportion is written as follows:

$\frac{4}{16} = \frac{1}{4}$ or 4:16::1:4

The preceding proportion example has all the answers in it; there is nothing to solve. In calculating dosages, mathematical proportions are used, but with one element unknown. We must solve for that unknown, or x. For example:

$\frac{4}{16} = \frac{1}{x}$

Always in a proportion, we solve the problem by *cross-multiplication*. Do not confuse this with plain multiplication. If you see an equals sign (=) between two fractions, it indicates that the equation is to be *cross-multiplied*.

$4 \times x = 16 \times 1$

Therefore

$4x = 16$

We know what $4x$ equals, but next we must find what $1x$, or x, equals. To determine the value of x, we must find a way to leave x (or $1x$) alone on one side of the equation. We can change $4x$ to $1x$ by dividing the number 4 by itself:

$4x \div 4 = 1x$

But what we do on one side of an equation, we must do on the other side, or the equation will not be equal anymore. Therefore we divide 16 by 4:

$16 \div 4 = 4$ Therefore $x = 4$ and $\frac{4}{16} = \frac{1}{4}$

Directions: Solve for x and compare the two fractions.

Show your work here.

1. $3 : 4 = x : 12$
2. $1 : 2 = x : 6$
3. $2 : 5 = x : 100$

4. 2 : 6 = x : 12

5. 1 : 3 = x : 75

Part VII. Calculating Dosages

Standard Formula:

$$\frac{\text{Available strength}}{\text{Ordered strength}} = \frac{\text{Available amount}}{\text{Amount to give}}$$

Procedure: Rewrite the formula, replacing unknown values with known quantities from the label and the doctor's order. The unknown, when you solve for x, will be the amount you actually give.

Let's Practice: The doctor orders 200 mg of medication. The label reads 100 mg per tablet. How many tablets do you give?

$$\frac{100 \text{ mg}}{200 \text{ mg}} = \frac{1 \text{ tablet}}{x}$$

Cross-multiply: 100 mg times x = 200 mg times 1 tablet

Divide both sides by 100 to leave x by itself on the left side.

What is the result? How many tablets do you give?

Another way to complete the same problem is to use a formula:

$$\text{Pediatric Dose} = \frac{\text{Child's Age in Months}}{150 \text{ months}} \times \text{Adult Dose}$$

$$\frac{200 \text{ mg}}{100 \text{ mg}} \times 1 \text{ tablet}$$

What is the result? How many tablets do you give?

Practice calculations 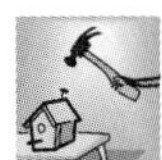

Directions: Calculate the following:

Doctor's Order	Label Reads	Amount to Give	Practice Charting
Keflex 500 mg	250-mg capsule		
Lasix 40 mg	20-mg tablet		
Zoloft 75 mg	25-mg tablet		
Claritin 30 mg	10-mg tablet		
Prilosec 40 mg	10-mg capsule		
Celebrex 200 mg	100-mg capsule		
Vioxx 12.5 mg	25 mg		
Lanoxin .125 mg	.25-mg tablet		

Doctor's Order	Label Reads	Amount to Give	Practice Charting
Coumadin 20 mg	5-mg tablet		
Augmentin 250 mg	500 mg per 5 ml		
Prednisone 40 mg	5-mg tablet		
Prozac 20 mg	10-mg capsule		
Synthroid .44 mg	88 μg per tablet		
Zocor 60 mg	20-mg tablet		
Glucophage 1 g	500-mg tablet		
Zestril 2.5 mg	5-mg tablet		
Norvasc 10 mg	2.5-mg tablet		
Cipro 750 mg	250-mg tablet		
Zyrtec syrup 4 mg	5 mg/5 ml		
Zovirax 200 mg	400-mg tablet		

Part VIII. Pediatric Dosages

Directions: Complete the following:

Fried's Law

$$\text{Pediatric Dose} = \frac{\text{Child's Age in Months}}{\text{150 months}} \times \text{Adult Dose}$$

Order	Adult Dose	Child's Age	Amount to Give
Penicillin	100,000 U	18 mo	
Benadryl	50 mg	5 yr	
Tylenol	500 mg	2 yr	
Sudafed	60 mg	10 mo	

Clark's Rule

$$\text{Pediatric Dose} = \frac{\text{Child's Weight in Pounds}}{\text{150 pounds}} \times \text{Adult Dose}$$

Order	Adult Dose	Child's Weight	Amount to Give
Penicillin	100,000 U	22 lb	
Benadryl	50 mg	13 lb	
Tylenol	500 mg	54 lb	
Sudafed	60 mg	37 lb	

West's Nomogram

$$\text{Pediatric Dose} = \frac{\text{Body Surface Area (BSA) of Child in Square Meters} \times \text{Adult Dose}}{1.7\ m^2 \text{ (Average Adult BSA)}}$$

Order	Adult Dose	Child's BSA	Amount to Give
Penicillin	100,000 U	.5 m^2	
Benadryl	50 mg	.3 m^2	
Tylenol	500 mg	.6 m^2	
Sudafed	60 mg	.7 m^2	

Part IX. Putting It All Together

Directions: Use Fried's Law, Clark's Rule, or West's Nomogram to answer the following questions.

1. A child weighs 42 lb. The doctor orders 1 mg of medication per kilogram. How many kilograms does the child weigh? How many milligrams of medication do you need to give? ______________
2. A 5-year-old needs cough medicine. The adult dose is 20 mg. According to Fried's Law, what is the pediatric dose? ______________
3. An infant weighs 14 lb. The adult dose is 100 mg. When Clark's Rule is used, how much is the pediatric dose? ______________
4. The doctor orders 5 mg of medication per kilogram of body weight. The patient weighs 145 lb. How many milligrams do you give? ______________

5. The child has a BSA of .9 m^2 and the adult dose is 200 mg. According to West's nomogram, what is the pediatric dose? ________________

6. The nurse practitioner orders 250 mg of Rocephin to be given by injection. The vial contains Rocephin at a concentration of 500 mg/ml. How much medication will the medical assistant draw into the syringe? ________________

7. The patient takes 5000 U of heparin by injection each day. The vial contains heparin, 10,000 U/ml. How much heparin does the home health nurse need to draw up into the syringe?

   ____

8. The patient weighs 163 lb. The order is for 2 mg/kg. How much medicine does the patient need? ________________

9. The doctor orders Phenergan 12.5 mg by mouth. You have Phenergan syrup that has a concentration of 25 mg/5 ml. How many milliliters will you give? ________________

10. You need to give a 500 injection of vitamin B_{12}. You have on hand vitamin B_{12} at a concentration unit of 1000 unit/ml. How much will you measure in the syringe? ________________

Part X. Extra for Experts

Directions: Use the Internet or a drug reference book to collect information and make index cards for the drugs that were discussed in Chapters 30 and 31.

BRAND NAME:
GENERIC NAME:
TYPE OF DRUG:
USUAL DOSE:
USES:

Chapter 31 Quiz

Name: ______________________________

1. One cup equals ______________ ounces.

2. One teaspoon equals ______________ ml.

3. There are ______________ ml in one ounce.

4. A grain is part of the ______________ system.

   a. metric

   b. household

   c. apothecary

5. A liter is a unit of

   a. weight

   b. volume

   c. length

   ____

6. Milliliters are sometimes called ______________.

7. The Roman numeral for four is ______________.

8. There are ______________ teaspoons in one tablespoon.

9. True or False: Clark's rule uses a child's age to calculate dosage.

   ____

10. There are ______________ pounds in one kilogram.

CHAPTER 32

Administering Medications

Part I. Vocabulary

Directions: Match the following terms and definitions.

1. _____ Angled tip of a needle
2. _____ Narrowing of the bronchiole tubes
3. _____ Abnormal accumulation of fluid in the interstitial spaces of tissues
4. _____ A coating added to an oral medication that resists the effects of stomach juices; designed so medicine is absorbed in the small intestine
5. _____ Sealed so that no air is allowed to enter
6. _____ Low blood pressure
7. _____ Administering repeated injections of diluted extracts of the substance that causes an allergy; also called *desensitization*
8. _____ An abnormally hard, inflamed area
9. _____ Administering a double dose for the first dose of the medication; usually done with antibiotic therapy to reach therapeutic blood levels quickly
10. _____ Surgical removal of the breast; usually includes excision of lymph nodes in the axillary region
11. _____ The curved formation of liquids in a container
12. _____ Excretion of an unusually large amount of urine
13. _____ Drug in pill form manufactured with an indentation for division through the center
14. _____ Increase in the diameter of a blood vessel
15. _____ The quality of being thick; property of resistance to flow in a fluid
16. _____ Referring to an explosive substance's capacity to vaporize at a low temperature
17. _____ Localized area of edema or a raised lesion

A. bevel
B. scored tablet
C. hypotension
D. polyuria
E. volatile
F. wheal
G. viscosity
H. vasodilation
I. immunotherapy
J. loading dose
K. edema
L. meniscus
M. bronchoconstriction
N. induration
O. enteric-coated
P. mastectomy
Q. hermetically sealed

Part II.

Directions: List the seven rights of drug administration.

1. ______________________________
2. ______________________________
3. ______________________________
4. ______________________________
5. ______________________________
6. ______________________________
7. ______________________________

Solid Oral Forms

Directions: Define the following.

1. Scored ______________________________
2. Tablet ______________________________
3. Buffered ______________________________
4. Capsule ______________________________
5. Caplet ______________________________
6. Time-released ______________________________

Liquid Oral Forms

Directions: Define the following.

1. Syrup ______________________________
2. Aromatic waters ______________________________
3. Liquors ______________________________
4. Suspension ______________________________
5. Emulsion ______________________________
6. Gel/magma ______________________________
7. Tinctures ______________________________
8. Elixirs ______________________________

Mucous Membrane Forms

Directions: List the site of absorption for the following.

1. Buccal ______________________________
2. Sublingual ______________________________
3. Inhalation ______________________________

Topical Forms

Directions: Describe the following.

1. Lotion ______
2. Liniment ______
3. Ointment ______
4. Trandermal ______

Parenteral Forms

Directions: Define the following.

1. Vial ______
2. Ampule ______
3. Multi-use ______
4. Prefilled ______
5. Cartridge system ______

Directions: Indicate whether each item in the figure below is a vial or an ampule.

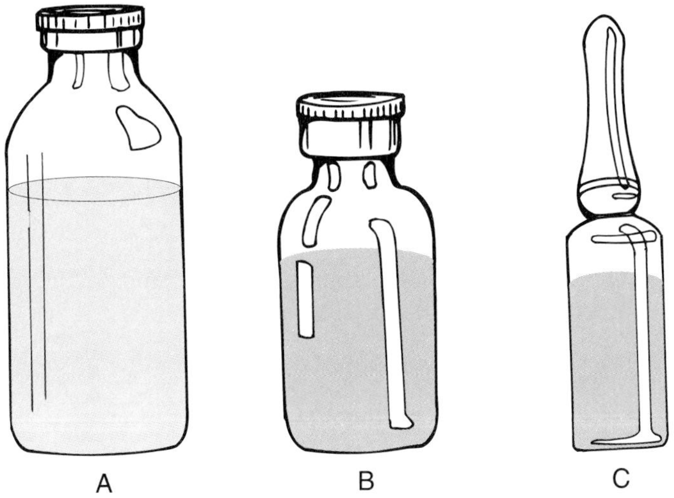

A B C

A. ______

B. ______

C. ______

Directions: Label the following statements as either "ampule" or "vial."

1. ______________ Has a rubber stopper.
2. ______________ Has sharp edges after it is opened.
3. ______________ Is always single-use.
4. ______________ Must have air injected into it before medicine can be removed.
5. ______________ Can be multi-use.
6. ______________ A filtered needle should be used to avoid getting glass in the syringe.
7. ______________ Has a vacuum after it is opened.
8. ______________ Extra care must be taken to avoid contamination.
9. ______________ Always disposed of in a sharps container.
10. ______________ Gauze or an unopened alcohol prep should be used to prevent injury as the neck breaks away.

Directions: List four routes of parenteral administration. Include approved abbreviations.

1. ______________________________
2. ______________________________
3. ______________________________
4. ______________________________

Parenteral Medication Equipment

Directions: Indicate which statements about needles are true (T) and which statements are false (F).

1. _____ Needles may be purchased separately or as part of a needle-syringe unit.
2. _____ The diameter or lumen size of a needle is called its *gauge*, and needle gauges range in size from 14 (the largest) to 28 (the smallest).
3. _____ The larger the gauge number, the smaller is the diameter of the needle.
4. _____ Gauges 25 and 26 are commonly used for subcutaneous injections.
5. _____ Larger needles (gauges 20 to 23) are usually necessary for intramuscular injections when the medication is thick (e.g., penicillin).
6. _____ Needles that are ½ or 5/8 inch long are used for intramuscular injections.
7. _____ Needles that are ½ or 5/8 inch long are used for subcutaneous injections.
8. _____ The contaminated needle should be immediately placed in a sharps container.
9. _____ The parts of the needle are the barrel, calibrated scale(s), plunger, and tip.
10. _____ Longer needles are necessary for depositing drugs intradermally.

Directions: Label the syringes in the figure below. 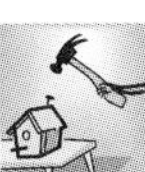

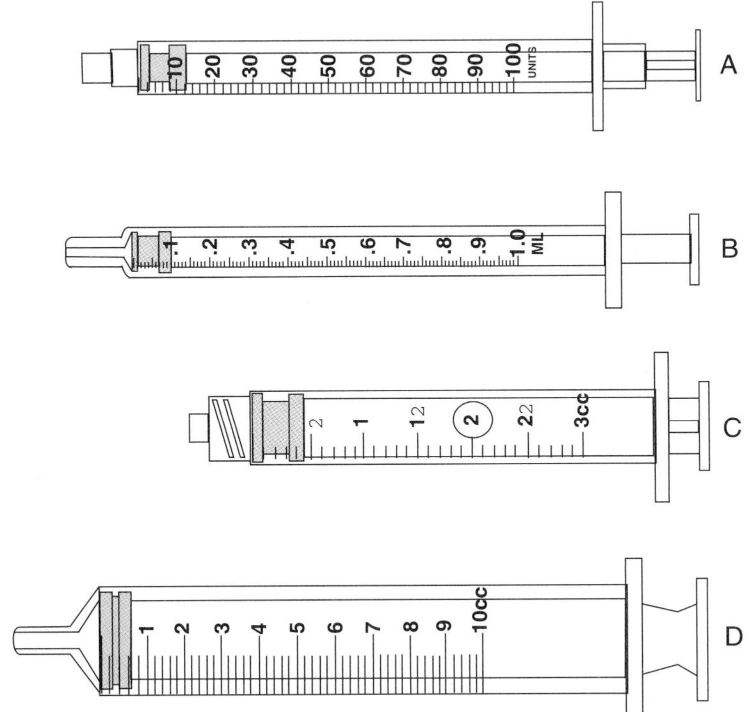

1. On the 10-cc slip-tip syringe, draw a line at 4.8 cc.
2. On the insulin syringe, draw a line at 62 units.
3. On the tuberculin syringe, draw a line at .3 cc.
4. On the 3-cc Luer-Lok syringe, draw a line at $^1/_2$ cc.

Part III. Injection Sites

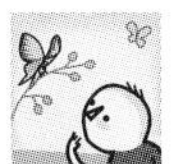

Directions: On the figure on p. 246, label the intramuscular, intradermal, and subcutaneous injection sites correctly.

A. Deltoid

B. Ventrogluteal

C. Vastus lateralis

D. Gluteal (dorsogluteal)

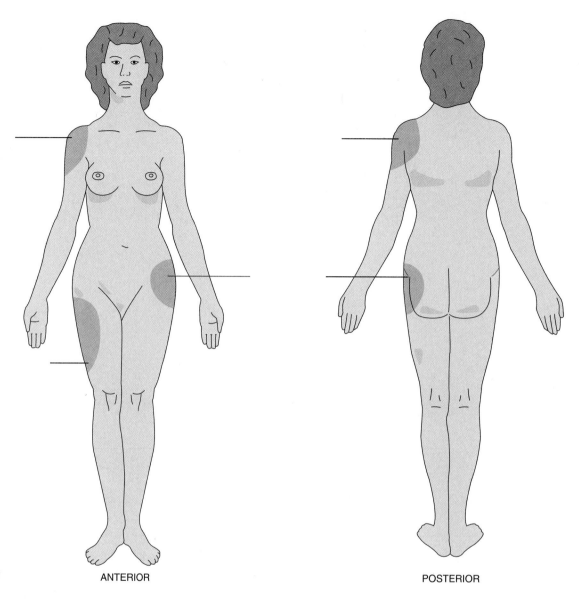

ANTERIOR

POSTERIOR

Pediatric Sites

Directions: On the figure below, label and name the appropriate injection site for a small child who is too young to walk.

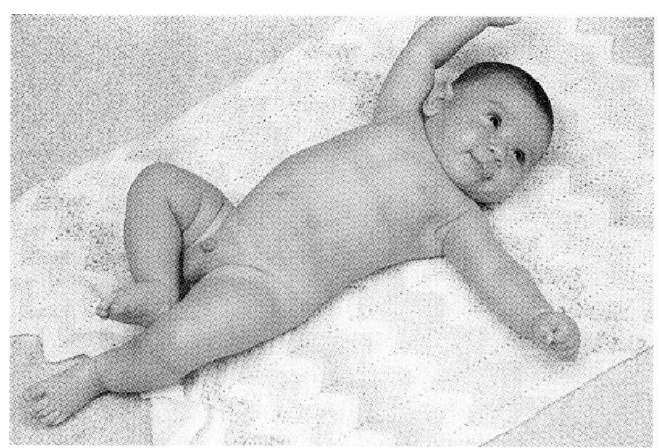

When instilling ear drops into an infant's ear, you must straighten the ear canal. On the figure below, draw an arrow to show which direction you pull the pinna.

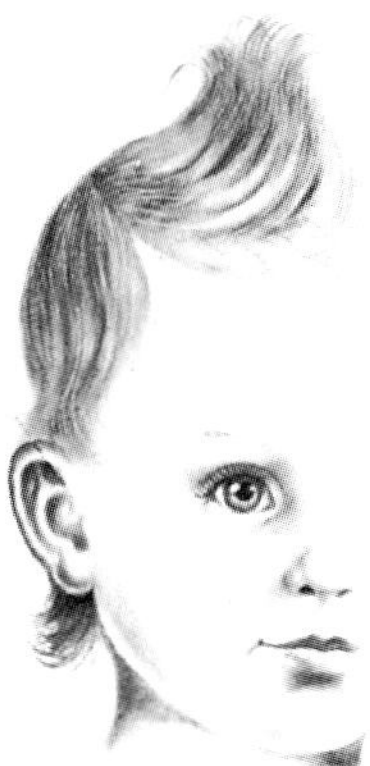
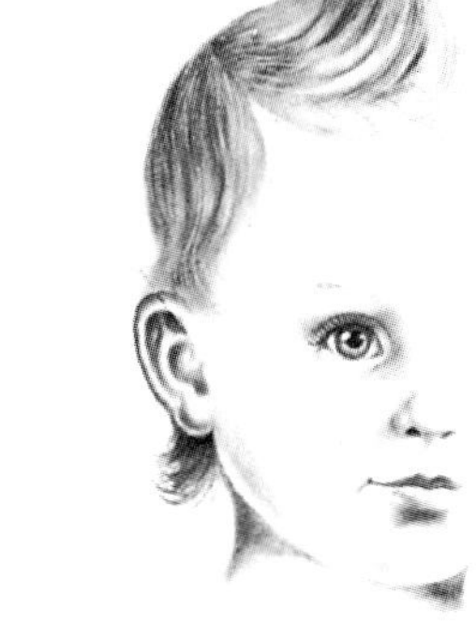

Part IV.

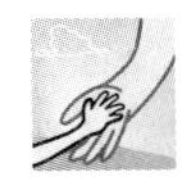
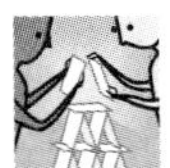

How do you feel about giving your first injection? How will you prepare for that experience? Discuss your thoughts with a classmate. Share your concerns with your instructor.

____

____

____

____

____

____

Extra for Experts

Directions: Visit a pharmacy and find out about each section of a written prescription. Label each part of the sample prescription below.

Superscription

Inscription

Subscription

Sig

Refills

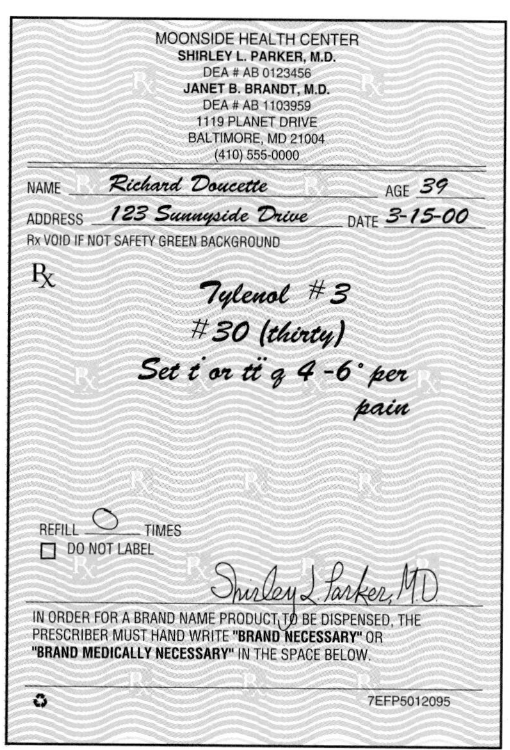

MOONSIDE HEALTH CENTER
SHIRLEY L. PARKER, M.D.
DEA # AB 0123456
JANET B. BRANDT, M.D.
DEA # AB 1103959
1119 PLANET DRIVE
BALTIMORE, MD 21004
(410) 555-0000

NAME Richard Doucette AGE 39

ADDRESS 123 Sunnyside Drive DATE 3-15-00

Rx VOID IF NOT SAFETY GREEN BACKGROUND

℞

Tylenol #3
#30 (thirty)
Sig: i or ii q 4-6° prn
pain

REFILL 0 TIMES

☐ DO NOT LABEL

Shirley L. Parker, MD

IN ORDER FOR A BRAND NAME PRODUCT TO BE DISPENSED, THE PRESCRIBER MUST HAND WRITE **"BRAND NECESSARY"** OR **"BRAND MEDICALLY NECESSARY"** IN THE SPACE BELOW.

7EFP5012095

Your patient asks you to explain what the doctor has written on the prescription. Explain the directions for taking Tylenol #3.

Spell out the following abbreviations.

1. q4h ____________________
2. tid ____________________
3. qid ____________________
4. bid ____________________
5. q3h ____________________
6. hs ____________________
7. ac ____________________
8. pc ____________________
9. prn ____________________
10. po ____________________
11. npo ____________________
12. pr ____________________
13. IV ____________________
14. SC (SQ) ____________________
15. IM ____________________
16. SL ____________________
17. qd ____________________
18. qod ____________________
19. qam ____________________
20. qpm ____________________

Chapter 32 Quiz

Name: ____________________

1. True or False: An 18-gauge needle is larger than a 23-gauge needle.

   ____

2. A tuberculin syringe holds ____________ ml (cc).

3. True or False: An ampule is multi-use.

   ____

4. One site of a subcutaneous injections is:
   a. Vastus lateralis
   b. Deltoid
   c. Gluteal (dorsogluteal)
   d. Abdomen

   ____

5. The safest site for an intramuscular injection on a small child is the:
   a. Vastus lateralis
   b. Deltoid
   c. Gluteal (dorsogluteal)

   ____

6. Milliliters are sometimes called ____________ on syringes.

7. The ____________ is the slanted part of a needle.

8. ____________ is the route for heparin and insulin.

9. True or False: Z-track is used for an intramuscular injection of an irritating substance.

   ____

10. True or False: Intradermal medication is usually given at a 90-degree angle.

    ____

CHAPTER 33

Assisting with Medical Emergencies

Part I. Vocabulary

A. **Directions:** Define the following.

1. cyanosis ______
2. dyspnea ______
3. ecchymosis ______
4. emetic ______
5. fibrillation ______
6. hematuria ______
7. mediastinum ______
8. myocardium ______
9. necrosis ______
10. photophobia ______
11. polydipsia ______
12. polyuria ______
13. transient ischemic attack ______

B. **Directions:** Fill in the blanks with the correct terms.

1. ______ ______ is defined as the immediate care given to a person who has been injured or has suddenly taken ill.
2. AED stands for ______.
3. CPR stands for ______.
4. CVA stands for ______.
5. TIA stands for ______.
6. MI stands for ______.
7. A heart attack, or ______, is usually caused by a blockage of the coronary arteries, which decreases the amount of blood being delivered to the myocardium. The most common signal of a heart attack is an uncomfortable pressure, squeezing, fullness, or pain in the center of the chest.

C. List five other symptoms of a heart attack.

1. ______________________________

2. ______________________________

3. ______________________________

4. ______________________________

5. ______________________________

D. List seven types of shock.

1. ______________________________

2. ______________________________

3. ______________________________

4. ______________________________

5. ______________________________

6. ______________________________

7. ______________________________

E. Sprains and strains are treated with:

1. ______________________________

2. ______________________________

3. ______________________________

4. ______________________________

F. Give five examples of situations in which patients with abdominal pain should be seen immediately.

1. ______________________________

2. ______________________________

3. ______________________________

4. ______________________________

5. ______________________________

Part II. Heat-Related Illnesses

Directions: Fill in the blanks with the correct terms.

1. ______________ ______________ is the most dangerous form of heat-related injury and results in a shutdown of body systems.

2. ______________ are the initial signs of a heat-related emergency, and heat exhaustion is a more serious condition.

3. Patients with ______________ ______________ appear flushed and report headaches, nausea, vertigo, and weakness.

Part III. Emergency Situations

Directions: Complete the table with appropriate triage questions and home care advice.

Situation	Triage Questions	Home Care Advice
Syncope	1. 2.	1. 2. 3.
Animal bites	1. 2. 3.	1. 2. 3.
Insect bites and stings	1. 2.	1. 2. 3.
Asthma	1. 2.	1.
Burns	1. 2. 3.	1. 2. 3. 4.

Situation	Triage Questions	Home Care Advice
Wounds	1. 2. 3. 4.	1. 2. 3. 4.
Head injury	1.	1.

Chapter 33 Quiz

Name: ______________________________

1. AED stands for ______________ ______________ ______________.

2. A ______________ ______________ seizure involves uncontrolled muscular contractions.

3. List three symptoms of a heart attack.
   a. ______________
   b. ______________
   c. ______________

4. Syncope means to ______________.

5. List three causes of shock.
   a. ______________
   b. ______________
   c. ______________

6. True or False: Epinephrine is a vasoconstrictor.
   ____

7. True or False: Accidental poisoning is the leading cause of death in children.
   ____

8. List two ways to treat lacerations.
   a. ______________
   b. ______________

9. During a life-threatening emergency, always call ______________.

10. ______________ means to sort patients.

CHAPTER 34

Assisting in Ophthalmology and Otolaryngology

Part I. Medical Terminology

Directions: Match the following terms and definitions.

1. _____ Adjustment of the eye for seeing various sizes of objects at different distances
2. _____ Reduction or dimness of vision with no apparent organic cause; often referred to as *lazy eye syndrome*
3. _____ An allied healthcare professional specializing in evaluation of hearing function, detection of hearing impairment, and determination of the anatomic site of impairment
4. _____ Structures found in the retina that make the perception of color possible
5. _____ A small pit in the center of the retina that is considered the center of clearest vision
6. _____ Any substance or medication that causes constriction of the pupil
7. _____ Region at the back of the eye where the optic nerve meets the retina; considered the blind spot of the eye because it contains only nerve fibers and no rods or cones and thus is insensitive to light
8. _____ Second cranial nerve that carries impulses for the sense of sight
9. _____ Formation of spongy bone in the labyrinth of the ear, often causing the auditory ossicles to become fixed and unable to vibrate when sound enters the ear
10. _____ A substance or medication that damages the eighth cranial nerve or the organs of hearing and balance
11. _____ Abnormal sensitivity to light

A. cones
B. accommodation
C. seborrhea
D. psoriasis
E. rods
F. audiologist
G. amblyopia
H. photophobia
I. optic nerve
J. otosclerosis
K. ototoxic
L. fovea centralis
M. optic disc
N. miotic

12. ______ Usually chronic, recurrent skin disease marked by bright red patches covered with silvery scales

13. ______ Structures located in the retina of the eye and forming the light-sensitive elements

14. ______ Excessive discharge of sebum from the sebaceous glands, forming greasy scales or cheesy plugs on the body

Part II. Spelling

1. Spell the name of the color blindness test. ____________________
2. Spell the name of the chart that is used for testing far vision. ________________
3. Spell the name of the chart used for testing near vision. ________________________

Part III. Anatomy and Physiology

A. **Directions:** On the figure below, label the structures of the outer eye.

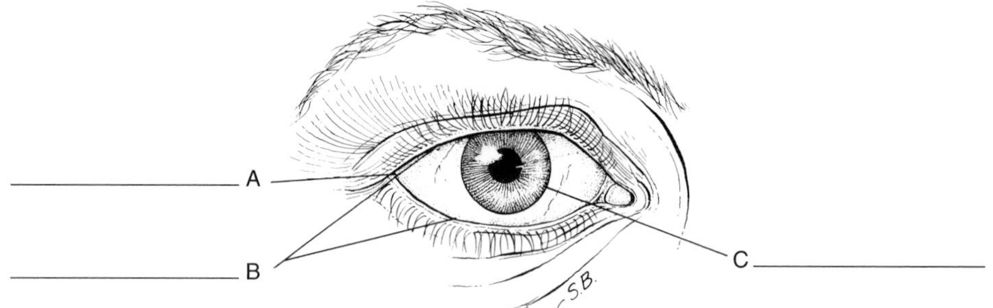

B. **Directions:** On the figure below, label the structures of the outer ear.

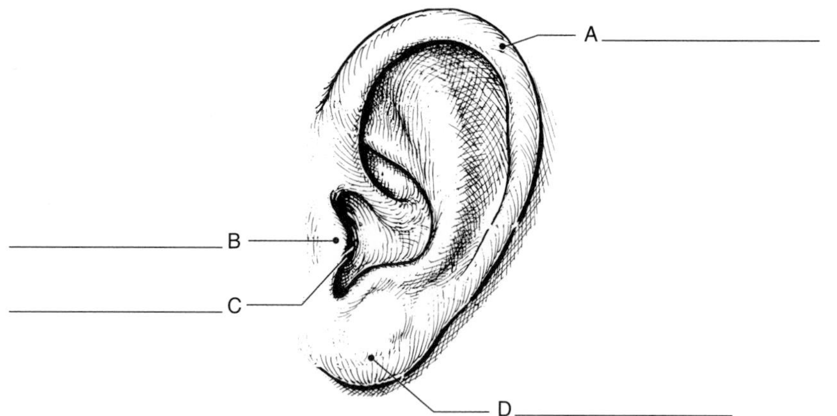

Part IV. Theory/Triage

A. **Directions:** Name the two disorders of the outer eye that are pictured below.

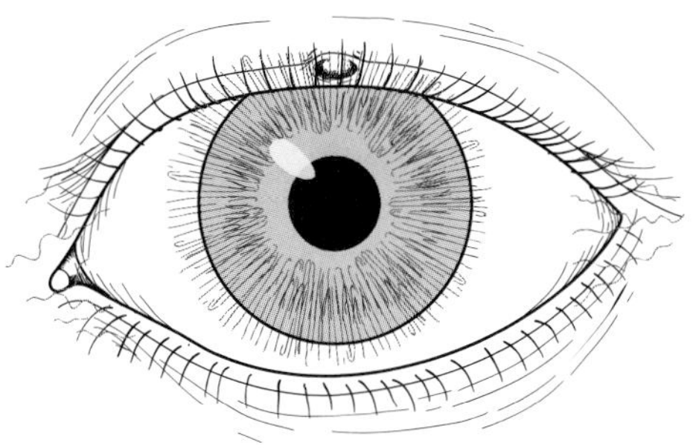

1. ______________________________

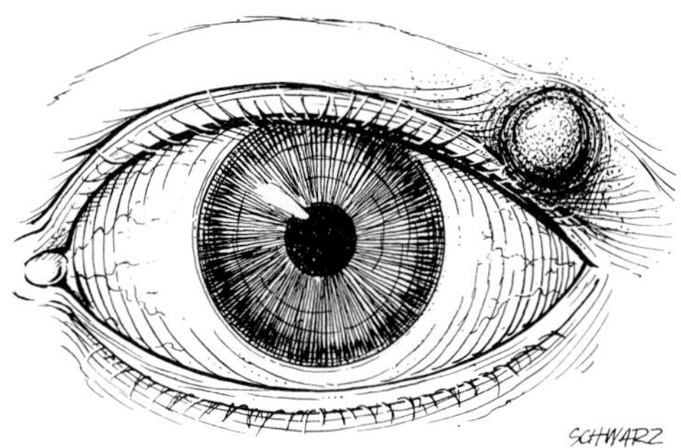

2. ______________________________

Part V. Documentation

Directions: Refer to the charts in the figure below to answer the questions.

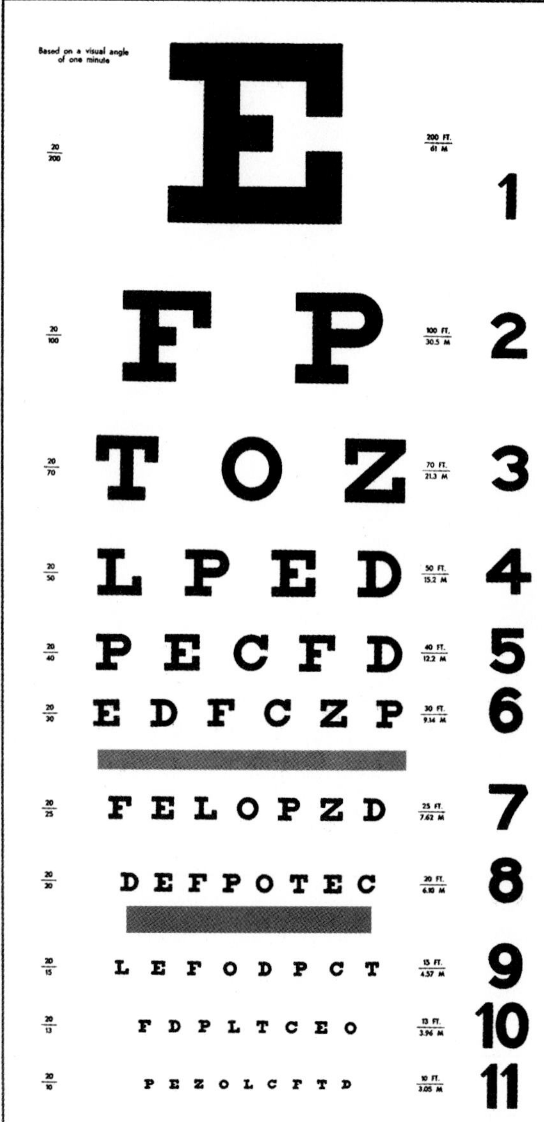

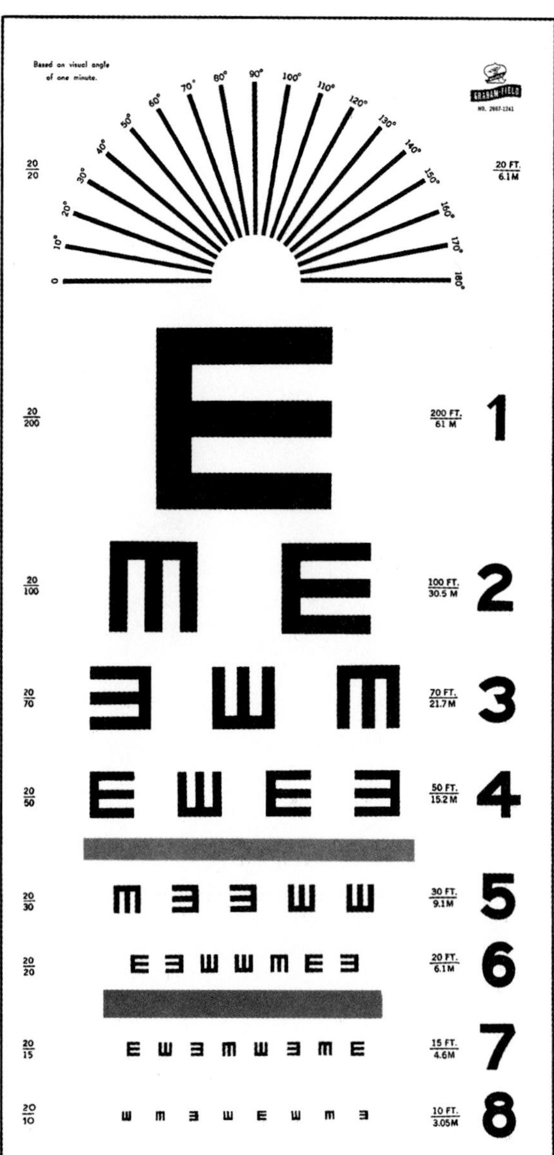

A. Your patient can read line number 8 with the right eye, number 9 with the left eye, and number 8 with both eyes on the Snellen chart. Document your findings on p. 263. Use appropriate abbreviations. Be sure to include the date and your signature. Correct mistakes by drawing one line. Use black ink.

Documentation

B. Your patient cannot read English. He indicates that he can see line number 6 with the right eye, number 5 with the left eye, and number 6 with both eyes on the E chart. How will you have your patient respond so that you know your findings are accurate?

Document your findings below. Use appropriate abbreviations. Be sure to include the date and your signature. Correct mistakes by drawing one line. Use black ink.

Documentation

Part VI. Drugs to Know

Directions: Use a drug reference book or the Internet to make drug cards for the following.

1. carbamide peroxide (Debrox)
2. Cortisporin otic
3. Pilocarpine ophthalmic
4. Betaoptic
5. Diamox
6. Acular
7. Livostin
8. Tobrex
9. Bleph-10
10. Timoptic

Part VII. Laboratory Tests and Diagnostic Tools to Know

A. **Directions:** Label the drawings with the names of these two hearing tests.

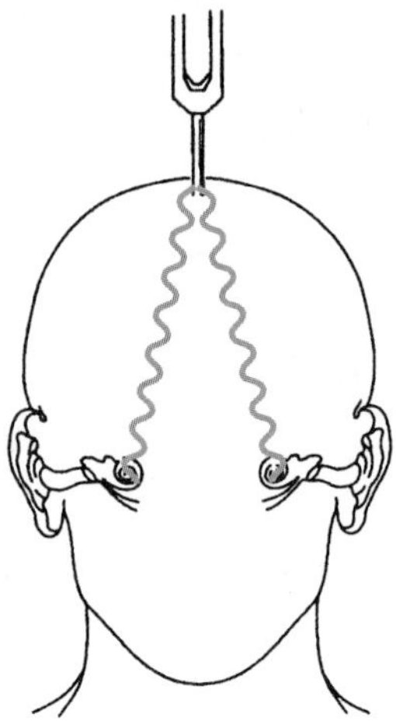

1. ______________________________

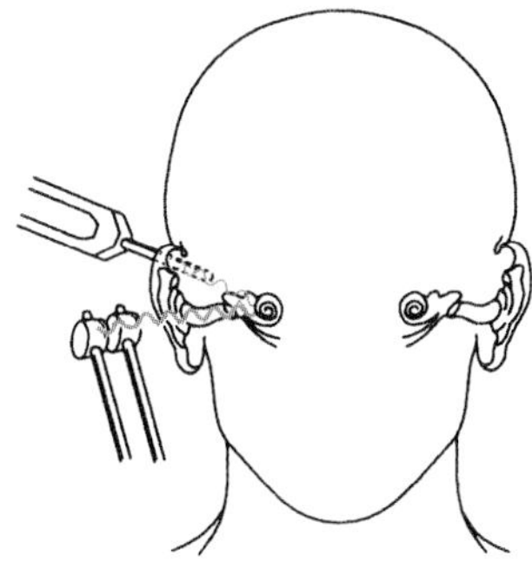

2. ______________________________

B. **Directions:** Hold the workbook 14 inches from your eyes and look at the figure below. What is the smallest line you can read clearly? On p. 266 document your near acuity in both eyes separately and together.

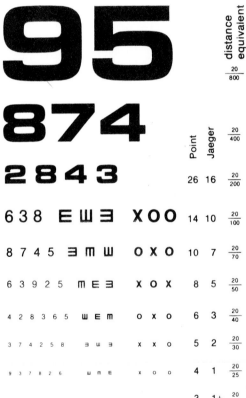

ROSENBAUM POCKET VISION SCREENER

			Point	Jaeger	distance equivalent
95					20/800
874					20/400
2843			26	16	20/200
638	E Ш Ǝ	X O O	14	10	20/100
8745	Ǝ m Ш	O X O	10	7	20/70
63925	m E Ǝ	X O X	8	5	20/50
428365	Ш E m	O X O	6	3	20/40
374258	Ǝ Ш Ǝ	X X O	5	2	20/30
937826	Ш m E	X O O	4	1	20/25
428739	E Ш m	O O X	3	1+	20/20

Card is held in good light 14 inches from eye. Record vision for each eye separately with and without glasses. Presbyopic patients should read thru bifocal segment. Check myopes with glasses only.

DESIGN COURTESY J. G. ROSENBAUM, M.D.

PUPIL GAUGE (mm.)

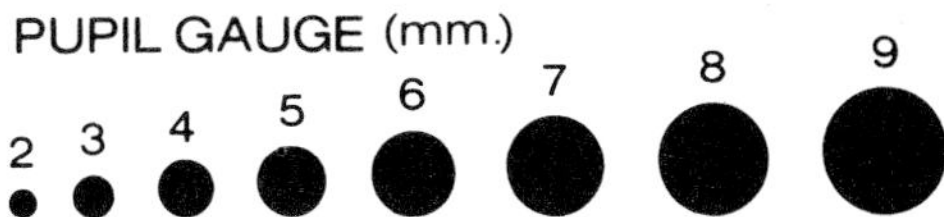

Documentation

Part IX. Transdisciplinary Skills

ICD-9 Coding

You have looked up *otitis* in the index of diseases, and you are confirming codes in the tabular index.

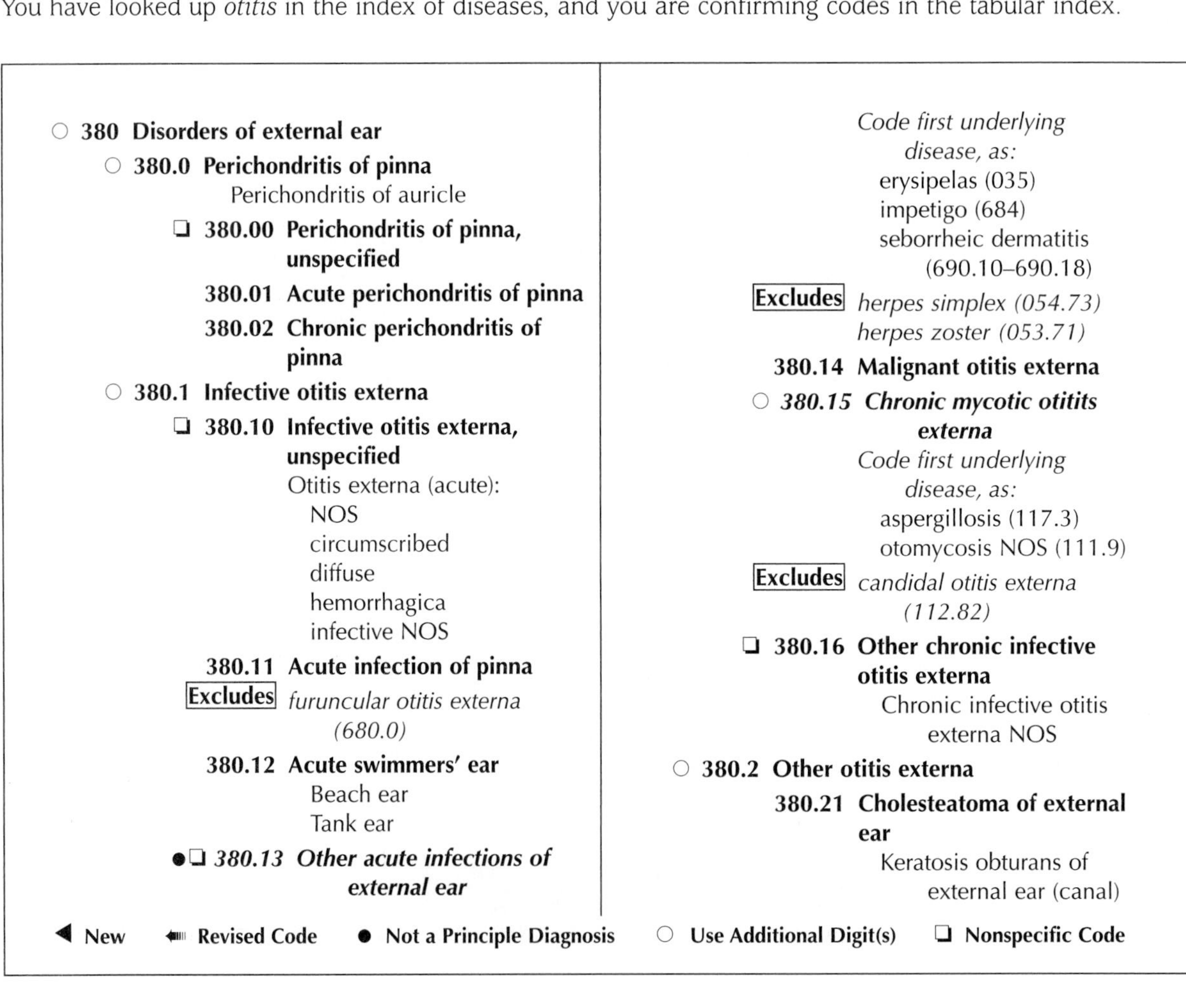

○ **380 Disorders of external ear**

○ **380.0 Perichondritis of pinna**
Perichondritis of auricle

❑ **380.00 Perichondritis of pinna, unspecified**

380.01 Acute perichondritis of pinna

380.02 Chronic perichondritis of pinna

○ **380.1 Infective otitis externa**

❑ **380.10 Infective otitis externa, unspecified**
Otitis externa (acute):
NOS
circumscribed
diffuse
hemorrhagica
infective NOS

380.11 Acute infection of pinna
Excludes *furuncular otitis externa (680.0)*

380.12 Acute swimmers' ear
Beach ear
Tank ear

●❑ ***380.13 Other acute infections of external ear***
Code first underlying disease, as:
erysipelas (035)
impetigo (684)
seborrheic dermatitis (690.10–690.18)
Excludes *herpes simplex (054.73)*
herpes zoster (053.71)

380.14 Malignant otitis externa

○ ***380.15 Chronic mycotic otitits externa***
Code first underlying disease, as:
aspergillosis (117.3)
otomycosis NOS (111.9)
Excludes *candidal otitis externa (112.82)*

❑ **380.16 Other chronic infective otitis externa**
Chronic infective otitis externa NOS

○ **380.2 Other otitis externa**

380.21 Cholesteatoma of external ear
Keratosis obturans of external ear (canal)

◀ New   ⬅ Revised Code   ● Not a Principle Diagnosis   ○ Use Additional Digit(s)   ❑ Nonspecific Code

Excludes *cholesteatoma NOS (385.30–385.35)*
postmastoidectomy (383.32)

❑ **380.22 Other acute otitis externa**
Acute otitis externa:
actinic
chemical
contact
eczematoid
reactive

❑ **380.23 Other chronic otitis externa**
Chronic otitis externa NOS

○ **380.3 Noninfectious disorders of pinna**

❑ **380.30 Disorder of pinna, unspecified**

380.31 Hematoma of auricle or pinna

380.32 Acquired deformities of auricle or pinna
Excludes *cauliflower ear (738.7)*

❑ **380.39 Other**
Excludes *gouty tophi of ear (274.81)*

380.4 Impacted cerumen
Wax in ear

○ **380.5 Acquired stenosis of external ear canal**
Collapse of external ear canal

❑ **380.50 Acquired stenosis of external ear canal, unspecified as to cause**

380.51 Secondary to trauma

380.52 Secondary to surgery

380.53 Secondary to inflammation

○ **380.8 Other disorders of external ear**

380.81 Exostosis of external ear canal

❑ **380.89 Other**

❑ **380.9 Unspecified disorder of external ear**

○ **381 Nonsuppurative otitis media and Eustachian tube disorders**

○ **381.0 Acute nonsuppurative otitis media**
Acute tubotympanic catarrh
Otitis media, acute or subacute:
catarrhal
exudative
transudative
with effusion
Excludes *otitic barotrauma (993.0)*

❑ **381.00 Acute nonsuppurative otitis media, unspecified**

381.01 Acute serous otitis media
Acute or subacute secretory otitis media

381.02 Acute mucoid otitis media
Acute or subacute seromucinous otitis media
Blue drum syndrome

381.03 Acute sanguinous otitis media

381.04 Acute allergic serous otitis media

381.05 Acute allergic mucoid otitis media

381.06 Acute allergic sanguinous otitis media

○ **381.1 Chronic serous otitis media**
Chronic tubotympanic catarrh

381.10 Chronic serous otitis media, simple or unspecified

❑ **381.19 Other**
Serosanguinous chronic otitis media

○ **381.2 Chronic mucoid otitis media**
Glue ear
Excludes *adhesive middle ear disease (385.10–385.19)*

381.20 Chronic mucoid otitis media, simple or unspecified

❑ **381.29 Other**
Mucosanguinous chronic otitis media

❑ **381.3 Other and unspecified chronic nonsuppurative otitis media**
Otitis media, chronic:
allergic
exudative
secretory
seromucinous
transudative
with effusion

❑ **381.4 Nonsuppurative otitis media, not specified as acute or chronic**
Otitis media:
allergic
catarrhal
exudative
mucoid
secretory
seromucinous
serous
transudative
with effusion

◀ New ⬅ Revised Code ● Not a Principle Diagnosis ○ Use Additional Digit(s) ❑ Nonspecific Code

Code the following diagnoses.

1. Swimmer's ear ______
2. Acute serous otitis media ______
3. Chronic fungal otitis externa ______
4. Chronic serous otitis media ______
5. Impacted ear wax ______

Part IX. Certification Review

A. Refractive errors include:

1. ______
2. ______
3. ______

B. Eye disorders can range from problems with eye movement, as in strabismus and nystagmus, to infections of the eye including:

1. ______
2. ______
3. ______
4. ______

C. Disorders of the eyeball include:

1. ______
2. ______
3. ______
4. ______

D. Examination of the nose and throat begins with examination of the nasal cavity and then visual examination of the throat and the nasopharynx.

1. In the drawing below, the physician is examining the ______.

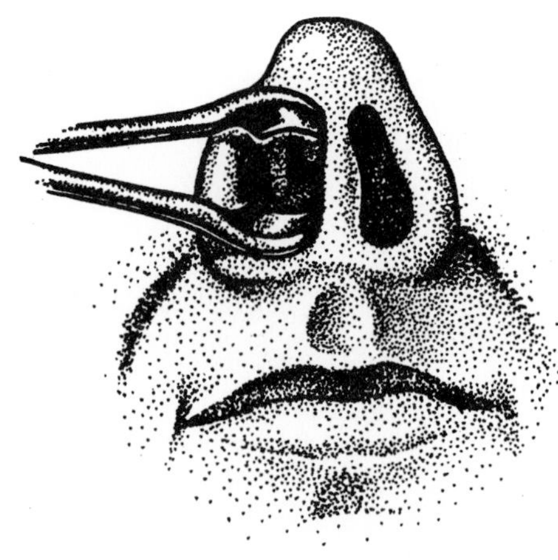

2. Name two instruments that would be needed for this exam.

   a. ____________________

   b. ____________________

E. Differentiate between otitis media and otitis externa.

____

____

____

____

F. Differentiate between hyperopia and myopia.

____

____

____

____

Chapter 34 Quiz

Name: ______________________________

1. Nearsightedness is called ____________.

2. OD means ____________

____________.

3. What is the name of the color blindness test?

____

4. OS means ____________

____________.

5. List two types of glaucoma:

 a. ____________

 b. ____________

6. Hyperopia means ____________

____________.

7. True or False: Another name for a stye is *hordeolum.*

____

8. List three refractive errors.

 a. ____________

 b. ____________

 c. ____________

9. Otic means ____________.

10. ____________ test air versus bone conduction of sound.

CHAPTER 35

Assisting in Dermatology

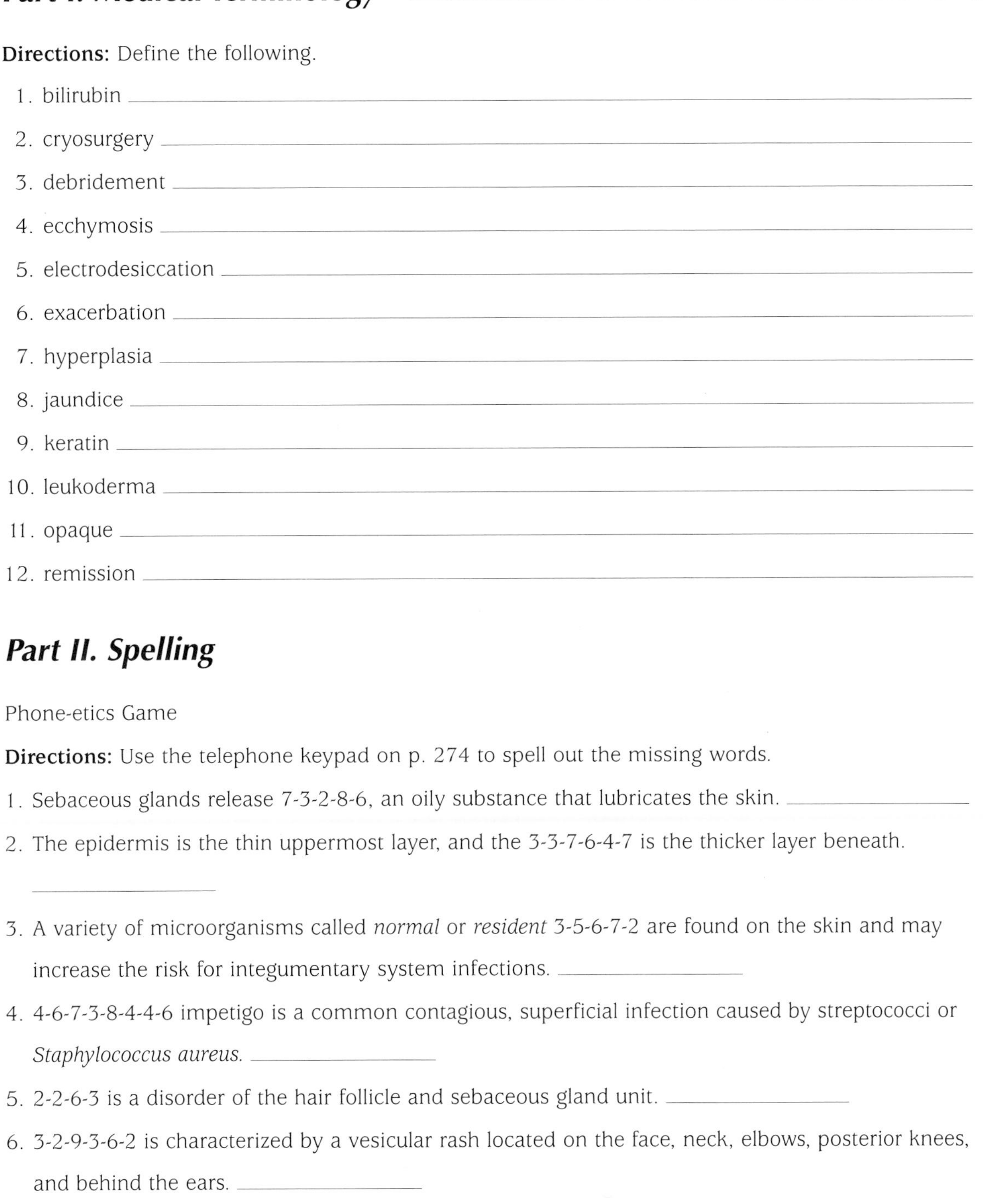

Part I. Medical Terminology

Directions: Define the following.

1. bilirubin ____________________
2. cryosurgery ____________________
3. debridement ____________________
4. ecchymosis ____________________
5. electrodesiccation ____________________
6. exacerbation ____________________
7. hyperplasia ____________________
8. jaundice ____________________
9. keratin ____________________
10. leukoderma ____________________
11. opaque ____________________
12. remission ____________________

Part II. Spelling

Phone-etics Game

Directions: Use the telephone keypad on p. 274 to spell out the missing words.

1. Sebaceous glands release 7-3-2-8-6, an oily substance that lubricates the skin. ____________
2. The epidermis is the thin uppermost layer, and the 3-3-7-6-4-7 is the thicker layer beneath. ____________
3. A variety of microorganisms called *normal* or *resident* 3-5-6-7-2 are found on the skin and may increase the risk for integumentary system infections. ____________
4. 4-6-7-3-8-4-4-6 impetigo is a common contagious, superficial infection caused by streptococci or *Staphylococcus aureus*. ____________
5. 2-2-6-3 is a disorder of the hair follicle and sebaceous gland unit. ____________
6. 3-2-9-3-6-2 is characterized by a vesicular rash located on the face, neck, elbows, posterior knees, and behind the ears. ____________

1	ABC 2	DEF 3
GHI 4	JKL 5	MNO 6
PRS 7	TUV 8	WXY 9
*	0	#

Part III. Anatomy and Physiology

Directions: Label the three layers of the skin in the drawing below.

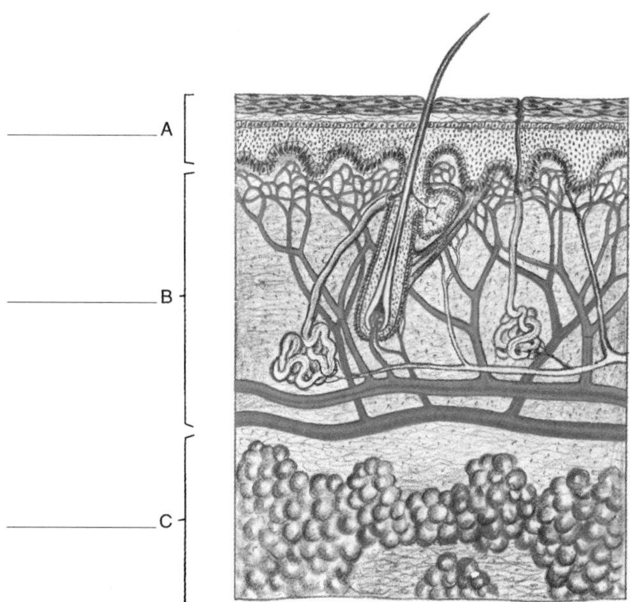

Part IV. Theory/Triage

Directions: Give a common name for each of these fungal (mycotic) infections.

1. tinea pedis ______
2. tinea cruris ______
3. tinea corporis ______
4. tinea unguium ______
5. scabies ______
6. pediculosis ______
7. verrucae ______
8. erysipelas ______

Part V. Documentation

A. Your patient has a red, flat rash with itching. Use the correct medical terminology to chart your findings. Use appropriate abbreviations. Be sure to include the date and your signature. Correct mistakes by drawing one line. Use black ink.

Documentation

B. Your patient has a red, raised rash with small blisters. Use the correct medical terminology to chart your findings. Use appropriate abbreviations. Be sure to include the date and your signature. Correct mistakes by drawing one line. Use black ink.

Documentation

Part VI. Drugs to Know

Directions: Fill in the blanks with the correct terms.

1. Antiacne medications include topical tretinoin (________________) gel and antibacterial creams such as ________________ peroxide.
2. Oral antibiotics, such as ________________ and erythromycin, at a maintenance dose of 250 mg once or twice daily, can be prescribed to control comedones and pustules.
3. Severe cystic acne can be treated with ________________, but it is a strong teratogen and should never be prescribed for pregnant women or those not using contraceptives.
4. Skin parasites are treated with 5% permethrin cream (________________) or 1% lindane lotion (________________).
5. Prednisone or methylprednisolone (Medrol) is used to treat ________________.
6. Supply a brand name for each of the following antifungal topical agents: clotrimazole (________________), ketoconazole (________________), Spectazole, or nystatin (________________).

7. An antiviral drug is acyclovir (________________).

8. Zyrtec and Allegra are used to treat ________________.

Part VII. Laboratory Tests and Diagnostic Tools to Know

A. Telephone Triage

A patient calls and states there is redness on her upper arm. What questions do you need to ask before scheduling the appointment?

____

____

____

____

____

B. List four ways to perform allergy testing.

1. ____
2. ____
3. ____
4. ____

C. Early warning signs of malignant melanoma are:

1. A ____
2. B ____
3. C ____
4. D ____

Part VIII. ICD-9 Coding

You have looked up *herpes* in the index of diseases, and you are confirming codes in the tabular index.

Code the following diagnoses.

1. Chicken pox ____
2. Herpes zoster ____
3. Varicella ____
4. Herpes simplex virus type I ____

○ **052 Chickenpox**
- **052.0 Postvaricella encephalitis**
  Postchickenpox encephalitis
- **052.1 Varicella (hemorrhagic) pneumonitis**
- ❑ **052.7 With other specified complications**
- ❑ **052.8 With unspecified complication**
- **052.9 Varicella without mention of complication**
  Chickenpox NOS
  Varicella NOS

○ **053 Herpes zoster**
Includes: shingles
zona
- **053.0 With meningitis**
- ○ **053.1 With other nervous system complications**
  - ❑ **053.10 With unspecified nervous system**
  - **053.11 Geniculate herpes zoster**
    Herpetic geniculate ganglionitis
  - **053.12 Postherpetic trigeminal neuralgia**
  - **053.13 Postherpetic polyneuropathy**
  - ❑ **053.19 Other**
- ○ **053.2 With ophthalmic complications**
  - **053.20 Herpes zoster dermatitis of eyelid**
    Herpes zoster ophthalmicus
  - **053.21 Herpes zoster kerato-conjunctivitis**
  - **053.22 Herpes zoster iridocyclitis**
  - ❑ **053.29 Other**
- ○ **053.7 With other specified complications**
  - **053.71 Otitis externa due to herpes zoster**
  - ❑ **053.79 Other**
- ❑ **053.8 With unspecified complication**
- **053.9 Herpes zoster without mention of complication**
  Herpes zoster NOS

○ **054 Herpes simplex**
Excludes *congenital herpes simplex (771.2)*
- **054.0 Eczema herpeticum**
  Kaposi's varicelliform eruption
- ○ **054.1 Genital herpes**
  - ❑ **054.10 Genital herpes, unspecified**
    Herpes progenitalis
  - **054.11 Herpetic vulvovaginitis**
  - **054.12 Herpetic ulceration of vulva**
  - **054.13 Herpetic infection of penis**
  - ❑ **054.19 Other**
- **054.2 Herpetic gingivostomatitis**
- **054.3 Herpetic meningoencephalitis**
  Herpes encephalitis
  Simian B disease
- ○ **054.4 With ophthalmic complications**
  - ❑ **054.40 With unspecified ophthalmic complication**
  - **054.41 Herpes simplex dermatitis of eyelid**
  - **054.42 Dendritic keratitis**
  - **054.43 Herpes simplex disciform keratitis**
  - **054.44 Herpes simplex iridocyclitis**
  - ❑ **054.49 Other**
- **054.5 Herpetic septicemia**
- **054.6 Herpetic whitlow**
  Herpetic felon
- ○ **054.7 With other specified complications**
  - **054.71 Visceral herpes simplex**
  - **054.72 Herpes simplex meningitis**
  - **054.73 Herpes simplex otitis externa**
  - ❑ **054.79 Other**
- ❑ **054.8 With unspecified complication**
- **054.9 Herpes simplex without mention of complication**

◀ **New** ⇐ **Revised Code** ● **Not a Principle Diagnosis** ○ **Use Additional Digit(s)** ❑ **Nonspecific Code**

5. Shingles ______________________________

6. Genital herpes ______________________________

7. Herpetic conjunctivitis and keratitis ______________________________

8. Herpes zoster of the external ear ______________________________

9. Simean B disease ______________________________

10. Herpes whitlow L index finger ______________________________

Part IX. Certification Review

A. **Directions:** Define and give an example of the following. Consult a medical dictionary and your text.

1. Macule

____

____

2. Papule

____

____

3. Plaque

____

____

4. Fissure

____

____

5. Pustule

____

____

6. Vesicle

____

____

7. Bulla

____

____

8. Cyst

____

____

9. Ulcer

____

____

10. Wheal

____

____

B. Name four bacterial infections of the skin.

1. _______________
2. _______________
3. _______________
4. _______________

C. List six inflammatory disorders of the skin.

1. _______________
2. _______________
3. _______________
4. _______________
5. _______________
6. _______________

List the seven warning signs of cancer.

1. C _______________
2. A _______________
3. U _______________
4. T _______________
5. I _______________
6. O _______________
7. N _______________

List three procedures for appearance modification.

1. _______________
2. _______________
3. _______________

Chapter 35 Quiz

Name: ______________________________

1. Herpes zoster is also called ______________.

2. HPV stands for ______________ ______________ ______________.

3. Tinea is another name for a ______________ infection.

4. Pruritus means ______________ ______________.

5. List three common fungal infections.
   a. ______________
   b. ______________
   c. ______________

6. Kwell is used to treat ______________ and ______________.

7. Another name for a bruise is ______________.

8. List three depths of burns.
   a. ______________
   b. ______________
   c. ______________

9. SLE is an abbreviation for ______________ ______________ ______________.

10. ______________ degree burns have blisters.

CHAPTER 36

Assisting in Gastroenterology

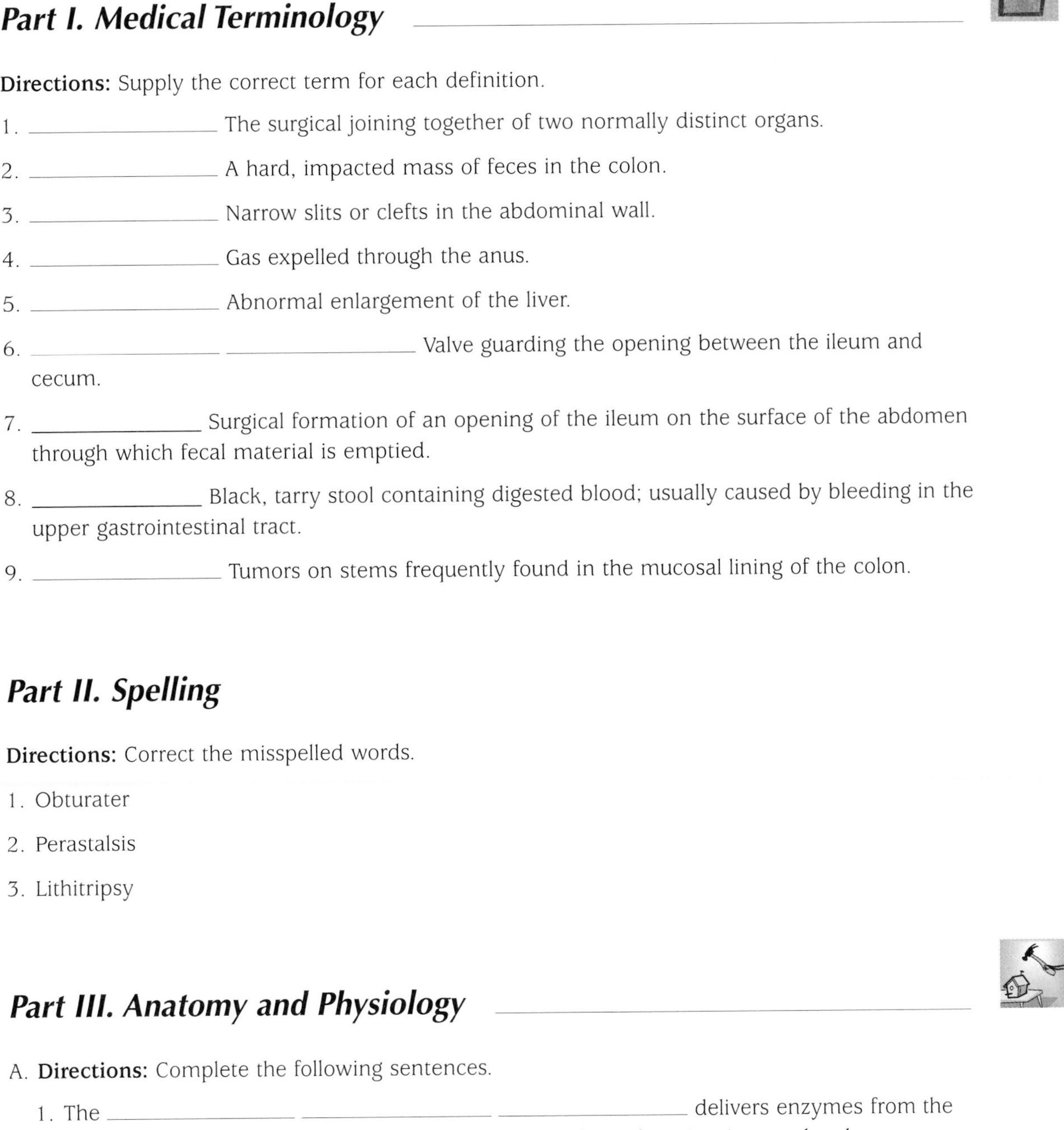

Part I. Medical Terminology

Directions: Supply the correct term for each definition.

1. ______________ The surgical joining together of two normally distinct organs.
2. ______________ A hard, impacted mass of feces in the colon.
3. ______________ Narrow slits or clefts in the abdominal wall.
4. ______________ Gas expelled through the anus.
5. ______________ Abnormal enlargement of the liver.
6. ______________ ______________ Valve guarding the opening between the ileum and cecum.
7. ______________ Surgical formation of an opening of the ileum on the surface of the abdomen through which fecal material is emptied.
8. ______________ Black, tarry stool containing digested blood; usually caused by bleeding in the upper gastrointestinal tract.
9. ______________ Tumors on stems frequently found in the mucosal lining of the colon.

Part II. Spelling

Directions: Correct the misspelled words.

1. Obturater
2. Perastalsis
3. Lithitripsy

Part III. Anatomy and Physiology

A. **Directions:** Complete the following sentences.

1. The ______________ ______________ ______________ delivers enzymes from the pancreas and bile from the liver to the duodenum where digestion is completed.

2. The ________________ intestine is made up of the duodenum, jejunum, and ileum.

3. The small intestine is lined with transverse folds of tissue called ________________.

B. **Directions:** List seven parts of the large intestine; start with the vermiform appendix.

1. ________________
2. ________________
3. ________________
4. ________________
5. ________________
6. ________________
7. ________________

C. **Directions:** Define the following terms.

1. peritoneum

____

____

2. mesentery

____

____

3. omentum

____

____

4. adhesions

____

____

D. **Directions:** Label the structures of the upper abdominal cavity on the figure below.

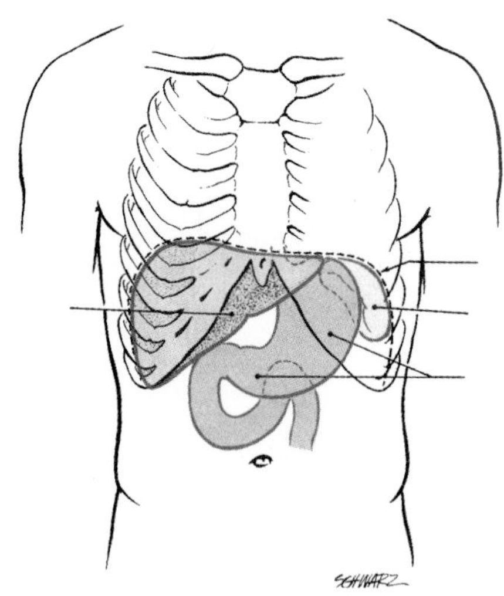

Part IV. Theory/Triage

Directions: Fill in the blanks with the correct terms.

1. ______________ are concerned with the diseases and disorders involving the stomach, small intestine, large intestine (colon), appendix, and the accessory organs of the liver, gallbladder, and pancreas.

2. List three disorders of the esophagus and stomach.

 a. ______________

 b. ______________

 c. ______________

3. List 10 disorders of the intestines.

 a. ______________

 b. ______________

 c. ______________

 d. ______________

 e. ______________

 f. ______________

 g. ______________

 h. ______________

 i. ______________

 j. ______________

4. List two disorders of the liver and gallbladder.

 a. ______________

 b. ______________

Directions: Complete the table below by listing the causes of each gastrointestinal complaint.

Gastrointestinal Complaint	
Vomiting (emesis)	Caused by:

Diarrhea	Caused by:
Constipation	Caused by:

Part V. Documentation

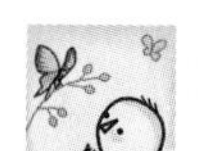

Directions: Complete the table below by listing the characteristics of abdominal pain that the medical assistant should report and record. Hint: Review Table 36-1 in your textbook.

Abdominal Pain	Important Characteristics That Should Be Reported and Recorded

Directions: Complete the table below by listing common sources of food poisoning.

Microorganism	Source
Staphylococcus aureus	
Escherichia coli	
Salmonella species	
Clostridium botulinum	

Part VI. Drugs to Know

Directions: Use a drug reference book or the Internet to make drug cards for the following. Include drug classification, generic name, usual dose for an adult, and drug form.

1. Imodium
2. Lomotil
3. Phenergan
4. Tigan
5. Anzemet
6. Zofran
7. Kytril
8. Bentyl
9. Levsin
10. Axid
11. Preacid
12. Prilosec
13. Tagamet
14. Zantac
15. Nexium
16. Protonix

Part VII. Laboratory Tests and Diagnostic Tools to Know

A. List four tests performed for patients with ulcers.

1. ______________________________
2. ______________________________
3. ______________________________
4. ______________________________

B. Complete this chart.

Hepatitis Type	Mode of Transmission	Incubation Period
A (Infectious hepatitis)		
B (Serum hepatitis)		
C (Non-A-non-B)		

Part VIII. Transdisciplinary Skills

A. You are making follow-up phone calls after scheduling patients for the following diagnostic tests. List the instructions that you will provide for each patient.

Patient	Test	Description and Purpose	Patient Preparation
Terry Smith	Barium swallow	X-ray or fluoroscopic examination of the pharynx and esophagus after swallowing of barium sulfate; used to diagnose hiatal hernia, esophageal varices, strictures, or tumors.	
Jill Fields	Upper gastrointestinal and small-bowel series	X-ray and fluoroscopic examination of esophagus, stomach, and small intestine after swallowing of barium sulfate; used to diagnose ulcers, tumors, regional enteritis, and malabsorption syndrome.	
Pam Gibbs	Barium enema	X-ray examination of large intestine after rectal instillation of barium sulfate; used to diagnose colorectal cancer; inflammatory disease of the colon; and to detect polyps, diverticula, or obstructions.	
Vince Wells	Oral cholecystography	X-ray examination of gallbladder after ingestion of contrast medium; x-ray films are obtained before and after ingestion of high-fat meal to visualize biliary system; used to detect cholelithiasis and diagnose cholecystitis or tumors.	

Patient	Test	Description and Purpose	Patient Preparation
Suzette Yi	Sigmoidoscopy	Endoscopic examination of distal sigmoid colon, rectum, and anal canal; used to diagnose inflammatory, infectious, and ulcerative bowel disease and tumors and to detect hemorrhoids, polyps, fissures, fistulas, abscesses in the rectum and anal canal. Biopsy specimens may be collected.	
Bobby Day	Colonoscopy	Endoscopic examination of the large intestine; used to detect or monitor inflammatory or ulcerative disease, to locate site of gastrointestinal bleeding, and to identify tumors or strictures.	

B. *ICD-9* Coding

You have looked up *diverticulitis* in the index of diseases, and you are confirming codes in the tabular index.

○ **562.0 Small intestine**

562.00 Diverticulosis of small intestine (without mention of hemorrhage)
Diverticulosis:
duodenum without mention of diverticulitis
ileum without mention of diverticulitis
jejunum without mention of diverticulitis

562.01 Diverticulitis of small intestine (without mention of hemorrhage)
Diverticulitis (with diverticulosis):
duodenum
ileum
jejunum
small intestine

562.02 Diverticulosis of small intestine with hemorrhage

562.03 Diverticulitis of small intestine with hemorrhage

○ **562.1 Colon**

562.10 Diverticulosis of colon (without mention of hemorrhage)
Diverticulosis without mention of diverticulitis:
NOS
intestine (large) without mention of diverticulitis
Diverticular disease (colon) without mention of diverticulitis

562.11 Diverticulitis of colon without mention of hemorrhage
Diverticulitis (with diverticulosis):
NOS
colon
intestine (large)

562.12 Diverticulosis of colon with hemorrhage

562.13 Diverticulitis of colon with hemorrhage

◀ **New** ⇐ **Revised Code** ● **Not a Principle Diagnosis** ○ **Use Additional Digit(s)** ❏ **Nonspecific Code**

Code the following diagnoses.

1. Diverticulosis of small intestine with hemorrhage ________________

2. Diverticulitis of small intestine ________________

3. Diverticulosis of colon with hemorrhage ________________

4. Diverticulitis of ileum ____________________

5. Diverticulosis of colon ____________________

Part IX. Certification Review

Directions: Fill in the blanks with the correct terms.

A. Groups at Risk for Hepatitis A, B, and C

1. Hepatitis ____________________: intravenous drug users, homosexual men, patients undergoing hemodialysis, patients with hemophilia, healthcare personnel, persons with multiple sexual partners.

2. Hepatitis ____________________: children and employees in day care centers, institutionalized residents, individuals traveling to infected areas.

3. Hepatitis ____________________: patients who receive frequent blood transfusions, homosexual men, intravenous drug users, and hospital personnel.

B. Abdominal Regions

1. The gallbladder is located in the ____________________ quadrant of the abdomen.

2. The appendix is located in the ____________________ quadrant of the abdomen.

3. The stomach is located in the ____________________ quadrant of the abdomen.

4. The liver is located in the ____________________ quadrant of the abdomen.

5. The pancreas is located in the ____________________ quadrant of the abdomen.

C. The organism related to ulcer formation is ____________________.

D. True or False: Biaxin and Zithromax are antibiotics used to treat ulcers. ____________________

E. The patient in the figure below is placed in ____________________ ____________________ position. What are the major concerns when this position is used?

____

____

____

____

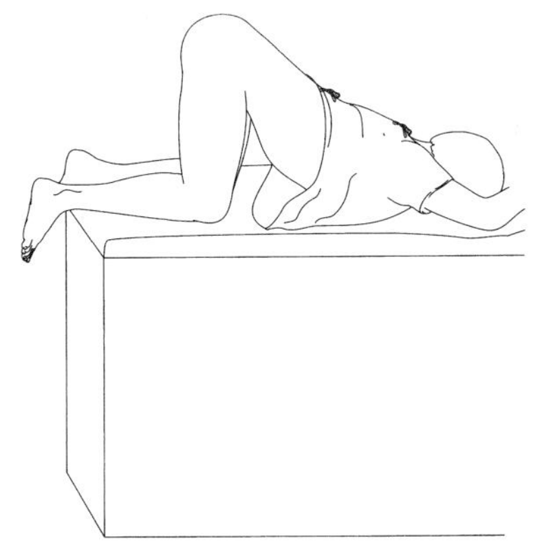

F. Name the position shown in the figure. ________________

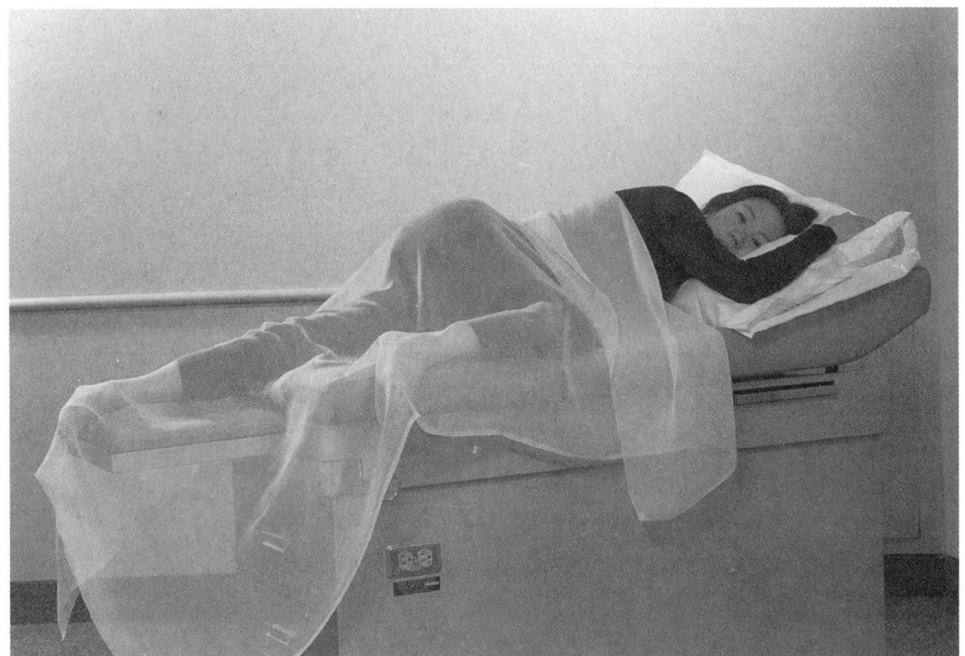

Chapter 36 Quiz

Name: ______________________________

1. The liver is located in the ______________ region.

2. The appendix is part of the ______________.

3. ______________ ______________, which is the narrowing and hardening of the pyloric sphincter at the distal end of the stomach, is typically seen as a congenital defect in infants.

4. Diverticulosis means: ______________________________.

5. List two foods to avoid before an occult blood screening.
   a. ______________
   b. ______________

6. Hepatitis ______________ is food-borne.

7. True or False: Hepatitis B is blood-borne.
   ____

8. List two causes of ulcers.
   a. ______________
   b. ______________

9. Cholelithiasis is ______________.

10. ______________ is a food-borne illness caused by eating raw eggs, poultry, or shellfish.

CHAPTER 37

Assisting in Urology and Male Reproduction

Part I. Medical Terminology

Directions: Define the following terms.

1. albuminuria

2. azotemia

3. casts

4. copulation

5. erythropoietin

6. urgency

7. urology

Part II. Spelling

Directions: Supply the correct spelling for four types of urinary tract infections.

1. ______________________ inflammation of the urethra.
2. ______________________ infection of the urinary bladder.
3. ______________________ an inflammation of the renal pelvis and kidney.
4. ______________________ degenerative inflammation of the glomeruli.

Part III. Anatomy and Physiology

Directions: Label the structures of the scrotum on the figure below.

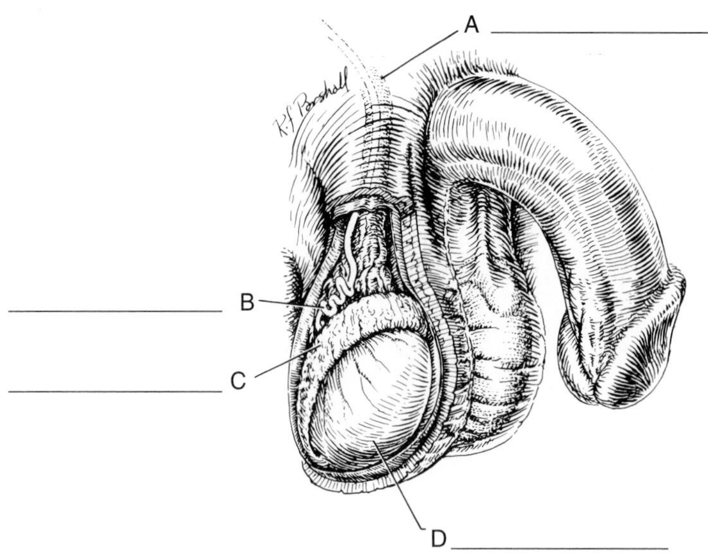

Part IV. Theory/Triage

List five reasons for performing a catheterization.

1. ______________________
2. ______________________
3. ______________________
4. ______________________
5. ______________________

Part V. Documentation

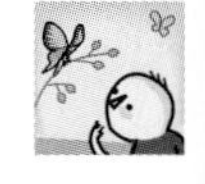

You performed a catheterization on a male patient for collection of a sterile urine specimen. The urine is dark orange but clear. The amount of urine was 460 cc. The patient appeared to be comfortable during the procedure. Document your findings on p. 297. Use appropriate abbreviations. Be sure to include the date and your signature. Correct mistakes by drawing one line. Use black ink.

Documentation

Part VI. Drugs to Know

A. **Directions:** Use a drug reference book or the Internet to make drug cards for the following. Include the drug classification, generic name, usual dose, and drug form.

1. Keflex
2. Bactrim
3. Viagra
4. Flomax
5. Hytrin
6. Detrol
7. Ditropan
8. Xylocaine

B. **Directions:** Review drugs that are used to treat sexually transmitted diseases and complete the table below.

Disease (Causative Organism)	Treatment
Chlamydia (*Chlamydia trachomatis*)	
Genital herpes simplex virus (HSV-2)	
Genital warts (human papillomavirus)	
Gonorrhea (*Neisseria gonorrhoeae* [bacteria])	
Syphilis (*Treponema pallidum* [spirochete bacteria])	
Trichomoniasis (*Trichomonas vaginalis* [protozoa])	

Part VII. Laboratory Tests and Diagnostic Tools to Know

A. **Directions:** Complete the table of common urinary system diagnostic tests.

Test	Description	Patient Preparation
Kidney-ureter-bladder x-ray examination (KUB)		

Test	Description	Patient Preparation
Renal scanning		
Cystography and voiding cystourethrogram		
Intravenous pyelography (IVP)		
Arteriography (angiography)		
Renal computed tomography		
Renal ultrasonography		
Cystoscopy		
Retrograde pyelography		

B. **Directions:** Describe the following.

1. Creatinine

2. BUN

3. UA

Part VIII. Transdisciplinary Skills

ICD-9 Coding

You have looked up *prostatitis* in the index of diseases, and you are confirming codes in the tabular index.

○ **600 Hyperplasia of prostate**
Use additional code to identify urinary incontinence (788.30–788.39)

600.0 Hypertrophy (benign) of prostate
Benign prostatic hypertrophy
Enlargement of prostate
Smooth enlarged prostate
Soft enlarged prostate

600.1 Nodular prostate
Hard, firm prostate
Multinodular prostate
Excludes *malignant neoplasm of prostate (185)*

600.2 Benign localized hyperplasia of prostate
Adenofibromatous hypertrophy of prostate
Adenoma of prostate
Fibroadenoma of prostate
Fibroma of prostate
Myoma of prostate
Polyp of prostate
Excludes *benign neoplasms of prostate (222.2)*
hypertrophy of prostate (600.0)
malignant neoplasm of prostate (185)

600.3 Cyst of prostate

❑ **600.9 Hyperplasia of prostate, unspecified**
Median bar
Prostatic obstruction NOS

○ **601 Inflammatory diseases of prostate**
Use additional code to identify organism, such as Staphylococcus (041.1), or Streptococcus (041.0)

601.0 Acute prostatitis

601.1 Chronic prostatitis

601.2 Abscess of prostate

601.3 Prostatocystitis

● ***601.4 Prostatitis in diseases classified elsewhere***
Code first underlying disease, as:
actinomycosis (039.8)
blastomycosis (116.0)
syphilis (095.8)
tuberculosis (016.5)
Excludes *prostatitis:*
gonococcal (098.12, 098.32)
monilial (112.2)
trichomonal (131.03)

❑ **601.8 Other specified inflammatory diseases of prostate**
Prostatitis:
cavitary
diverticular
granulomatous

❑ **601.9 Prostatitis, unspecified**
Prostatitis NOS

◀ **New** ⬅ **Revised Code** ● **Not a Principle Diagnosis** ○ **Use Additional Digit(s)** ❑ **Nonspecific Code**

Code the following diagnoses.

1. Stricture of prostate ________________
2. BPH ________________
3. Cyst of prostate ________________
4. Acute prostatitis ________________
5. Chronic prostatitis ________________

Part IX. Certification Review

A. **Directions:** Define the following terms.

1. Epididymis
2. Balanitis
3. Impotence
4. Infertility
5. Prostatitis
6. BPH
7. Cryptorchidism
8. Hydrocele

9. Enuresis

____

____

10. Renal calculi

____

____

B. In the figure below, the physician is examining the male patient for presence of a hernia. What region of the abdomen is he examining? ______________

Why are males at risk for developing a hernia in this area?

____

____

____

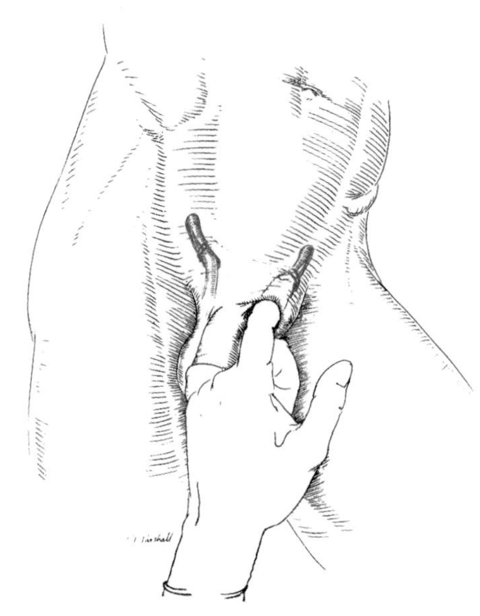

Chapter 37 Quiz

Name: ______________________________

1. Renin regulates ______________ ______________.

2. Erythropoietin controls the formation of ______________.

3. Cryptorchidism means ______________ ______________.

4. KUB stands for ______________________________.

5. List two drugs used to treat UTIs.

   a. ______________

   b. ______________

6. True or False: The urethra connects the kidneys to the bladder.

   ____

7. Enuresis means ______________ ______________.

8. List two types of dialysis.

   a. ______________

   b. ______________

9. IVP stands for ______________ ______________.

10. ______________ is the functional unit of the kidney.

CHAPTER 38

Assisting in Obstetrics and Gynecology

Part I. Medical Terminology

Directions: Define the following terms.

1. rectocele

2. uterine prolapse

3. cystocele

4. PID

5. endometriosis

6. dilation and curettage

7. abruptio placenta

8. placenta previa

9. hysterectomy

____

____

Part II. Spelling

Directions: Read each definition and supply the term with correct spelling.

1. Pertaining to women who have had two or more pregnancies ______________
2. Thin, yellow, milky fluid secreted by the mammary glands a few days before and after delivery ______________
3. An x-ray procedure to guide the insertion of a needle into a specific area of the breast ______________
4. Spotting or bleeding between menstrual cycles ______________
5. Excessive menstrual blood loss, such as a menses lasting longer than 7 days ______________
6. The absence of menstruation for a minimum of 6 months ______________
7. A woman who has not menstruated for a period of 35 days to 6 months is experiencing ______________

Part III. Anatomy and Physiology

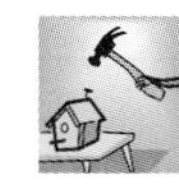

A. **Directions:** Fill in the blanks.

The 28-day cycle is divided into three phases: ______________ phase, ______________ phase, and ______________ phase.

B. **Directions:** Label the structures in the figure below.

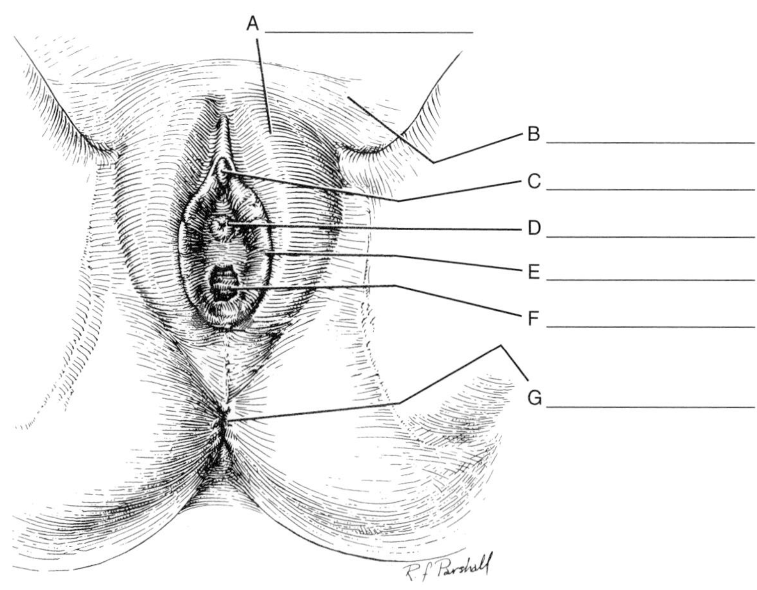

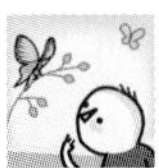

Part IV. Theory/Triage

A. You receive a telephone call from a female patient who is experiencing side effects from oral contraceptives. What symptoms will you ask about?

A ______

C ______

H ______

E ______

S ______

B. Name three bacterial STDs.

1. ______
2. ______
3. ______

C. Name an STD that is caused by protozoa.

______

D. Name two viral STDs.

1. ______
2. ______

E. Name three benign gynecological tumors.

1. ______
2. ______
3. ______

F. Name four gynecological cancers.

1. ______
2. ______
3. ______
4. ______

G. **Directions:** Labor is the physiologic process by which the uterus expels the fetus and the placenta. It is divided into three stages. Complete the following definitions:

1. Stage I: From onset of labor through complete ______ and ______ of the cervix
2. Stage II: From complete dilation and effacement of the cervix through the ______
3. Stage III: From the birth of the fetus through the expulsion of the ______

Part V. Documentation

Directions: List five types of naturally occurring abortions.

1. ______________________________
2. ______________________________
3. ______________________________
4. ______________________________
5. ______________________________

Part VI. Drugs to Know

A. **Directions:** Complete the table of various methods of contraception.

Type	Failure Rate	Contraindications	Side Effects
Condom (barrier method)			
Diaphragm or cervical cap (barrier method)			
Intrauterine device (IUD)			
Depo Provera (DMPA)			
Norplant			
Oral contraceptives (OCPs)			

B. **Directions:** Use a drug reference book or the Internet to make drug cards for the following. Include drug classification, generic name, usual dose, and drug form.

1. Tamoxifen
2. Premarin
3. Prempro
4. Methotrexate (for use in ectopic pregnancies)

Part VII. Laboratory Tests and Diagnostic Tools to Know

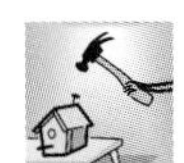

Directions: Define the following terms.

1. Ultrasonography

____

____

2. Chorionic villus sampling

____

____

3. Amniocentesis

____

____

4. Alpha-fetoprotein (AFP)

____

____

5. Mammography

____

____

6. Colposcopy

____

____

7. Cryosurgery

____

____

Part VIII. Transdisciplinary Skills

ICD-9 Coding

You have looked up *menorrhagia* in the index of diseases, and you are confirming codes in the tabular index.

○ **626 Disorders of menstruation and other abnormal bleeding from female genital tract**

Excludes *menopausal and premenopausal bleeding (627.0)*
pain and other symptoms associated with menstrual cycle (625.2–625.4)
postmenopausal bleeding (627.1)

626.0 Absence of menstruation
Amenorrhea (primary) (secondary)

626.1 Scanty or infrequent menstruation
Hypomenorrhea
Oligomenorrhea

626.2 Excessive or frequent menstruation
Heavy periods
Menometrorrhagia
Menorrhagia
Polymenorrhea

Excludes *premenopausal (627.0)*
that in puberty (626.3)

626.3 Puberty bleeding
Excessive bleeding associated with onset of menstrual periods
Pubertal menorrhagia

626.4 Irregular menstrual cycle
Irregular:
bleeding NOS
menstruation
periods

626.5 Ovulation bleeding
Regular intermenstrual bleeding

626.6 Metrorrhagia
Bleeding unrelated to menstrual cycle
Irregular intermenstrual bleeding

626.7 Postcoital bleeding

❑ **626.8 Other**
Dysfunctional or functional uterine hemorrhage NOS
Menstruation:
retained
suppression of

❑ **626.9 Unspecified**

◀ **New** ⇐ **Revised Code** ● **Not a Principle Diagnosis** ○ **Use Additional Digit(s)** ❑ **Nonspecific Code**

Code the following diagnoses.

1. amenorrhea ________________
2. metrorrhagia ________________
3. oligomenorrhea ________________
4. menorrhagia ________________
5. postcoital bleeding ________________

Part IX. Certification Review

A. Name the position used for female pelvic examinations that is pictured below.

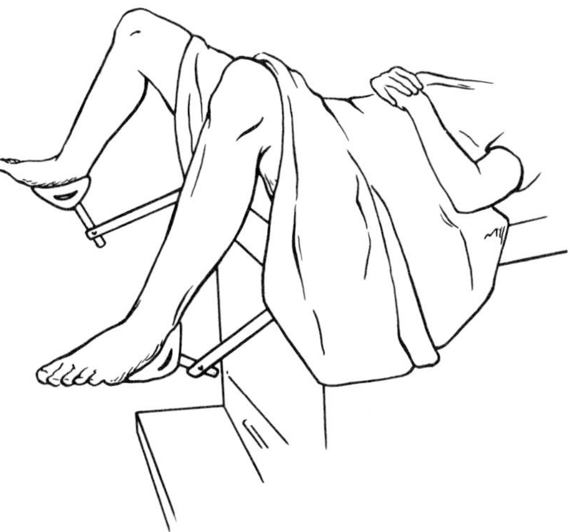

B. Name the instrument that is being used in the figure below.

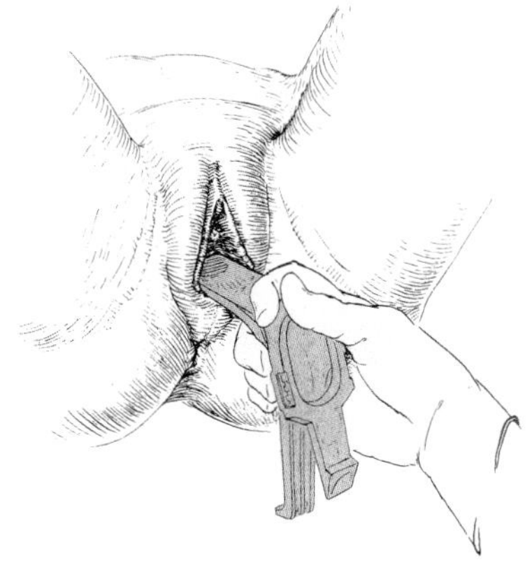

C. Name two supplies that will be needed to complete the bimanual exam illustrated below.

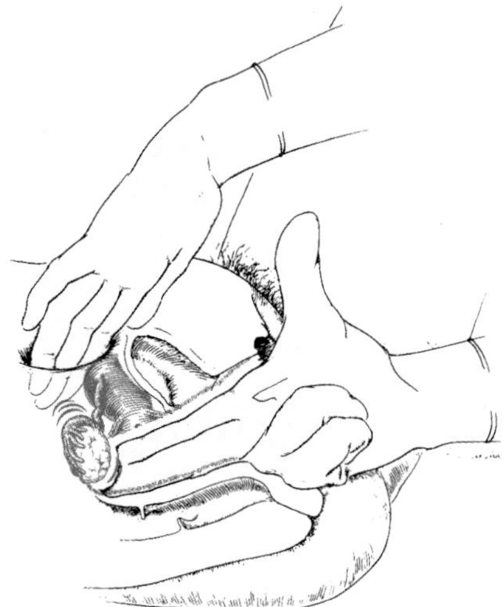

1. ____________________

2. ____________________

Chapter 38 Quiz

Name: ______________________________

1. *Candida albicans* causes ______________________

   ______________________.

2. Menorrhagia means ______________________.

3. Multiparous means ______________________

   ______________________.

4. PID stands for:

   ______________________________________.

5. List two common causes of PID.

   a. ______________________

   b. ______________________

6. True or False: AZT is used to help treat HIV.

   ____

7. Amenorrhea means

   ______________________________________.

8. List two ways to screen for breast cancer.

   a. ______________________

   b. ______________________

9. A Papanicolaou smear helps detect

   ______________________ ______________________.

10. One in ______________________ women are at risk for breast cancer.

CHAPTER 39

Assisting in Pediatrics

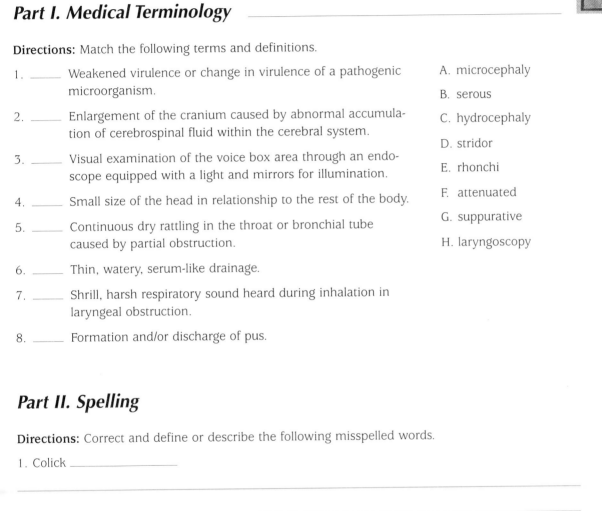

Part I. Medical Terminology

Directions: Match the following terms and definitions.

1. _____ Weakened virulence or change in virulence of a pathogenic microorganism.
2. _____ Enlargement of the cranium caused by abnormal accumulation of cerebrospinal fluid within the cerebral system.
3. _____ Visual examination of the voice box area through an endoscope equipped with a light and mirrors for illumination.
4. _____ Small size of the head in relationship to the rest of the body.
5. _____ Continuous dry rattling in the throat or bronchial tube caused by partial obstruction.
6. _____ Thin, watery, serum-like drainage.
7. _____ Shrill, harsh respiratory sound heard during inhalation in laryngeal obstruction.
8. _____ Formation and/or discharge of pus.

A. microcephaly
B. serous
C. hydrocephaly
D. stridor
E. rhonchi
F. attenuated
G. suppurative
H. laryngoscopy

Part II. Spelling

Directions: Correct and define or describe the following misspelled words.

1. Colick ____________

____

____

2. Diareah ____________

____

____

3. Rhinnitis ____________

____

____

4. Azthma ________________

5. Bronchialitus ________________

6. Influensa ________________

7. Diptherea ________________

8. Tetnus ________________

9. Mennengitis ________________

10. Hepetitus B ________________

11. Rye's Syndrone ________________

12. Systic Fibrosis ________________

13. Muscular Distrophy ________________

14. Rubellia ________________

15. Poleo ________________

Part III. Anatomy and Physiology

Directions: Fill in the blanks.

1. An infant's birth weight doubles by ________________.
2. By age ________________, the child has reached approximately 50% of his or her adult height.
3. Growth in height is fairly well complete by age ________________.

Part IV. Theory/Triage

A. **Directions:** Complete the following statements about developmental patterns.

1. By the age of 3 years, a child can:

____

____

____

____

2. During the preschool stage:

____

____

____

____

3. The school-aged child has perfected:

____

____

____

____

4. The adolescent, or transition, stage is when the individual attempts to:

____

____

____

____

B. **Directions:** Complete the table of action principles for telephone triage.

Complaint	Triage Questions
Pain	
Gastrointestinal	
Respiratory	

Part V. Documentation

Directions: A child weighs 20 pounds. You are asked to record the weight in kilograms. There are 2.2 pounds per kilogram. Show your work. Chart the weight below.

Part VI. Drugs to Know

Directions: Use a drug reference book or the Internet to make drug cards for the following. Include drug classification, generic name, usual pediatric dose, and drug form.

1. Amoxicillin
2. Ceclor
3. Cipro
4. Augmentin
5. EryPed
6. Septra

Part VII. Laboratory Tests and Diagnostic Tools to Know

Directions: Give examples of how each of the following is assessed in children.

1. Gross motor skills: ____________________

2. Language skills: ____________________

3. Fine motor–adaptive skills: ______

4. Personal skills: ______

Part VIII. Transdisciplinary Skills

Teaching Injury Prevention

A. **Directions:** List 10 safety guidelines for parents with small children.

1. ______
2. ______
3. ______
4. ______
5. ______
6. ______
7. ______
8. ______
9. ______
10. ______

B. **Directions:** Complete the following statement.

The Federal Child Abuse Prevention and Treatment Act states that ______

Part IX. Certification Review

1. What is a BRAT diet?

2. What is an MMR?

3. What is DPT?

---

4. Can you name the defect in the spine shown below?

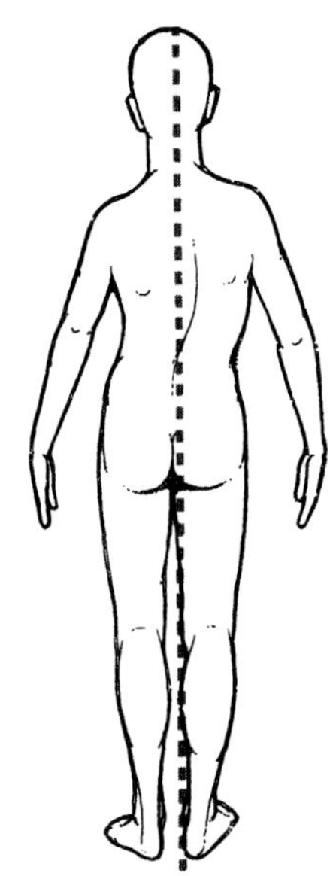

Chapter 39 Quiz

Name: ____

1. __________ is a respiratory condition with bronchospasms and inflammation.

2. __________ is a viral disorder with cough and stridor.

3. Chickenpox is another name for ______________________________ .

4. Inflammation of the brain and spinal cord is called ____________________ .

5. MMR stands for ________________, ______________ and ____________ .

6. The medical specialty that deals with children is ____________________ .

7. Average birth weight is __________ .

8. By age ___________, a child has reached 50% of its adult height and weight.

9. ____________________ is a disorder that is characterized by abdominal pain during infancy.

10. A common cold (rhinitis) is a ________________________ illness.

CHAPTER 40

Assisting in Orthopedic Medicine

Part I. Medical Terminology

Directions: Define the following terms.

1. kyphosis

2. lordosis

3. luxation

4. subluxation

5. thoracic

6. tendon

7. ligament

Part II. Spelling

Directions: Correct and define the misspelled words.

1. crepatation ________________

____

____

2. epiphisis ________________

____

____

3. cortisosteroeids ________________

____

____

4. gonometer ________________

____

____

5. ligiment ________________

____

____

Part III. Anatomy and Physiology

A. **Directions:** In the figure below, label the bones of the extremities.

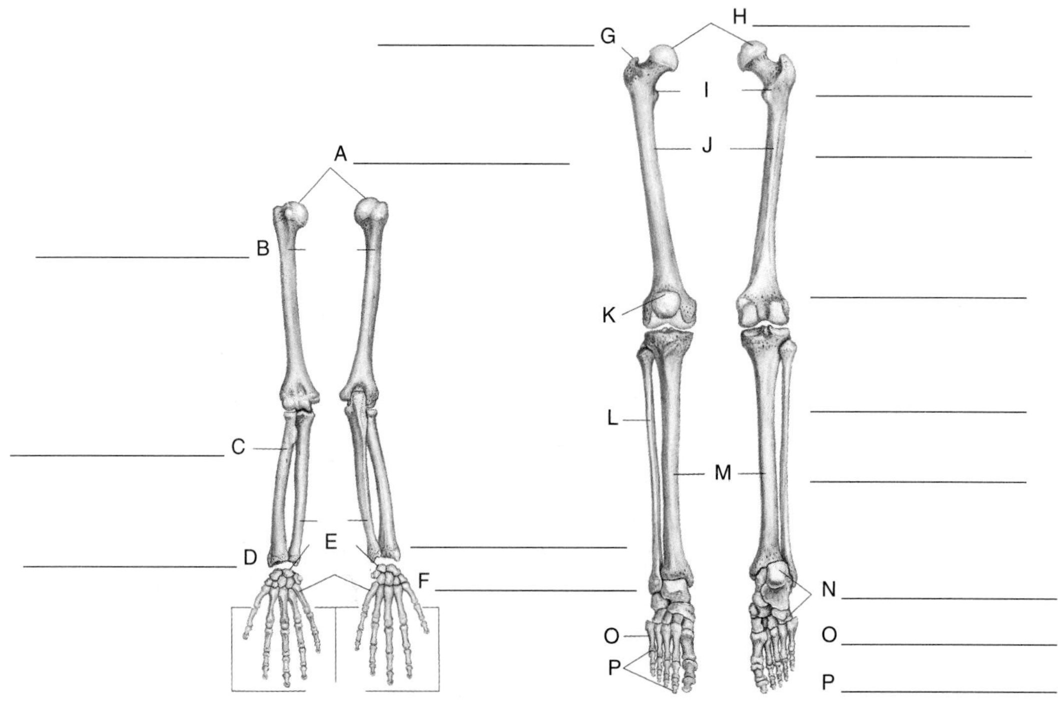

B. **Directions:** Label the drawing below with muscle, tendons, insertion, and origin.

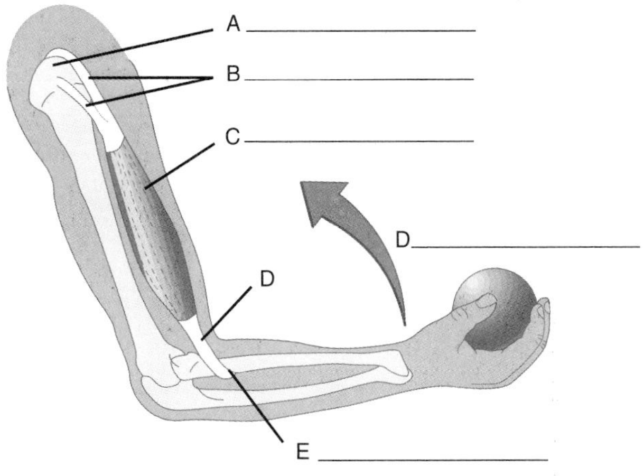

C. **Directions:** Label the three types of muscles shown in the figure below.

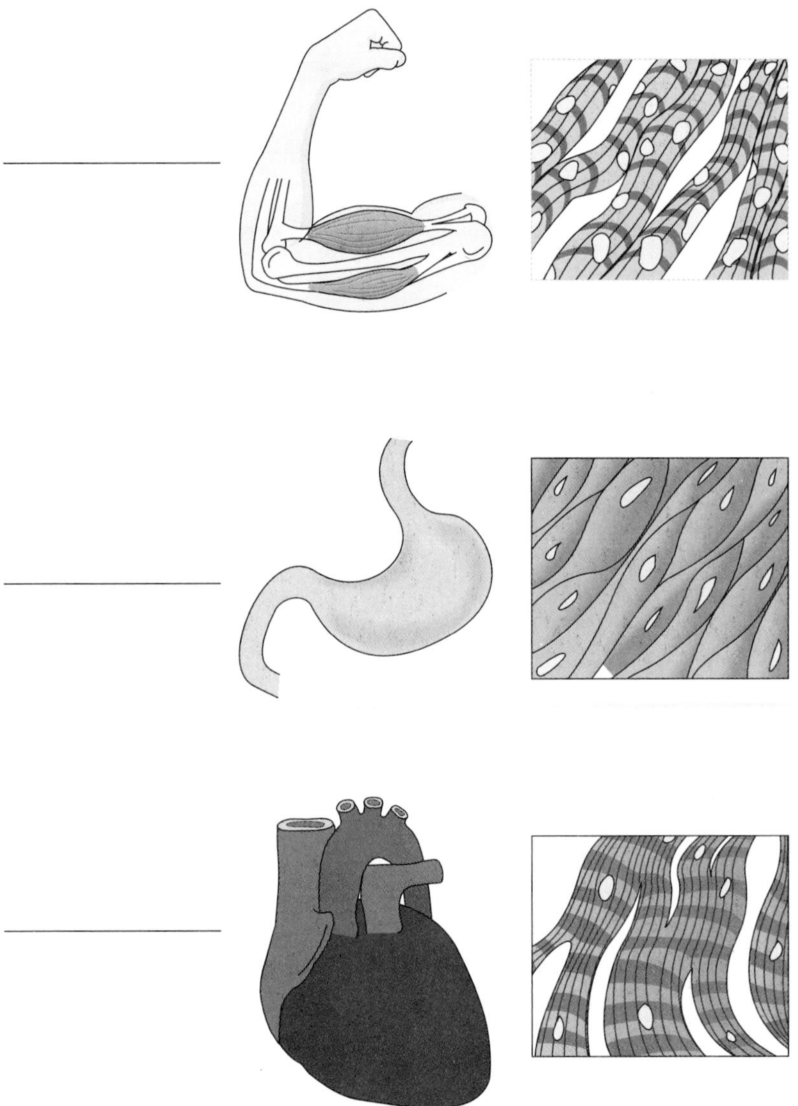

D. **Directions:** Indicate which statements are true (T) and which statements are false (F).

1. _____ The tibia is distal to the femur.
2. _____ The patella is superior to meta carpals.
3. _____ The radius is lateral to the ulna.
4. _____ The tibia is medial to the fibula.
5. _____ The metatarsals are inferior to the tarsals.

Part IV. Theory/Triage

A. **Directions:** Label each type of range of motion.

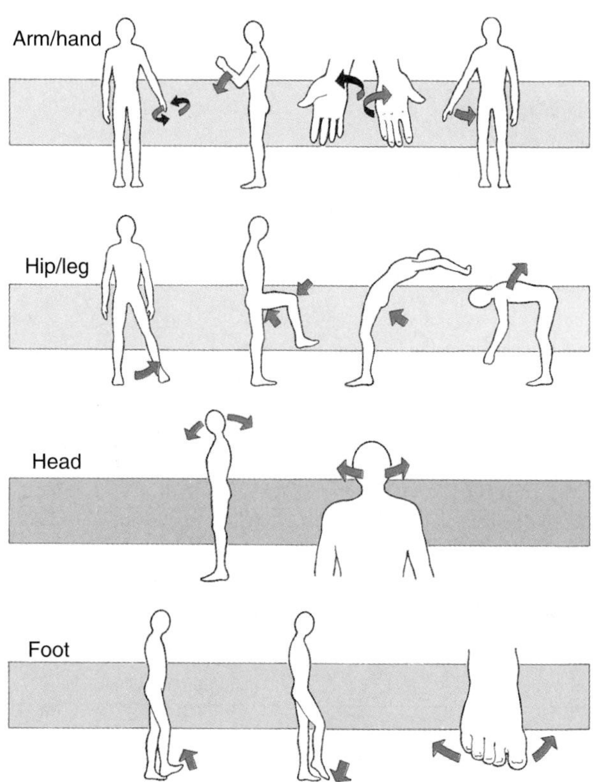

B. **Directions:** Differentiate among gout, osteoarthritis, and rheumatoid arthritis.

____

____

____

____

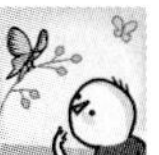

Part V. Documentation

Directions: A patient comes in with pain, tenderness, and deformity of fingers. What questions should you ask? What medications will you ask about?

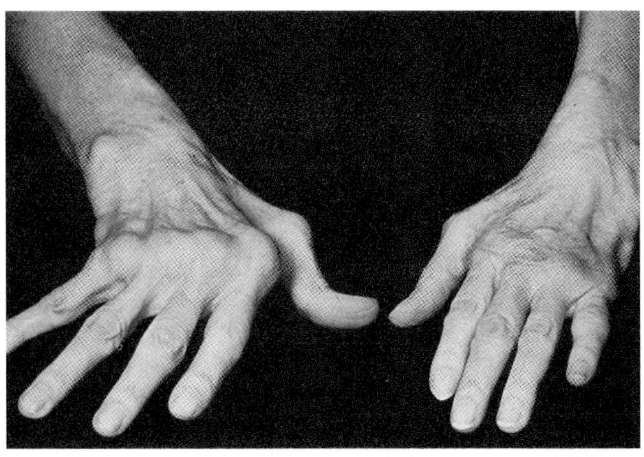

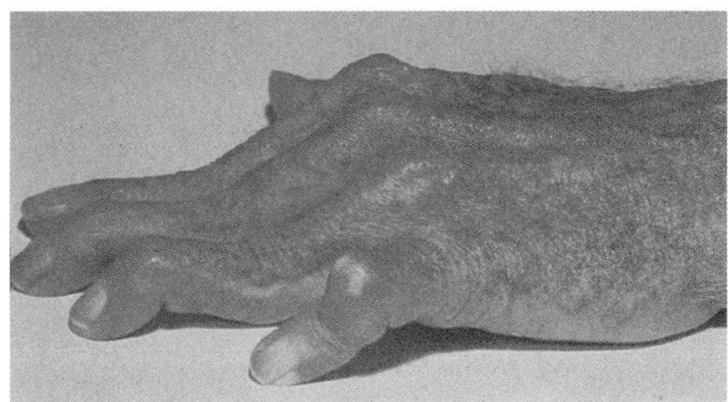

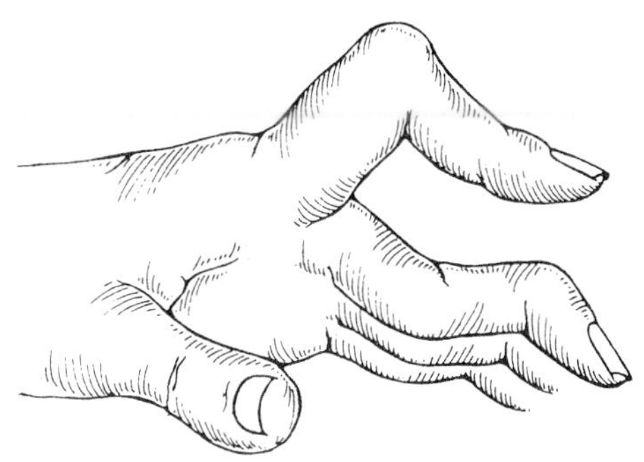

Part VI. Drugs to Know

Directions: Use a drug reference book or the Internet to make drug cards for the following. Include drug classification, generic name, usual adult dose, and drug form.

1. Aspirin
2. Motrin
3. Prednisone
4. Zyloprim
5. Colchicine
6. Anaprox
7. Cataflam
8. Relafen
9. Toradol
10. Voltaren
11. Naprosyn
12. Orudis
13. Vioxx
14. Celebrex
15. Acetaminophen

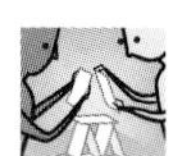

Part VII. Laboratory Tests and Diagnostic Tools to Know

Directions: Discuss and record your responses to the following questions.

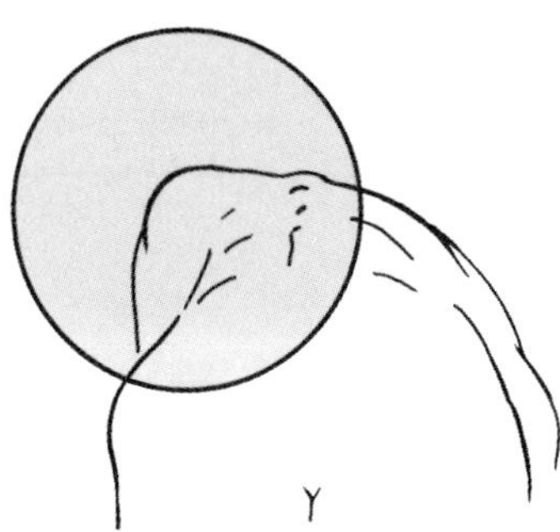

A. Discuss the procedure and findings for scoliosis assessment.

B. Define ESR.

Part VIII. Transdisciplinary Skills

ICD-9 Coding

You have looked up *backache* in the index of diseases, and you are confirming codes in the tabular index.

○ **724 Other and unspecified disorders of back**
Excludes *collapsed vertebra (code to cause, e.g., osteoporosis, 733.00–733.09)*
conditions due to:
intervertebral disc disorders (722.0–722.9)
spondylosis (721.0–721.9)

○ **724.0 Spinal stenosis, other than cervical**
❑ **724.00 Spinal stenosis, unspecified region**
724.01 Thoracic region
724.02 Lumbar region
❑ **724.09 Other**

724.1 Pain in thoracic spine

724.2 Lumbago
Low back pain
Low back syndrome
Lumbalgia

724.3 Sciatica
Neuralgia or neuritis of sciatic nerve
Excludes *specified lesion of sciatic nerve (355.0)*

❑ **724.4 Thoracic or lumbosacral neuritis or radiculitis, unspecified**
Radicular syndrome of lower limbs

❑ **724.5 Backache, unspecified**
Vertebrogenic (pain) syndrome NOS

724.6 Disorders of sacrum
Ankylosis, lumbosacral or sacroiliac (joint)
Instability, lumbosacral or sacroiliac (joint)

○ **724.7 Disorders of coccyx**
❑ **724.70 Unspecified disorder of coccyx**
724.71 Hypermobility of coccyx
❑ **724.79 Other**
Coccygodynia

❑ **724.8 Other symptoms referable to back**
Ossification of posterior longitudinal ligament NOS
Panniculitis specified as sacral or affecting back

❑ **724.9 Other unspecified back disorders**
Ankylosis of spine NOS
Compression of spinal nerve root NEC
Spinal disorder NOS
Excludes sacroiliitis *(720.2)*

◀ **New** ⬅ **Revised Code** ● **Not a Principle Diagnosis** ○ **Use Additional Digit(s)** ❑ **Nonspecific Code**

Code the following diagnoses.

1. Sciatica ______________
2. Lumbar spinal stenosis ______________
3. Lumbago ______________
4. Thoracic pain ______________
5. Unspecific disorder of coccyx ______________

Part IX. Certification Review

Directions: Review and label the fractures shown in the figure below. Match the name of the fracture with the letter corresponding to the illustration of the fracture in the figure below.

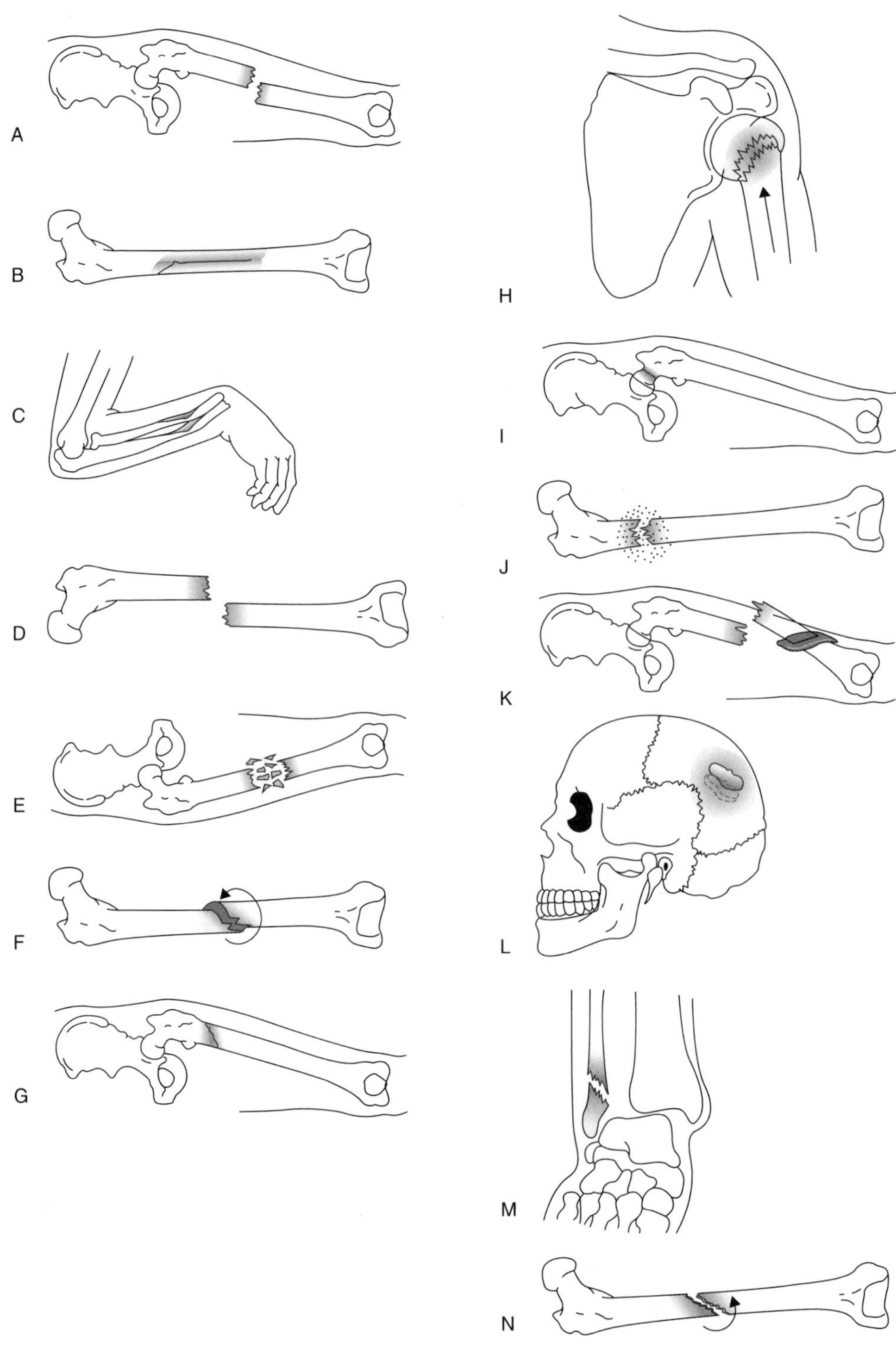

1. _____ transverse
2. _____ spiral
3. _____ simple
4. _____ pathologic
5. _____ oblique
6. _____ longitudinal
7. _____ intracapsular
8. _____ impacted
9. _____ greenstick
10. _____ extracapsular
11. _____ fracture/dislocation
12. _____ depressed
13. _____ compound
14. _____ comminuted

Chapter 40 Quiz

Name: ____

1. ____________ is the large bone of the lower leg.

2. There are ____________ bones in the thoracic spine.

3. An __________ fracture is where the skin is broken.

4. SLE stands for _______________ _______________ _______________ .

5. _______________ arthritis is an autoimmune disease that attacks the synovial fluid and results in deformity.

6. The long part of the bone is the _______________________________ .

7. Inflammation of the joint is called _______________________________ .

8. _____________ connects muscle to bone.

9. ______________ connects bones at a joint.

10. The elbow joints flex and _______________________________ .

CHAPTER 41

Assisting in Neurology and Mental Health

Part I. Medical Terminology

Directions: Define the following terms.

1. anoxia

2. ataxia

3. atrophy

4. coma

5. diplopia

6. gait

Part II. Spelling

Directions: Correct and define the misspelled words.

Ideopathic ____

Ipselateral ____________________

____

____

Controlateral ____________________

____

____

Part III. Anatomy and Physiology ________________________________

A. **Directions:** Label the functional structures and lobes of the brain on the figure below.

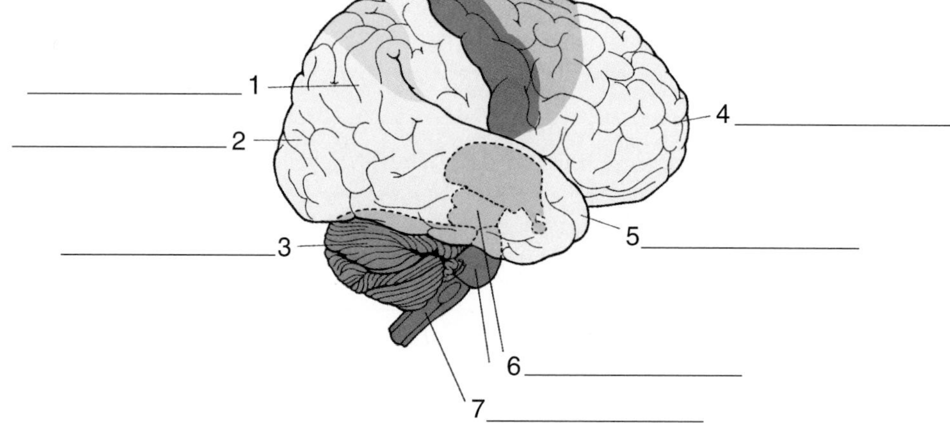

B. **Directions:** List the functions of each of the following.

1. CSF

____

____

2. cerebellum

____

____

3. brain stem

____

____

4. hypothalamus

____

____

5. cerebrum

____

____

6. spinal nerves

____

____

7. cranial nerves

____

____

8. autonomic nerves

____

____

C. **Directions:** Label the cranial nerves on the figure below.

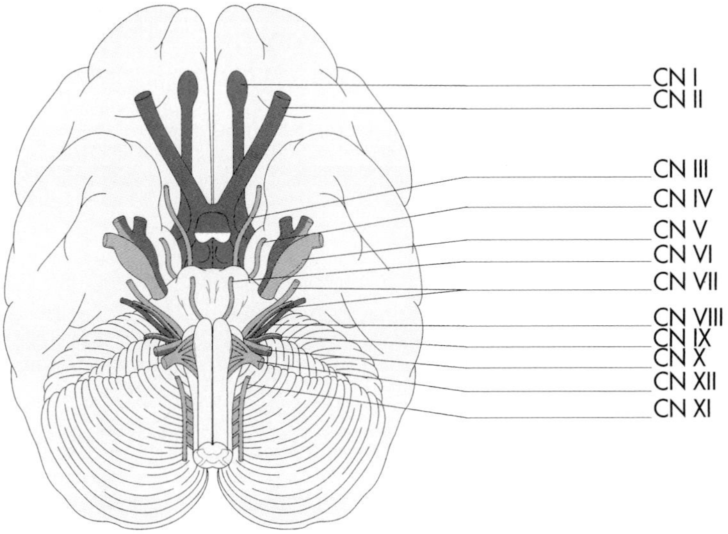

CN I ____

CN II ____

CN III ____

CN IV ____

CN V ____

CN VI ____

CN VII ____

CN VIII ____

CN IX ____

CN X ____

CN XI ____

Part IV. Theory/Triage

Directions: Fill in the blanks or indicate whether statements are true or false.

A. Differentiate between a thrombus and an embolus.

____

____

B. True or False: The cause of Alzheimer's disease remains unknown and there is no known cure.

____

C. CVA is commonly referred to as ______________ or brain attack.

D. True or False: Transient ischemic attacks (TIAs) are also called *mini strokes.* ______________

E. An ______________ consists of some form of visual disturbance, such as dark lines across or spots within the visual field.

F. Absence or ______________ ______________ seizures are a less serious form of seizure consisting of momentary clouding of consciousness and loss of contact with reality.

G. The typical presentation of ______________ includes muscular rigidity, unilateral pill-rolling tremor of the hand, high-pitched monotone voice, and a ______________-like facial expression. The patient has a bent-forward posture with the head bowed. Muscular tremors and ______________ increase. The cause is unknown, but some research indicates that it sometimes occurs after a remote earlier ______________ infection. There is a deficiency of the neurotransmitter ______________ in the brain.

H. ______________ ______________ results from the progressive inflammation and deterioration of these myelin sheaths, leaving the nerve fibers uncovered.

I. ______________, or Lou Gehrig's disease, is a progressive, destructive neurologic disease that results in muscle atrophy.

J. ______________ ______________ affects the seventh cranial nerve of the face. It occurs suddenly and usually subsides spontaneously over several weeks to several months.

K. Carpal tunnel syndrome results from a compression or entrapment of the ______________ nerve as it courses past the carpal bones of the ______________ toward the hand.

Part V. Documentation

PTSS stands for ____.

ADD stands for ____.

LD stands for ____.

List six symptoms of depression.

a. ____

b. ____

c. ____

d. ______________________________

e. ______________________________

f. ______________________________

Part VI. Drugs to Know

Directions: Use a drug reference book or the Internet to make drug cards for the following. Include drug classification, generic name, usual adult dose, and drug form.

1. Coumadin
2. Plavix
3. Aspirin
4. Heparin
5. methysergide maleate
6. sumatriptan succinate
7. L-dopa
8. Dilantin
9. phenobarbital
10. valproic acid
11. Prozac
12. Paxil

Part VII. Laboratory Tests and Diagnostic Tools to Know

Directions: Define the following.

1. MRI

____

____

2. CT

____

____

3. EEG

____

____

4. Lumbar puncture

____

____

Part VIII. Transdisciplinary Skills

A. **Direction:** If you have a *CPT* coding book in your classroom or library, try to code the four diagnostic tests in the previous exercise.

1. MRI of wrist ____________________
2. CT of head without contrast ____________________
3. EEG (standard) ____________________
4. Lumbar puncture ____________________

B. *ICD-9* Coding

Directions: You have looked up *hemiplegia* in the index of diseases, and you are confirming codes in the tabular index.

○ **342 Hemiplegia and hemiparesis**

Note: This category is to be used when hemiplegia (complete) (incomplete) is reported without further specification, or is stated to be old or long-standing but of unspecified cause. The category is also for use in multiple coding to identify these types of hemiplegia resulting from any cause.

Excludes *congenital (343.1)*
hemiplegia due to late effect of cerebrovascular accident (438.20–438.22)
infantile NOS (343.4)

The following fifth digits are for use with codes 342.0–342.9

❑ **0 affecting unspecified side**
1 affecting dominant side
2 affecting nondominant side

○ **342.0 Flaccid hemiplegia**
○ **342.1 Spastic hemiplegia**
❑ ○ **342.8 Other specified hemiplegia**
❑ ○ **342.9 Hemiplegia, unspecified**

○ **343 Infantile cerebral palsy**

Includes: cerebral:
palsy NOS
spastic infantile paralysis
congenital spastic paralysis (cerebral)
Little's disease
paralysis (spastic) due to birth injury:
intracranial
spinal

Excludes *hereditary cerebral paralysis, such as:*
hereditary spastic paraplegia (334.1)
Vogt's disease (333.7)
spastic paralysis specified as noncongenital or noninfantile (344.0–344.9)

343.0 Diplegic
Congenital diplegia
Congenital paraplegia

343.1 Hemiplegic
Congenital hemiplegia

Excludes *infantile hemiplegia NOS (343.4)*

343.2 Quadriplegic
Tetraplegic

343.3 Monoplegic

343.4 Infantile hemiplegia
Infantile hemiplegia (postnatal) NOS

❑ **343.8 Other specified infantile cerebral palsy**

❑ **343.9 Infantile cerebral palsy, unspecified**
Cerebral palsy NOS

◀ **New** ⬅ **Revised Code** ● **Not a Principle Diagnosis** ○ **Use Additional Digit(s)** ❑ **Nonspecific Code**

Code the following diagnoses with all five digits.

1. spastic hemiplegia, unspecified ____________

2. flaccid hemiplegia, dominant side ____________

3. hemiplegia ____________

4. spastic hemiplegia, nondominant side ____________

5. flaccid hemiplegia, nondominant side ____________

Part IX. Certification Review

Directions: Name the following abbreviations and define the conditions.

1. CVA

2. ALS

3. MS

4. PTSD

5. ADD

6. TIA

Chapter 41 Quiz

Name: ____

1. The brain receives ____________ of the body's blood supply.

2. The ______________ is the largest part of the brain.

3. The ______________________ controls balance and coordination.

4. The first cranial nerve deals with the sense of ______________________ .

5. The ____________________ nervous system slows everything down.

6. ____________ is another name for stroke.

7. A TIA is a ________________________ ________________________________ .

8. A disease that causes muscle rigidity, tremors, unusual gait, and facial expression is ____________________ .

9. A disease that causes deterioration of the myelin sheaths is ______________ ________________________________ .

10. Temporary paralysis of the facial nerve is ______________ ______________ .

CHAPTER 42

Assisting in Endocrinology

Part I. Medical Terminology

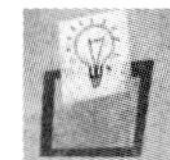

Directions: Match the following terms and definitions.

1. _____ a hormone produced by the alpha cells of the pancreatic islets; it stimulates the liver to convert glycogen into glucose.
2. _____ the abnormal presence of glucose in the urine.
3. _____ the sugar (starch) formed from glucose and stored mainly in the liver.

A. glucosuria
B. glycogen
C. glucagon

Part II. Spelling

Phone-etics Game

Directions: Use the telephone keypad on p. 348 to spell out the missing words.

1. 7-6-5-9-3-4-7-7-4-2 is excessive thirst. ______________________
2. 2-2-8-4 is a hormone that stimulates the production and secretion of glucocorticoids; it is released by the anterior pituitary gland. ______________________
3. 4-6-7-8-5-4-6 is a hormone secreted by the beta cells of the pancreatic islets in response to increased levels of glucose in the blood. ______________________
4. 5-3-8-6-7-4-7 means abnormal production of ketone bodies in the blood and tissues, resulting from fat catabolism in cells. Ketones accumulate in large quantities when fat, instead of, sugar is used as fuel for energy in cells. ______________________
5. 8-7-4 is a hormone secreted by the anterior lobe of the pituitary gland that stimulates the secretion of hormones produced by the thyroid gland. ______________________
6. 7-6-5-9-7-4-2-4-4-2 means increased appetite. ______________________
7. 2-3-4 is a hormone secreted by the posterior pituitary gland; it causes water retention in the kidneys and an elevation in blood pressure. It is also known as *vasopressin*. ______________________
8. 7-6-5-9-8-7-4-2 is excessive urine production.

1	ABC 2	DEF 3
GHI 4	JKL 5	MNO 6
PRS 7	TUV 8	WXY 9
*	0	#

Part III. Anatomy and Physiology ______

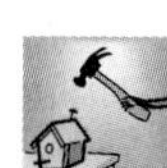

Directions: Fill in the blanks.

1. The posterior pituitary gland secretes ______ and ______.
2. The hormones released by the anterior pituitary gland are:
   a. ______
   b. ______
   c. ______
   d. ______
   e. ______
   f. ______
3. Three conditions related to alterations in growth hormone are:
   a. ______
   b. ______
   c. ______

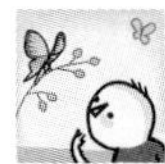

Part IV. Theory/Triage

A. **Directions:** Complete the chart of endocrine diseases by writing in common signs and symptoms.

Location	Disease	Common Signs/Symptoms
Adrenal gland	Addison's disease	
	Cushing's disease	
	Pheochromocytoma	
Pancreas	Diabetes mellitus	
	Hyperinsulinism	
Pituitary gland (anterior lobe)	Acromegaly	
	Gigantism	
	Dwarfism	
Pituitary gland (posterior lobe)	Diabetes insipidus	
Thyroid gland	Hyperthyroidism	
	Hypothyroidism	

B. **Directions:** Differentiate between type 1 and type 2 diabetes.

____

____

____

____

C. **Directions:** Differentiate between diabetic coma and insulin shock.

____

____

____

____

D. **Directions:** Name and define the three "poly" conditions of diabetes.

1. _______________

____

____

2. _______________

____

____

3. _______________

____

____

Directions: Fill in the blanks.

E. People with diabetes are _______________ times more likely to have heart disease or _______________. The destruction of the blood vessels is from atherosclerosis. _______________ _______________ _______________ (CAD) occurs at a quicker rate in both patients with type 1 and those with type 2 diabetes. It affects women as often as men and is often fatal. In individuals with diabetes, _______________ _______________ is strongly associated with an increased risk of CAD.

F. Diabetes is a leading cause of _______________ _______________ in people 20 to 74 years of age, which is often a result of 8 to 10 years of poorly controlled diabetes.

G. _______________ disease is present in 10% to 21% of all patients with diabetes.

Part V. Documentation

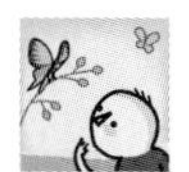

A. A patient with diabetes has come to your office because of a sore on the right big toe. He states that he was trimming a corn a week ago and the area has become painful. You notice that the area is red and warm to the touch. Pedal pulses are weak. The patient is wearing beach sandals. The patient's fasting blood sugar (FBS) is 348. Oral temperature is 100.9. The blood pressure is 182/110 and pulse is 88.

Directions: Use the correct medical terminology to chart your findings. Use appropriate abbreviations. Be sure to include the date and your signature. Correct mistakes by drawing one line. Use black ink.

Documentation

Part VI. Drugs to Know

Directions: Describe a use for each of the following drugs.

Synthroid	
Hydrocortisone	
DDAVP	
DiaBeta	
Glucophage	
Glynase	
Micronase	
Glucovance	
Avandia	
Actos	

Part VII. Laboratory Tests and Diagnostic Tools to Know

A. **Directions:** Describe each of the following laboratory tests.

1. Thyroid stimulating hormone (TSH)

2. Sodium

3. Potassium

4. Fasting blood sugar (FBS)

5. Glucose tolerance test (GTT)

6. Glycohemoglobin or hemoglobin A_{1c}

○ **250 Diabetes mellitus**

Excludes *gestational diabetes (648.8)*
hyperglycemia NOS (790.6)
neonatal diabetes mellitus (775.1)
nonclinical diabetes (790.2)

The following fifth-digit subclassification is for use with category 250:

0 type II [non-insulin dependent type] [NIDDM type] [adult-onset type] or unspecified type, not stated as uncontrolled
Fifth-digit 0 is for use for type II, adult-onset, diabetic patients, even if the patient requires insulin

1 type I [insulin dependent type] [IDDM] [juvenile type], not stated as uncontrolled

2 type II [non-insulin dependent type] [NIDDM type] [adult-onset type] or unspecified type, uncontrolled
Fifth-digit 2 is for use for type II, adult-onset, diabetic patients, even if the patient requires insulin

3 type I [insulin dependent type] [IDDM] [juvenile type], uncontrolled

○ **250.0 Diabetes mellitus without mention of complication**
Diabetes mellitus without mention of complication or manifestation classifiable to 250.1–250.9
Diabetes (mellitus) NOS

○ **250.1 Diabetes with ketoacidosis**
Diabetic:
acidosis without mention of coma
ketosis without mention of coma

○ **250.2 Diabetes with hyperosmolarity**
Hyperosmolar (nonketotic) coma

○ **250.3 Diabetes with other coma**
Diabetic coma (with ketoacidosis)
Diabetic hypoglycemic coma
Insulin coma NOS

Excludes *diabetes with hyperosmolar coma (250.2)*

○ **250.4 Diabetes with renal manifestations**
Use additional code to identify manifestation, as:
diabetic:
nephropathy NOS (583.81)
nephrosis (581.81)
intercapillary glomerulosclerosis (581.81)
Kimmelstiel-Wilson syndrome (581.81)

○ **250.5 Diabetes with ophthalmic manifestations**
Use additional code to identify manifestation, as:
diabetic:
blindness (369.00–369.9)
cataract (366.41)
glaucoma (365.44)
retinal edema (362.83)
retinopathy (362.01–362.02)

○ **250.6 Diabetes with neurological manifestations**
Use additional code to identify manifestation, as:
diabetic:
amyotrophy (358.1)
mononeuropathy (354.0–355.9)
neurogenic arthropathy (713.5)
peripheral autonomic neuropathy (337.1)
polyneuropathy (357.2)

○ **250.7 Diabetes with peripheral circulatory disorders**
Use additional code to identify manifestation, as:
diabetic:
gangrene (785.4)
peripheral angiopathy (443.81)

❑ ○ **250.8 Diabetes with other specified manifestations**
Diabetic hypoglycemia
Hypoglycemic shock
Use additional code to identify manifestation, as:
any associated ulceration (707.10–707.9)
diabetic bone changes (731.8)
Use additional E code to identify cause, if drug-induced

❑ ○ **250.9 Diabetes with unspecified complication**

◀ **New** ⬅ **Revised Code** ● **Not a Principle Diagnosis** ○ **Use Additional Digit(s)** ❑ **Nonspecific Code**

Part VIII. Transdisciplinary Skills

ICD-9 Coding

Directions: You have looked up *diabetes* in the index of diseases, and you are confirming codes in the tabular index.

Code the following diagnoses with five digits.

1. Hypoglycemia, insulin, juvenile, shock (uncontrolled) ________________
2. Ketoacidosis, NIDDM (uncontrolled) ________________
3. Hyperosmolar nonketotic coma, insulin dependent (uncontrolled) ________________
4. Controlled juvenile diabetes ________________
5. Uncontrolled noninsulin-dependent diabetes ________________
6. Diabetes type 2 ________________
7. Controlled adult-onset diabetes ________________
8. Uncontrolled IDDM ________________
9. Diabetic cataract, controlled, juvenile onset ________________ ________________
10. Diabetic renal failure, NIDDM (uncontrolled) ________________

Part IX. Certification Review

Directions: Fill in the blanks or indicate whether statements are true or false.

1. True or False: Type 1 diabetes is insulin dependent. ________________
2. True or False: Ketoacidosis can occur if blood sugar gets too low. ________________
3. Cushing's disease in an ________________ in cortisol.
4. Graves' disease is an excess of ________________ hormones.
5. True or False: A simple goiter is any thyroid enlargement that has not been caused by an infection or neoplasm. ________________

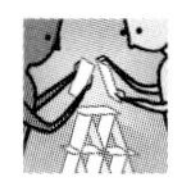

Part X. Class Project

Directions: Evaluate the sample daily food plan for a patient with diabetes. With a partner, see whether you can follow the diet for 24 hours. Read labels to determine calories. Be careful to monitor serving sizes. If you need to estimate, allow 100 calories for one serving of fruit, bread, cereal, and egg. At the end of 24 hours, evaluate the experience. Note: **Any dietary changes should be approved by your doctor.**

Breakfast
- one piece of fruit
- small bowl of unsweetened cereal
- one slice of whole wheat bread or toast
- one egg
- coffee or tea with skim milk

Snack
one piece of fruit
coffee or tea with skim milk

Lunch
one slice of whole wheat bread
one medium serving of fish, lean meat, or low-fat cheese
small salad
one piece of fruit
coffee or tea with skim milk

Snack
one piece of fruit
coffee or tea with skim milk

Dinner
small serving of vegetable or clear soup
medium serving of fish, lean meat, or chicken
one potato or one serving of corn or rice
three servings of vegetables
coffee or tea with skim milk

Snack
one piece of fruit or three plain crackers

Food Choice	Calories	Personal Thoughts
Breakfast		
Snack		
Lunch		
Snack		
Dinner		
Snack		
No. of glasses of water =	Total calories	

Ideas to share with the class about the diabetic diet experience.

Chapter 42 Quiz

Name: ______________________________

1. The posterior pituitary gland secretes:

   a. ______________

   b. ______________

2. Too much growth hormone causes

   ______________.

3. Another term for hyperthyroidism is

   ______________ *disease*.

4. Cortisol ______________ blood sugar levels.

5. List two types of diabetes mellitus.

   a. ______________

   b. ______________

6. True or False: Insulin shock occurs when the blood sugar level is too low.

   ____

7. Diabetic coma occurs with a very

   ______________ blood glucose level.

8. Older adults are at risk for:

   a. type 1 diabetes

   b. type 2 diabetes

   ____

9. A hemoglobin A_{1c} test can detect

   ______________.

10. True or False: Iodine deficiency is related to simple goiter formation. ______________

CHAPTER 43

Assisting in Pulmonary Medicine

Part I. Medical Terminology

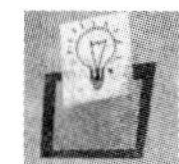

A. **Directions:** Define the following terms.

Medical Term	Definition
Apnea	
Atelectasis	
Dyspnea	
Empyema	
Hemoptysis	
Hemothorax	
Hypercapnia	
Hyperpnea	
Hypoxemia	
Orthopnea	
Pleurisy	
Pneumothorax	
Pyothorax	
Rhinoplasty	
Rhinorrhea	
Tachypnea	
Thoracotomy	

Part II. Spelling

Phone-etics Game

Directions: Use the telephone keypad on p. 360 to spell out the missing words.

1. 5-8-6-4 cancer is the leading cause of cancer-related deaths for both men and women in the United States. ________________

2. A positive 6-2-6-8-6-8-9 reaction indicates the possibility of active or dormant tuberculosis or exposure to the disease. ________________

3. Pulse 6-9-4-6-3-8-7-9 is a noninvasive method of evaluating the oxygen saturation of hemoglobin in arterial blood, as well as the pulse rate. ____________

4. Bronchoscopy provides an 3-6-3-6-7-2-6-7-4-2 view of the larynx, trachea, and bronchi.

____

1	ABC 2	DEF 3
GHI 4	JKL 5	MNO 6
PRS 7	TUV 8	WXY 9
*	0	#

Part III. Anatomy and Physiology

A. **Directions:** Label the drawing below with the anatomical landmarks: anterior, posterior, and mid-axillary lines.

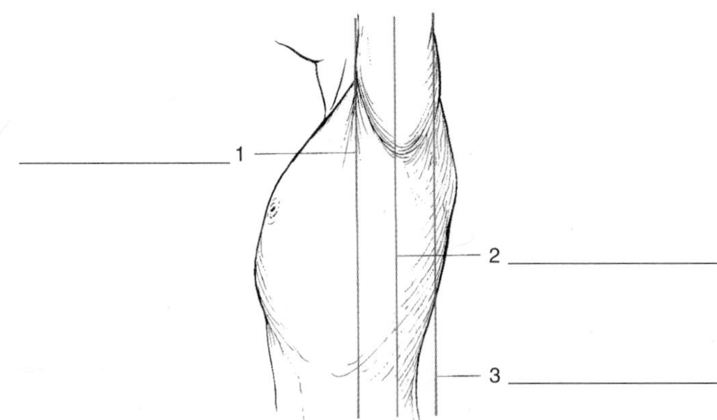

B. **Directions:** On the figure below, label the structures of the respiratory system, head, and chest.

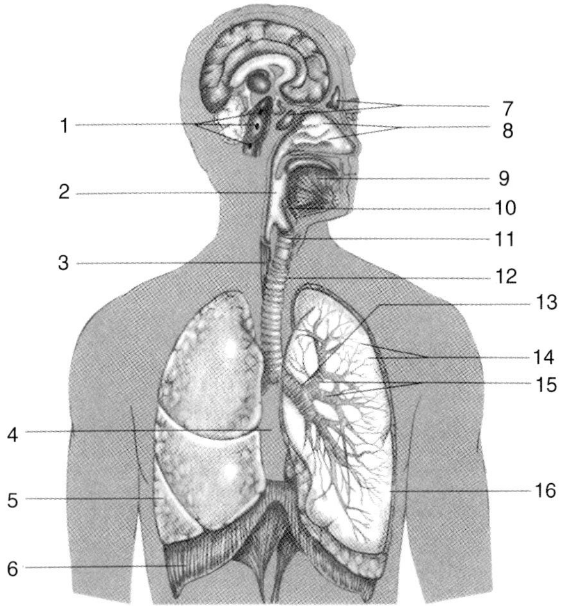

1. ______________________
2. ______________________
3. ______________________
4. ______________________
5. ______________________
6. ______________________
7. ______________________
8. ______________________
9. ______________________
10. ______________________
11. ______________________
12. ______________________
13. ______________________
14. ______________________
15. ______________________
16. ______________________

C. **Directions:** Label the lobes of the lungs on the figure below.

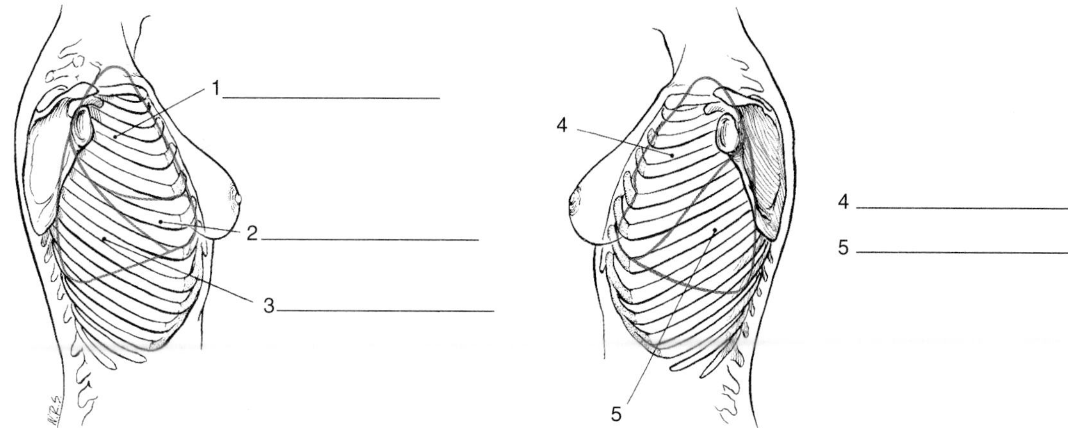

Part IV. Theory/Triage

Directions: Indicate whether each statement is true (T) or false (F).

1. _____ In asthma and/or emphysema, the individual has difficulty in getting the air out of the lungs, and accessory muscles in the chest are needed to assist the intercostal and diaphragm muscles for complete exhalation.

2. _____ Cigarette smoking is the primary contributing factor to emphysema; however, patients in whom emphysema develops at an early age may have a genetic predisposition to the disease.

Directions: Match the following occupations with the associated lung diseases.

1. _____ stone cutting or sand blasting
2. _____ insulation and shipbuilding
3. _____ coal mining

A. anthracosis
B. silicosis
C. asbestosis

Part V. Documentation

A. Your patient has had a fever and cough for four days. Oral temperature is 102.4°F. You hear a high-pitched, musical sound on expiration when you auscultate the posterior chest near the left side of the neck.

Directions: Use the correct medical terminology to chart your findings. Use appropriate abbreviations. Be sure to include the date and your signature. Correct mistakes by drawing one line. Use black ink.

Documentation

Part VI. Drugs to Know

A. **Directions:** Complete the chart below.

Drug	Use
Oxygen	
INH	
Allergra	
Rifampin	
Zyrtec	
Prednisone	
Ventolin	
Azmacort	

B. Identify the oxygen delivery devices shown in the figure below as simple face mask, non-rebreathing mask, or nasal cannula.

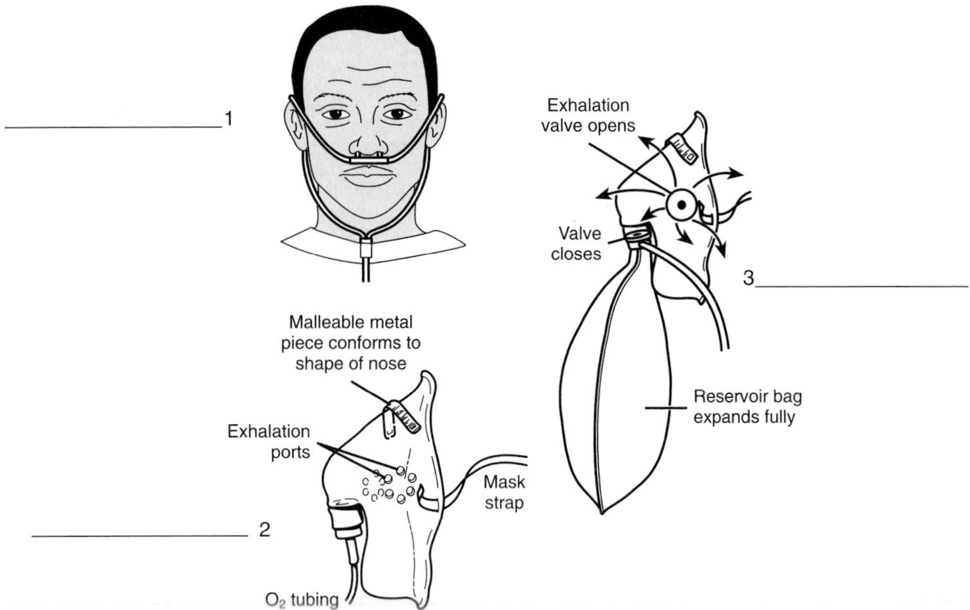

Part VII. Laboratory Tests and Diagnostic Tools to Know

A. **Directions:** Describe the condition shown in the figure below.

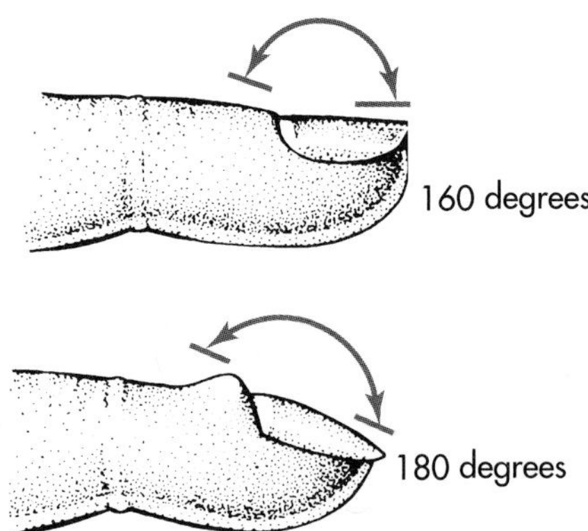

B. **Directions:** Describe the following.

1. Complete blood cell count

2. Chest radiographs

3. Spirometric evaluation

Part VIII. Transdisciplinary Skills

ICD-9 Coding

You have looked up *COPD* in the index of diseases, and you are confirming codes in the tabular index.

❑ **490 Bronchitis, not specified as acute or chronic**
Bronchitis NOS:
catarrhal
with tracheitis NOS
Tracheobronchitis NOS
Excludes *bronchitis:*
allergic NOS (493.9)
asthmatic NOS (493.9)
due to fumes and vapors (506.0)

○ **491 Chronic bronchitis**
Excludes *chronic obstructive asthma (493.2)*

491.0 Simple chronic bronchitis
Catarrhal bronchitis, chronic
Smokers' cough

491.1 Mucopurulent chronic bronchitis
Bronchitis (chronic) (recurrent):
fetid
mucopurulent
purulent

○ **491.2 Obstructive chronic bronchitis**
Bronchitis:
asthmatic, chronic
emphysematous
obstructive (chronic) (diffuse)
Bronchitis with:
chronic airway obstruction
emphysema
Excludes *asthmatic bronchitis (acute) (NOS) 493.9*
chronic obstructive asthma 493.2

491.20 Without mention of acute exacerbation
Chronic asthmatic bronchitis
Emphysema with chronic bronchitis

491.21 With acute exacerbation
Acute bronchitis with chronic obstructive pulmonary disease [COPD]
Acute and chronic obstructive bronchitis
Acute exacerbation of chronic obstructive pulmonary disease [COPD]
Chronic asthmatic bronchitis with acute exacerbation
Emphysema with acute and chronic bronchitis
Excludes *chronic obstructive asthma with acute exacerbation (493.22)* ◀

❑ **491.8 Other chronic bronchitis**
Chronic:
tracheitis
tracheobronchitis

❑ **491.9 Unspecified chronic bronchitis**

○ **492 Emphysema**

492.0 Emphysematous bleb
Giant bullous emphysema
Ruptured emphysematous bleb
Tension pneumatocele
Vanishing lung

❑ **492.8 Other emphysema**
Emphysema (lung or pulmonary):
NOS
centriacinar
centrilobular
obstructive
panacinar
panlobular
unilateral
vesicular
MacLeod's syndrome
Unilateral hyperlucent lung
Excludes *emphysema:*
with both acute and chronic bronchitis (491.21)
with chronic bronchitis (491.20)
compensatory (518.2)
due to fumes and vapors (506.4)
interstitial (518.1)
newborn (770.2)
mediastinal (518.1)
surgical (subcutaneous) (998.81)
traumatic (958.7)
with chronic bronchitis (491.20)

○ **493 Asthma** ⬅
The following fifth-digit subclassification is for use with catergory 493:
0 without mention of status asthmaticus or acute exacerbation or unspecified
1 with status asthmaticus
2 with acute exacerbation
Excludes *wheezing NOS (786.07)*

○ **493.0 Extrinsic asthma**
Asthma:
allergic with stated cause
atopic
childhood
hay
platinum
Hay fever with asthma

◀ **New** ⬅ **Revised Code** ● **Not a Principle Diagnosis** ○ **Use Additional Digit(s)** ❑ **Nonspecific Code**

Excludes *asthma:*
allergic:
allergic NOS (493.9)
detergent (507.8)
miners' (500)
wood (495.8)

○ **493.1 Intrinsic asthma**
Late-onset asthma

○ **493.2 Chronic obstructive asthma**
Asthma with chronic obstructive pulmonary disease (COPD)
Excludes *acute bronchitis (466.0)* ◀
chronic asthmatic bronchitis (491.2)
chronic obstructive bronchitis (491.2)

❑ ○ **493.9 Asthma, unspecified**
Asthma (bronchial) (allergic NOS)
Bronchitis:
allergic asthmatic

○ **494 Bronchiectasis**
Bronchiectasis (fusiform) (postinfectious) (recurrent)
Bronchiolectasis
Excludes *congenital (748.61)*
tuberculous bronchiectasis (current disease) (011.5)

494.0 Bronchiectasis without acute exacerbation

494.1 Bronchiectasis with acute exacerbation
Acute bronchitis with bronchiectasis

◀ **New** ⇐ **Revised Code** ● **Not a Principle Diagnosis** ○ **Use Additional Digit(s)** ❑ **Nonspecific Code**

Code the following diagnoses.

1. Emphysema ________________
2. Chronic bronchitis (smoker's cough) ________________
3. Chronic tracheitis ________________
4. Asthma (unspecified) ________________
5. Intrinsic asthma ________________
6. Bronchitis ________________
7. Hay fever with asthma (extrinsic) ________________
8. Bronchiectasis with exacerbation ________________

Part IX. Certification Review

Directions: Fill in the blanks or indicate whether statements are true or false.

1. True or False: *Mycobacterium tuberculosis* is the bacterium that causes tuberculosis (TB). _____
2. Name three ways to screen for TB.
   a. ________________
   b. ________________
   c. ________________
3. The lungs are part of the ________________ airway.
4. The upper respiratory tract transports air from the atmosphere to the lungs and includes the:
   a. ________________
   b. ________________
   c. ________________

Chapter 43 Quiz

Name: ______________________________

1. COPD includes:
   a. ____________
   b. ____________

2. Apnea means ____________
____________.

3. Another term for sore throat is
____________.

4. The ____________ are part of the lower airway.

5. List two types upper respiratory infections.
   a. ____________
   b. ____________

6. True or False: Allegra and Zyrtec are used to treat allergies and hay fever. ________

7. Laryngitis means ____________.

8. Coughing up blood is:
   a. hemothorax
   b. hemoptysis
   c. atelectasis

   ____

9. Rhinorrhea means ____________
____________.

10. Another name for the windpipe is the
____________.

CHAPTER 44

Assisting in Cardiology

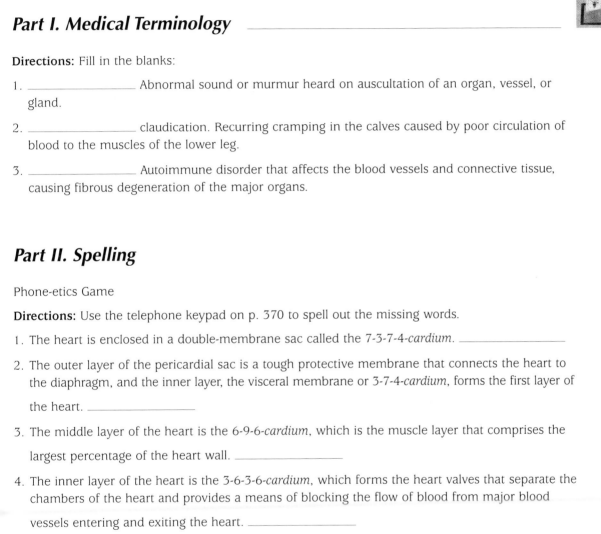

Part I. Medical Terminology

Directions: Fill in the blanks:

1. ________________ Abnormal sound or murmur heard on auscultation of an organ, vessel, or gland.
2. ________________ claudication. Recurring cramping in the calves caused by poor circulation of blood to the muscles of the lower leg.
3. ________________ Autoimmune disorder that affects the blood vessels and connective tissue, causing fibrous degeneration of the major organs.

Part II. Spelling

Phone-etics Game

Directions: Use the telephone keypad on p. 370 to spell out the missing words.

1. The heart is enclosed in a double-membrane sac called the 7-3-7-4-*cardium*. ________________
2. The outer layer of the pericardial sac is a tough protective membrane that connects the heart to the diaphragm, and the inner layer, the visceral membrane or 3-7-4-*cardium*, forms the first layer of the heart. ________________
3. The middle layer of the heart is the 6-9-6-*cardium*, which is the muscle layer that comprises the largest percentage of the heart wall. ________________
4. The inner layer of the heart is the 3-6-3-6-*cardium*, which forms the heart valves that separate the chambers of the heart and provides a means of blocking the flow of blood from major blood vessels entering and exiting the heart. ________________

1	ABC 2	DEF 3
GHI 4	JKL 5	MNO 6
PRS 7	TUV 8	WXY 9
*	0	#

Part III. Anatomy and Physiology

Directions: Label the parts of the heart on the figure below.

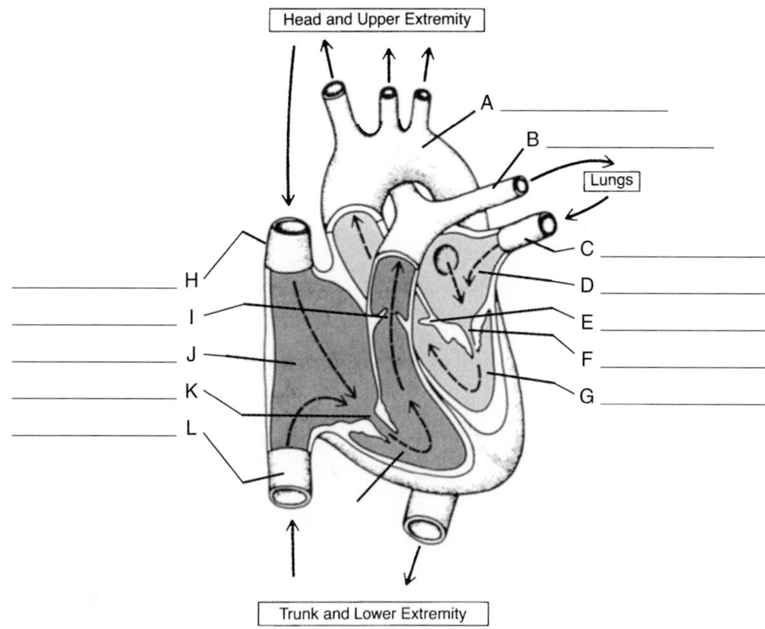

Part IV. Theory/Triage

A. CAD stands for ____________ ____________ ____________.

B. List five symptoms of myocardial infarction in women:

1. ____________
2. ____________
3. ____________
4. ____________
5. ____________

C. Telephone screening for chest pain

List five situations in which the medical assistant should activate emergency medical services.

1. ____________
2. ____________
3. ____________
4. ____________
5. ____________

D. List five conditions that can result from hypertension.

1. ____________
2. ____________
3. ____________
4. ____________
5. ____________

E. A myocardial infarction is

____

____

____

F. Identify the causes of the various types of shock.

Type	Definition	Causes
Cardiogenic		
Hypovolemic		
Neurogenic		

Type	Definition	Causes
Anaphylactic		
Septic (septicemia)		

Part V. Documentation

A. Your patient has congestive heart failure and complains of swelling of both legs. When you press on the pre-tibia area of the leg, you notice that your finger leaves a 6-mm indention.

Directions: Use the correct medical terminology to chart your findings. Use appropriate abbreviations. Be sure to include the date and your signature. Correct mistakes by drawing one line. Use black ink.

Documentation

Part VI. Drugs to Know

Directions: Look up the generic names of these drugs. Make a drug card for each one. What do you notice about the generic names within each category?

1. beta blockers (Tenormin, Lopressor, or Inderal)

   generic names ________________ ________________ ________________

2. angiotensin-converting enzyme (ACE) inhibitors (Lotensin, Capoten, or Vasotec)

   generic names ____________ ____________ ____________

3. anticholesterol agents (Lipitor, Mevacor, or Zocor)

   generic names ____________ ____________ ____________

4. anticoagulants (Coumadin)

   generic name ____________

5. cardiac glycosides (Lanoxin)

   generic name ____________

6. diuretics (HCTZ, Lasix, or Dyazide)

   generic names ____________ ____________ ____________

Part VII. Laboratory Tests and Diagnostic Tools to Know ____________

Directions: Research and describe the following.

1. ECG

____

____

2. CPK and LDH

____

____

3. ESR

____

____

Part VIII. Transdisciplinary Skills

ICD-9 Coding

You have looked up *rheumatic fever* in the index of diseases, and you are confirming codes in the tabular index.

390 Rheumatic fever without mention of heart involvement
Arthritis, rheumatic, acute or subacute
Rheumatic fever (active) (acute)
Rheumatism, articular, acute or subacute
Excludes *that with heart involvement (391.0–391.9)*

○ **391 Rheumatic fever with heart involvement**
Excludes *chronic heart diseases of rheumatic origin(393.0–398.9) unless rheumatic fever is also present or there is evidence of recrudescence or activity of the rheumatic process*

391.0 Acute rheumatic pericarditis
Rheumatic:
fever (active) (acute) with pericarditis
pericarditis (acute)
Any condition classifiable to 390 with pericarditis
Excludes *that not specified as rheumatic (420.0–420.9)*

391.1 Acute rheumatic endocarditis
Rheumatic:
endocarditis, acute
fever (active) (acute) with endocarditis or valvulitis
valvulitis, acute
Any condition classifiable to 390 with endocarditis or valvulitis

391.2 Acute rheumatic myocarditis
Rheumatic fever (active) (acute) with myocarditis
Any condition classifiable to 390 with myocarditis

❑ **391.8 Other acute rheumatic heart disease**
Rheumatic:
fever (active) (acute) with other or multiple types of heart involvement
pancarditis, acute
Any condition classifiable to 390 with other or multiple types of heart involvement

❑ **391.9 Acute rheumatic heart disease, unspecified**
Rheumatic:
carditis, acute
fever (active) (acute) with unspecified type of heart involvement
heart disease, active or acute
Any condition classifiable to 390 with unspecified type of heart involvement

◀ **New** ⬅ **Revised Code** ● **Not a Principle Diagnosis** ○ **Use Additional Digit(s)** ❑ **Nonspecific Code**

Code the following diagnoses.

1. Acute rheumatic myocarditis ________________
2. Acute rheumatic endocarditis ________________
3. Acute rheumatic pericarditis ________________
4. Rheumatic fever, active ________________
5. Rheumatic valvulitis ________________

Part IX. Certification Review

Directions: Fill in the blanks or indicate whether statement is true or false.

1. The heart is divided into four chambers. The ______________, the top chambers, receive blood, and the ______________, the bottom chambers, pump the blood out.
2. The cardiac impulse originates in specialized muscle tissue called the ______________ node.
3. ______________ ______________ ______________ occurs when the myocardium is unable to pump an adequate amount of blood to meet the needs of the body.
4. ______________ heart failure, when the left ventricle cannot completely empty, causes a backup of blood in the lungs resulting in pulmonary edema, a collection of fluid in the lungs.
5. ______________-sided heart failure, when the ventricle cannot maintain complete output, causes a backup of blood in the ______________ atrium, which prevents complete emptying of the vena cava and results in systemic edema, especially in the legs and feet.
6. True or False: The most common valve defect is mitral valve prolapse (MVP), an incompetence in the mitral valve. ______________

Chapter 44 Quiz

Name: ______________________________

1. Name two diuretics.

   a. ______________

   b. ______________

2. A common name for MI is a

   ______________.

3. What generic names end in "pril"?

   a. ACE inhibitors

   b. beta blockers

   c. calcium channel blockers

   ____

4. What does MVP mean? ______________

   ______________ ______________

5. Describe two types of valve disorders.

   a. ______________

   b. ______________

6. What is another name for right-sided heart failure? ______________________

   ____

7. ______________-sided heart failure causes lung congestion.

8. What generic names end in "lol"?

   a. ACE inhibitors

   b. beta blockers

   c. calcium channel blockers

   ____

9. Lasix, KCL, and ______________ are the drugs that are used commonly for CHF.

10. List four different types of shock.

    a. ______________

    b. ______________

    c. ______________

    d. ______________

CHAPTER 45

Assisting in Geriatrics

Part I. Theory/Triage

Directions: List five myths and stereotypes about aging.

1. ______________________________
2. ______________________________
3. ______________________________
4. ______________________________
5. ______________________________

Part II.

Directions: Complete the table of health promotion and body system changes associated with aging.

Body System	Age-Related Changes	Health Promotion
Cardiovascular		
Central nervous system		
Endocrine		
Gastrointestinal		

Body System	Age-Related Changes	Health Promotion
Musculoskeletal		
Pulmonary		
Sensory organs		
Urinary		
Sexuality		

Part III.

List six suggestions for helping the elderly prevent and treat dry skin.

1. __________
2. __________
3. __________
4. __________
5. __________
6. __________

Part IV.

List six suggestions for helping the older adult with mobility, dexterity, and balance.

1. __________
2. __________
3. __________
4. __________

5. ______

6. ______

Part V.

List eight suggestions for preventing falls.

1. ______
2. ______
3. ______
4. ______
5. ______
6. ______
7. ______
8. ______

Part VI.

List seven risk factors for cognitive decline.

1. ______
2. ______
3. ______
4. ______
5. ______
6. ______
7. ______

Part VII.

Describe the stages of Alzheimer's disease.

First Stage:

______

______

Second Stage:

______

______

Terminal Stage:

______

______

Part VIII.

Describe the guidelines for effective patient education with older adults.

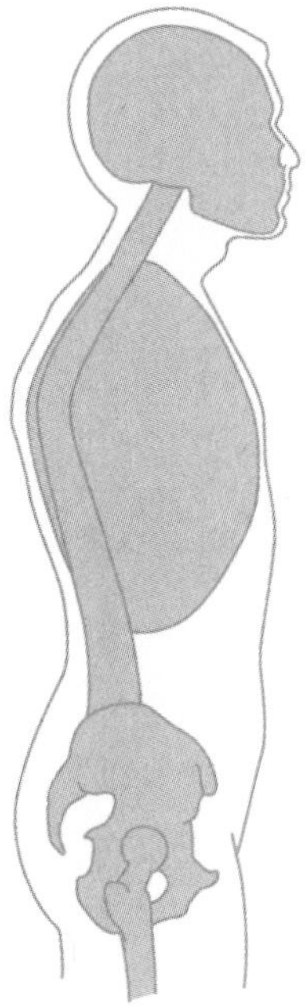

Part IX.

Describe the patient's stooped posture and possible causes. Who is at risk for this condition? What can be done to prevent this condition?

Chapter 45 Quiz

Name: ____________________

1. Describe two skin changes in the elderly:
   a. ____________
   b. ____________

2. Alopecia means ____________
____________.

3. Older adults frequently have problems with:
   a. diarrhea
   b. constipation
   c. vomiting
   ____

4. Presbycusis means ____________
____________.

5. Describe glaucoma.
____

6. What is a cataract? ____________
____________.

7. ____________ cause the greatest number of injuries in the elderly.

8. DNR stands for ____________
____________ ____________.

9. ____________ is used to treat impotence.

10. PLMD stands for ____________
____________ ____________
____________.

CHAPTER 46

Principles of Electrocardiography

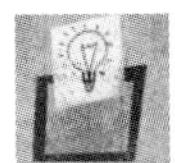

Part I. Medical Terminology

Directions: Match the following terms and definitions.

1. _____ bradycardia
2. _____ bundle of His
3. _____ cardiac arrest
4. _____ cardioversion
5. _____ defibrillator
6. _____ dyspnea
7. _____ hypertension
8. _____ infarction
9. _____ ischemic
10. _____ myocardial
11. _____ myocardium
12. _____ orthopnea
13. _____ sinoatrial (SA) node
14. _____ tachycardia

A. Complete cessation of cardiac contractions

B. Use of an electroshock to convert an abnormal cardiac rhythm to a normal one

C. Heart muscle

D. Heart rate of less than 60 beats per minute

E. Fibers that conduct electrical impulses from AV node to ventricular myocardium

F. Heart rate greater than 100 beats per minute

G. Area of tissue that has died because of lack of blood supply

H. Temporary interruption in blood supply to a tissue or organ

I. Pertaining to the heart muscle

J. Difficulty breathing when in supine position

K. Pacemaker of the heart located in the right atrium

L. Machine used to deliver an electroshock to the heart through electrodes placed on the chest wall

M. difficulty breathing

N. High blood pressure in which the diastolic pressure is greater than 90 mm Hg

Part II. Spelling

Phone-etics Game

Directions: Use the telephone keypad below to spell out the missing words. Write the corresponding numbers in the blanks provided.

_______________ The two upper chambers of the heart

_______________ The two lower chambers of the heart

_______________ Dizziness

_______________ Divide from one into two branches

1	ABC 2	DEF 3
GHI 4	JKL 5	MNO 6
PRS 7	TUV 8	WXY 9
*	0	#

Part III. Visual Aids

Directions: Use the figures on p. 387 to answer the following questions.

1. Describe the conduction pathways of the heart and label the structures of the heart on the following figure.

____

____

____

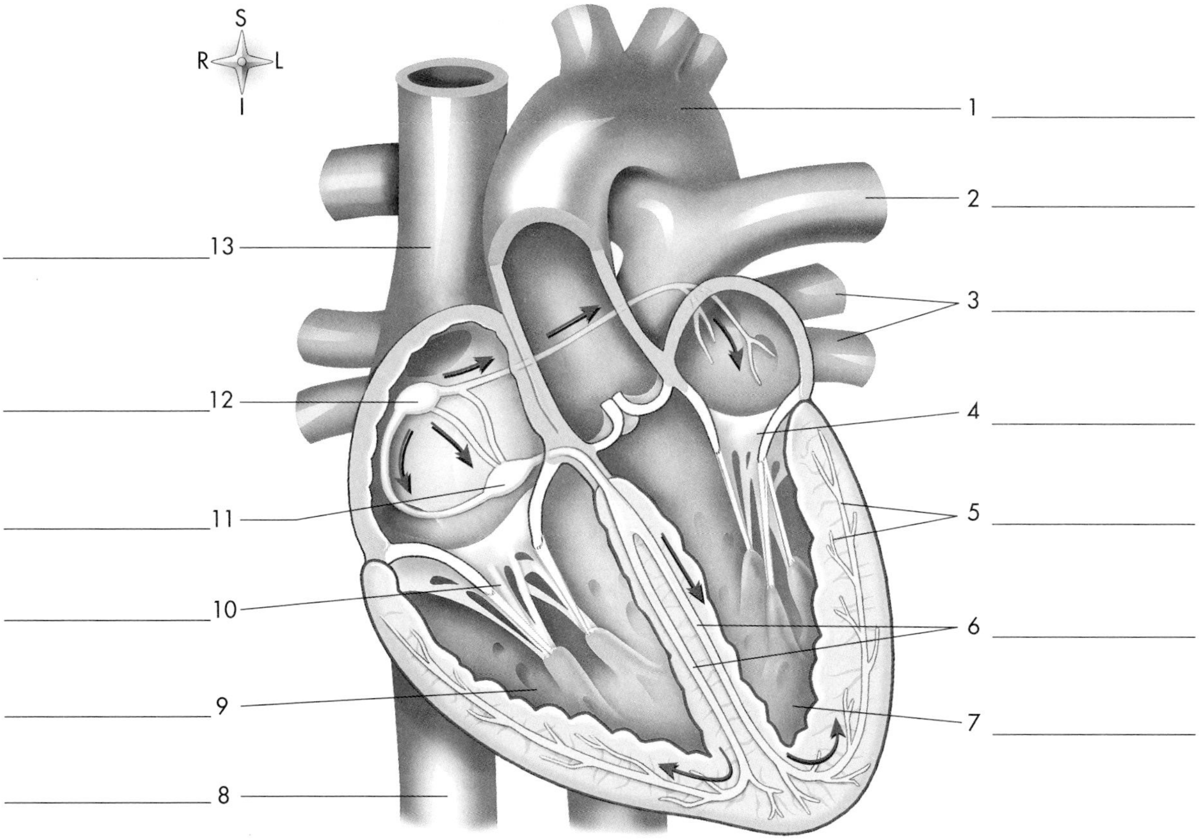

S
R
L
I
1 ____________
2 ____________
3 ____________
4 ____________
5 ____________
6 ____________
7 ____________
____________ 13
____________ 12
____________ 11
____________ 10
____________ 9
____________ 8

2. Label the precordial leads on the drawing below.

B ____________
C ____________
____________ A
D ____________
____________ E
F ____________

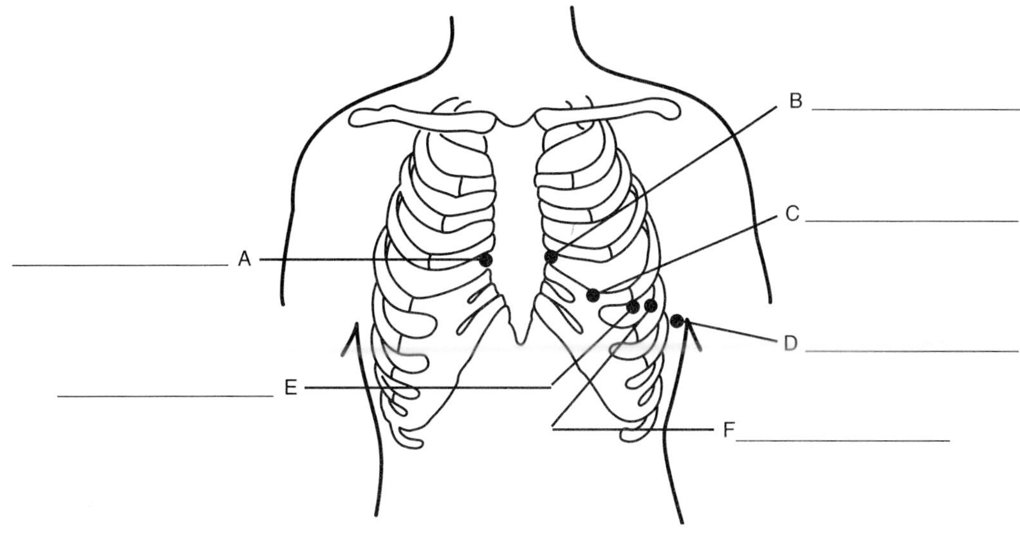

3. Draw in correct placement of leads for a 12-lead electrocardiogram (ECG). ____________

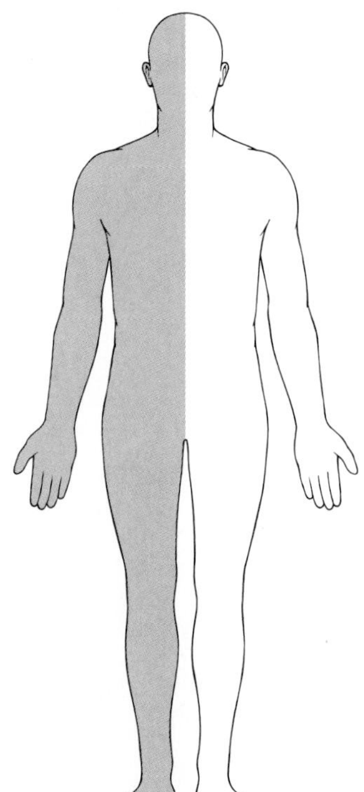

4. Name the rhythm shown below. ____________

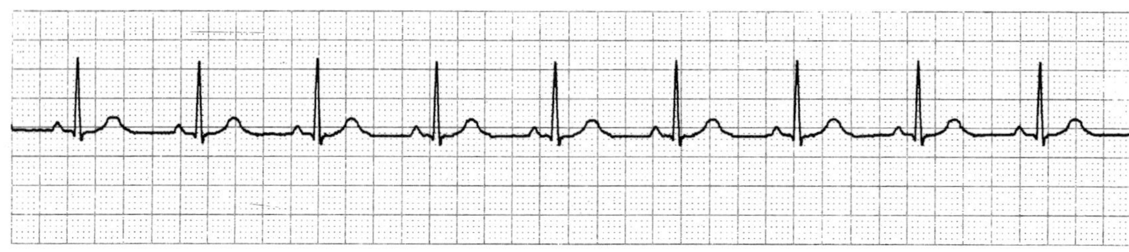

5. Name the rhythm shown below. ____________

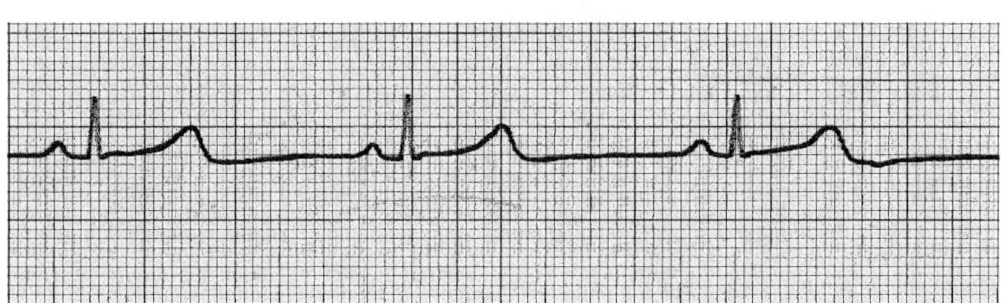

6. Name the rhythm shown below. ____________________

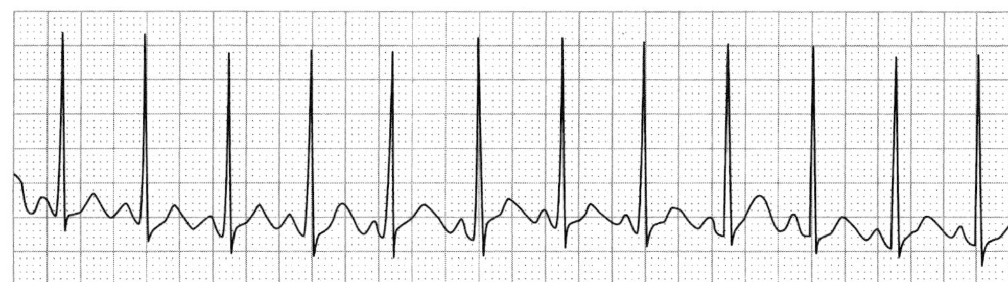

7. Name the rhythm shown below. ____________________

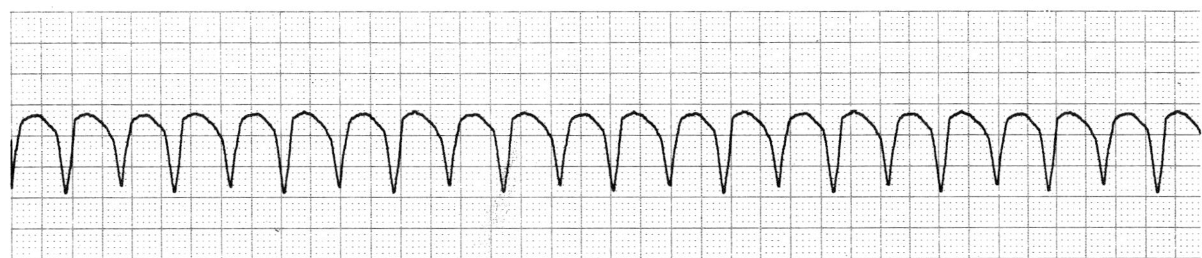

8. Name the rhythm shown below. ____________________

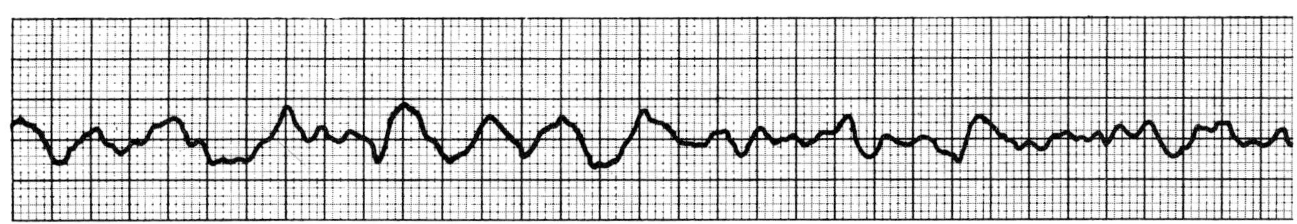

9. Name the rhythm shown below. ____________________

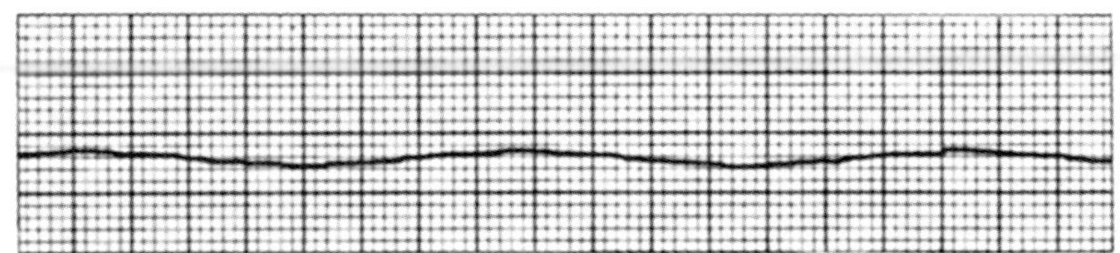

10. Describe the procedure shown in the drawing below.

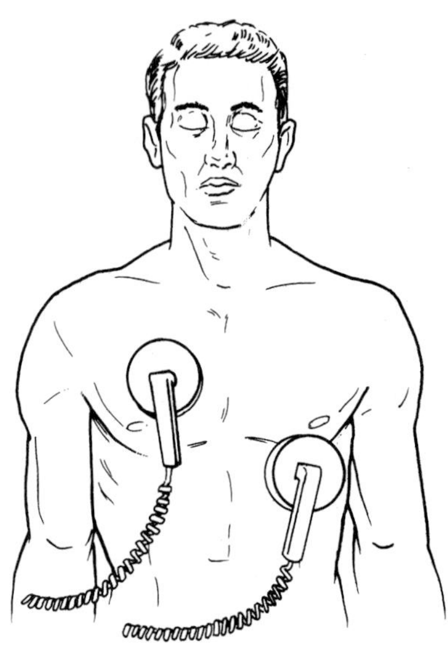

____

____

____

____

Part IV. Theory

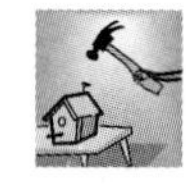

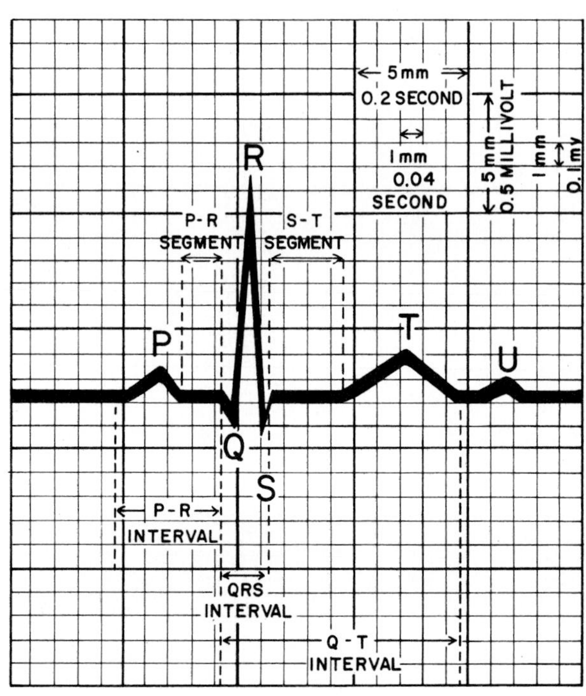

1. The ______________ wave occurs during the contraction of the atria and shows the beginning of cardiac depolarization.

2. The ______________ complex shows the contraction of both ventricles and also reflects the completion of cardiac depolarization.

3. The ________________ interval is the time from the beginning of atrial contraction to the beginning of ventricular contraction.

4. The T wave indicates ventricular recovery or ________________ of the ventricles.

5. ECG paper has horizontal and vertical lines at ________________ mm intervals.

6. When running at normal speed, one small, 1-mm square passes the stylus every ________________ seconds.

7. One large 5-mm square passes the stylus every ________________ seconds.

8. Lead I records the electrical activity between the ________________ arm and the ________________ arm.

9. Lead ________________ records the electrical activity between the right arm and the left leg.

10. Lead III records the electrical activity between the ________________ arm and the left leg.

11. ________________ records the activity from midway between the left leg and the left arm to the right arm.

12. ________________ records the activity from midway between the right arm and the left leg to the left arm.

13. ________________ records the activity from midway between the right arm and the left arm to the left leg.

14. The standardization button should cause the stylus to make a ________________ mm deflection or two large squares when the sensitivity is set at 1.

15. With the ________________ baseline, the stylus gradually shifts away from the center of the paper.

16. ________________ ________________ shows up on the recording as jagged peaks of irregular height and spacing and a shifting baseline.

17. ________________ ________________ occurs when the electric connection has been interrupted.

18. ________________ interference appears as a series of uniform small spikes on the paper.

19. Cardiac ________________ testing is conducted to observe and record the patient's cardiovascular response to measured exercise challenges.

20. A ________________ monitor is a portable system for recording the cardiac activity of a patient over a 24-hour period or longer.

Part V. Documentation

Refer to Table 46-2 in the text and complete the following statements.

A. On some older machines, standard marking codes for limb leads are indicated by:

____

B. Augmented leads are indicated by:

____

C. Precordial leads are indicated by:

____

Part VI. Transdisciplinary Skills

Procedural Coding

You have looked up ECG in the index, and you are confirming codes in the Medicine Section below. Answer the questions for the Cardiography subsection.

Cardiography

93000	Electrocardiography, routine ECG with at least 12 leads: with interpretation and report
93005	tracing only without interpretation and report
93010	interpretation only
93230	Electrocardiographic monitoring for 24 hours by continuous waveform recoding and storage....
93225	recording (includes hook-up, recording and disconnection)
93226	scanning analysis with report
93227	physician review and interpretation

1. You work for a cardiologist that reads 12 Lead ECGs for the local hospital. How would you code for the interpretation? ________________
2. A patient comes in with chest pain, and the physician orders a 12-lead ECG and makes a diagnosis of acute MI. What procedure code would you use? ________________
3. You are placing a Holter monitor on a patient. What *CPT* code would you choose?

   ____
4. When the Holter is taken off the next day and interpreted by the physician, which code would be placed on the HCFA 1500 form? ________________

Part VII. Certification Review

1. Limb leads are
   a. unipolar
   b. bipolar
2. Precordial leads are placed on the ________________.
3. Precordial leads are
   a. unipolar
   b. bipolar
4. What is the standard speed of ECG paper? ________________
5. Which leads are recorded from a midpoint? ________________
6. Name the limb leads.
   a. ________________
   b. ________________
   c. ________________

7. Name the augmented leads.

   a. ____________________

   b. ____________________

   c. ____________________

8. Name the precordial leads.

   a. ____________________

   b. ____________________

   c. ____________________

   d. ____________________

   e. ____________________

   f. ____________________

9. What does a p-wave represent? ____________________

10. PVC stands for ____________________ ____________________ ____________________.

Chapter 46 Quiz

Name: ____

1. A p-wave represents atrial __________ .

2. Ventricular depolarization is represented by the ________________ complex.

3. The ventricle recovers in the ____________________ complex.

4. The small square on the ECG represents __________ mm.

5. Standard limb leads are __________ leads.

6. The ____________ node is located in the right atrium.

7. A fast heart rate is called __________ .

8. ______________ is a slow heart rate.

9. An irregular cardiac rhythm is an ____________________ .

10. True or False: An ECG is an invasive procedure. ______________

CHAPTER 47

Assisting in Diagnostic Imaging

Part I. Medical Terminology

Directions: Fill in the blanks with the correct terms.

1. ________________ refers to the making of x-ray images called *radiographs*.
2. X-rays can penetrate most substances to some degree, but some substances, such as metals and bones, are more difficult to penetrate and are said to be ________________.
3. ________________ is a technique performed with special equipment that permits the radiologist to view x-ray images in motion.
4. The ________________ scanner consists of a movable table with remote control, a circular gantry structure that supports the x-ray tube and detectors, an operator console with a monitor, and the supporting computer system.
5. ________________ medicine scans do not provide clear images of anatomical structures. They are used to obtain information about the function of organs and tissues.

Anatomical Position Matching

Directions: Match the following terms and definitions.

1. _____ Forward or front portion of the body or body part
2. _____ Pertaining to the head; toward the head
3. _____ Away from the head; the opposite of cephalad
4. _____ Away from the source or point of origin; for example, the wrist is distal to the elbow; being farther from the point of origin of the arm, which is the shoulder
5. _____ To the outside, at or near the surface of the body or a body part
6. _____ Below, farther from the head
7. _____ Deep, near the center of the body or a part; the opposite of external
8. _____ Referring to the side; away from the center to the left or right
9. _____ Toward the center of the body or of a body part; the opposite of lateral
10. _____ Referring to the palm (anterior surface) of the hand

A. distal
B. internal
C. plantar
D. medial or mesial
E. palmar
F. external
G. anterior
H. inferior
I. lateral
J. posterior
K. cephalic, cephalad
L. caudal, caudad
M. superior
N. proximal
O. superior

11. _____ Referring to the sole of the foot

12. _____ Backward or back portion of the body or body part; the opposite of anterior

13. _____ Toward the source or point of origin; the opposite of distal

14. _____ Above, toward the head; the opposite of inferior

Part II. Spelling

Phone-etics Game

Directions: Use the telephone keypad below to spell out the missing words. Write the corresponding numbers in the blanks provided.

1. The _______________ gantry houses the magnet and the main radiographic/fluoroscopic (R/F) coil.
2. Ultrasound or _______________ uses high-frequency sound waves to produce echoes within the body.
3. _______________ projections are those in which the sagittal plane of the body or body part is parallel to the film. Lateral projections are always named for the side of the patient that is nearest the film.
4. _______________ projections are those in which the body or part is rotated so that the projection is neither frontal nor lateral.
5. _______________ projections are radiographs taken with a longitudinal angulation of the x-ray beam.

1	ABC 2	DEF 3
GHI 4	JKL 5	MNO 6
PRS 7	TUV 8	WXY 9
*	0	#

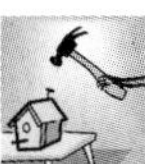

Part III. Visual Aids

Directions: Name the directions and planes of the body shown in the figure below.

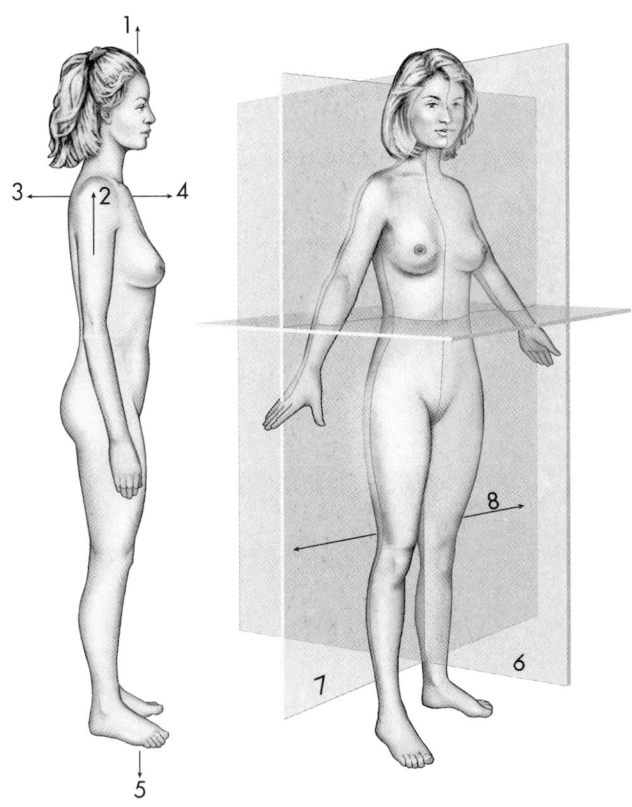

1. ______________________________
2. ______________________________
3. ______________________________
4. ______________________________
5. ______________________________
6. ______________________________
7. ______________________________
8. ______________________________

Part IV. Theory

Directions: Indicate which statements are true and which statements are false. For other statements, fill in the blanks.

1. True or False: Cardiac pacemakers are a particular hazard, and patients with pacemakers cannot have MRI examinations.

2. True or False: Radiation control regulations do not require that female patients of childbearing age be advised of potential radiation hazards before x-ray examination. _____
3. True or False: If the patient is supine, or facing the x-ray tube, the projection is said to be anteroposterior (AP). _____
4. The radiographer then selects the correct cassette and places a ________________ ________________ marker on it to identify the patient's right or left side.
5. The ________________ (R) is the conventional unit of radiation exposure that represents a measurement of radiation intensity and is determined by the interaction of the x-ray beam with air.
6. To measure both therapeutic radiation doses and specific tissue doses received in diagnostic applications, the conventional unit is the ________________, which stands for "radiation absorbed dose."
7. To measure occupational dose or other exposure that may involve more than one type of radiation, the dose equivalent unit used is the ________________, which stands for "roentgen equivalent in man."
8. True or False: X-rays do not linger in the room after the exposure, and they are not capable of making the objects in the room radioactive. _____

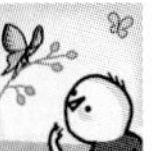

Part V. Workplace Applications

Directions: Identify each type of x-ray in the pictures below.

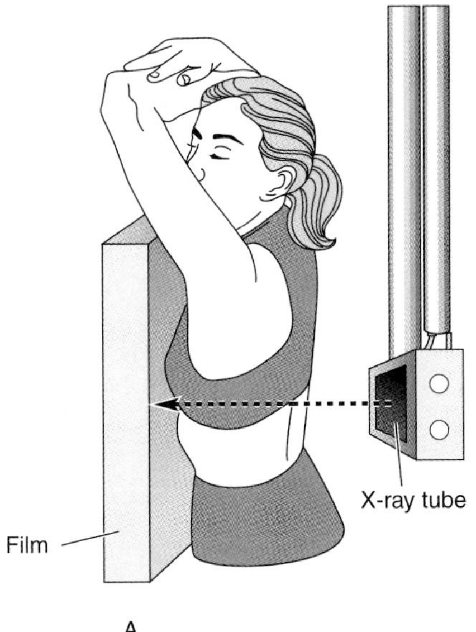

A ______________________

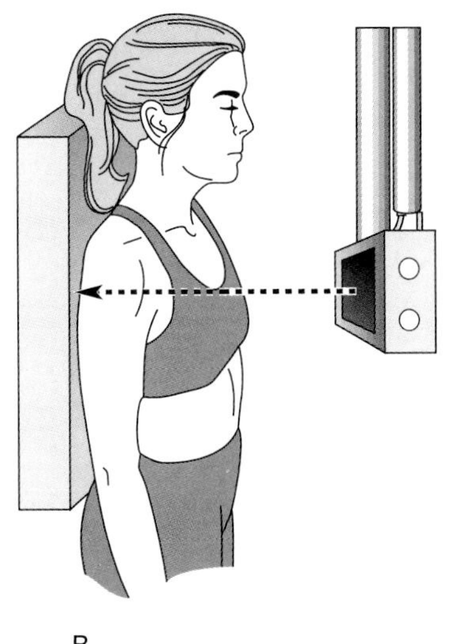

B ______________________

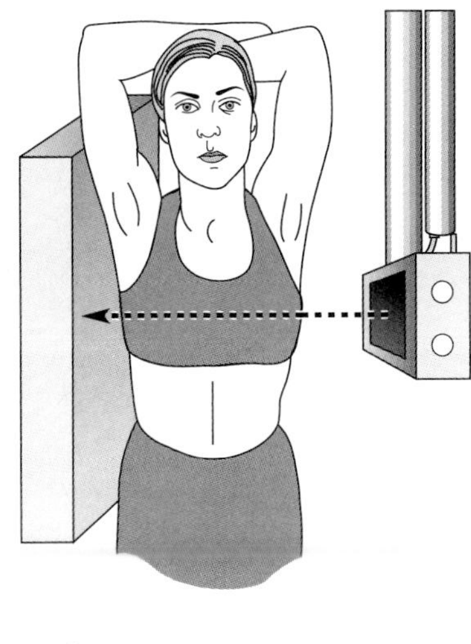

C ______________________

Part VI. Transdisciplinary Skills

Procedural Coding

You have looked up *chest x-ray* in the *CPT* index, and you are confirming codes in the Radiology Section below. Answer the questions for the diagnostic studies.

Radiology

71010	Radiologic examination, chest, single view, frontal
71015	stereo, frontal
71020	Radiologic examination, chest, two views, frontal and lateral
71021	with apical lordotic posture
71022	with oblique view
71023	with fluoroscopy
71250	Computerized axial tomography, thorax, with contrast material
71260	with contrast material
71550	Magnetic Resonance Imaging, chest, without contrast material
71551	with contrast material

1. What is the *CPT* code for chest CT with contrast? ________________
2. What code do you use for anteroposterior (AP) and lateral chest x-ray? ________________
3. What is the *CPT* code for magnetic resonance imaging of the chest without contrast?

   ____

4. A portable chest x-ray examination that only has one view would need which *CPT* code?

   ____

Part VII. Certification Review

Directions: Fill in the blanks by choosing the correct terms from the list below.

recumbent

upright

prone

lateral recumbent

supine

dorsal recumbent

ventral recumbent

1. Lying face down is known as the ________________ position.
2. Lying down is referred to as ________________.

3. Lying on the back, supine is called ________________ ________________.
4. Lying on the side would be ________________.
5. Lying face down, prone is called ________________ ________________.
6. Lying face up is known as the ________________ position.
7. Having an x-ray examination while standing or seated would be called an ________________ view.

Chapter 47 Quiz

Name: ____________________

1. An x-ray in motion is ______________ .

2. Imaging of blood vessels is __________ .

3. An AP view is when the patient is ______________ the x-ray tube.

4. During ______________ projection the sagittal plane of the body is parallel to the film.

5. The ______________ plane divides the body into superior and inferior portions.

6. Another name for an x-ray is a ______________ .

7. A ______________ is a computerized image that pictures slices of the body.

8. An x-ray of the breast is a __________ .

9. An imaging technique that uses a large magnet is a ______________ .

10. A material that is used to fill in hollow organs for better visualization during a radiography procedure is called ______________ ______________ .

CHAPTER 48

Assisting in the Clinical Laboratory

Part I. Medical Terminology

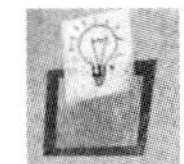

Directions: Write the correct term in the space provided.

1. ______________ A term used to describe a blood sample in which the red blood cells have ruptured.
2. ______________ A cylindrical glass or plastic tube used to deliver fluids.
3. ______________ The substance or chemical being analyzed or detected in a specimen.
4. ______________ A sample of body fluid, waste product, or tissue that is collected for analysis.
5. ______________ A substance that is known to cause cancer.
6. ______________ The ability of the eye to distinguish two objects that are very close together; the sharpness of an image.
7. ______________ A portion of a well-mixed sample removed for testing.
8. ______________ A substance that burns or destroys tissue by chemical action.
9. ______________ A liquid used to dilute a specimen or reagent.
10. ______________ A chemical added to the blood after collection to prevent clotting.
11. ______________ An order found on a laboratory requisition indicating that the test must be done immediately (from the Latin word statin, meaning "at once").
12. ______________ A substance that is known to cause birth defects.
13. ______________ Fluids with a high concentration of protein and cellular debris that have escaped from the blood vessels and been deposited in tissues or on tissue surfaces.
14. ______________ A sac filled with blood that may be the result of trauma.
15. ______________ ______________ Fluid within the subarachnoid space, the central canal of the spinal cord, and the four ventricles of the brain.
16. ______________ Substances added to a specimen to prevent deterioration of cells or chemicals.
17. ______________ ______________ Private or hospital-based laboratories that perform a wide variety of tests, many of them specialized. Physicians often send specimens collected in the office to one of these for testing.

Part II. Spell It Out

Phone-etics Game

Directions: Use the telephone keypad to spell out the acronyms for the following agencies beside their laboratory certifications. Write the corresponding letters in the blanks provided.

1. (2-7-2-7) MT, MLT ________________
2. (2-6-8) MT, MLT ________________
3. (2-2-6-2) CMA ________________
4. (2-2-4-3-7) RMA ________________

1	ABC 2	DEF 3
GHI 4	JKL 5	MNO 6
PRS 7	TUV 8	WXY 9
*	0	#

Part III. Visual Aids

Accuracy and Precision

Directions: Read the following scenario and answer the questions in the space provided.

1. One blood glucose meter always reads 10% too high. Another meter reads anywhere between 5% and 9% too high. Which one is the most precise? Which one is the most accurate? How is accuracy different from precision?

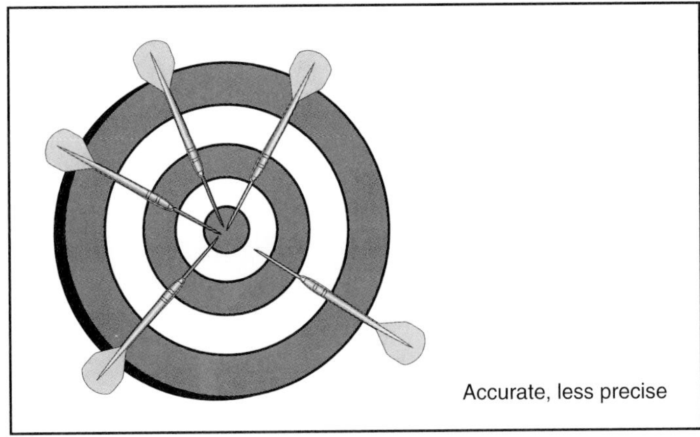
Accurate, less precise

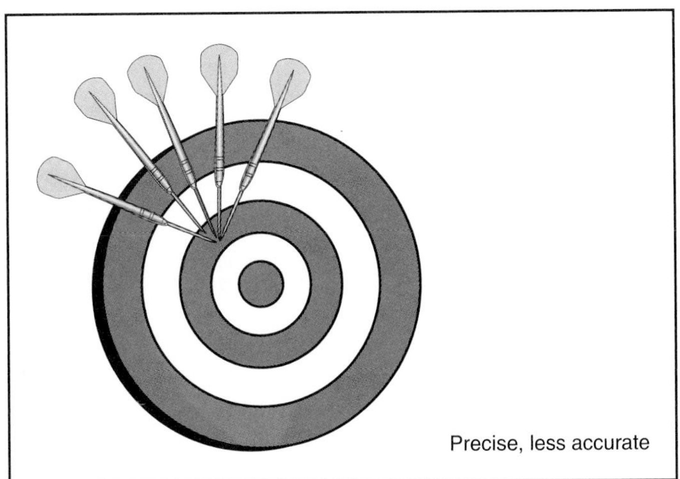
Precise, less accurate

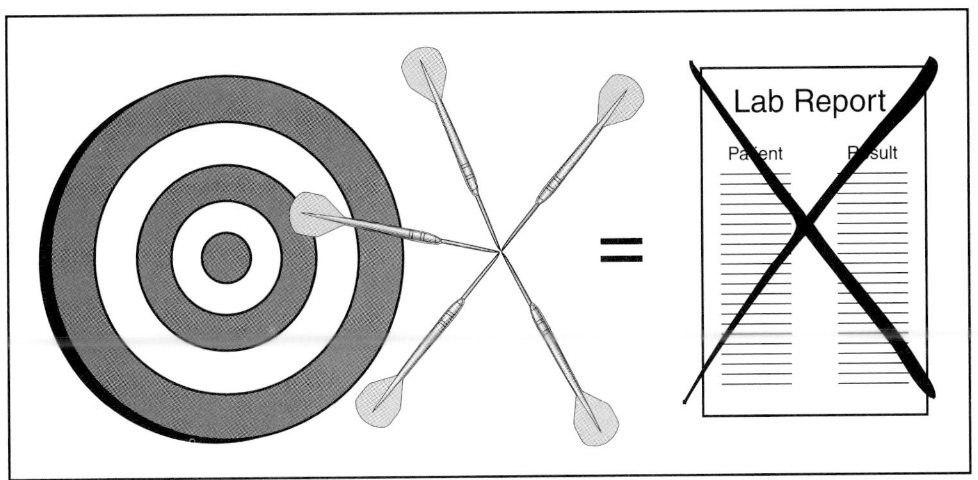
Lab Report
Patient
Result

2. Look at the clock below and write the military time for both afternoon and morning for the time shown.

   a. PM ________________

   b. AM ________________

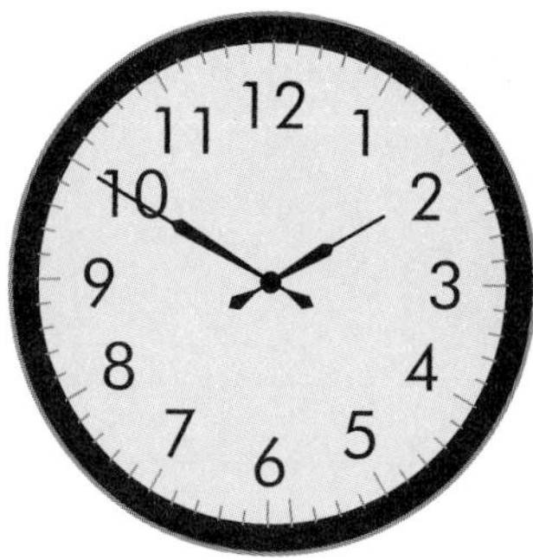

3. Label the parts of a microscope in the figure below.

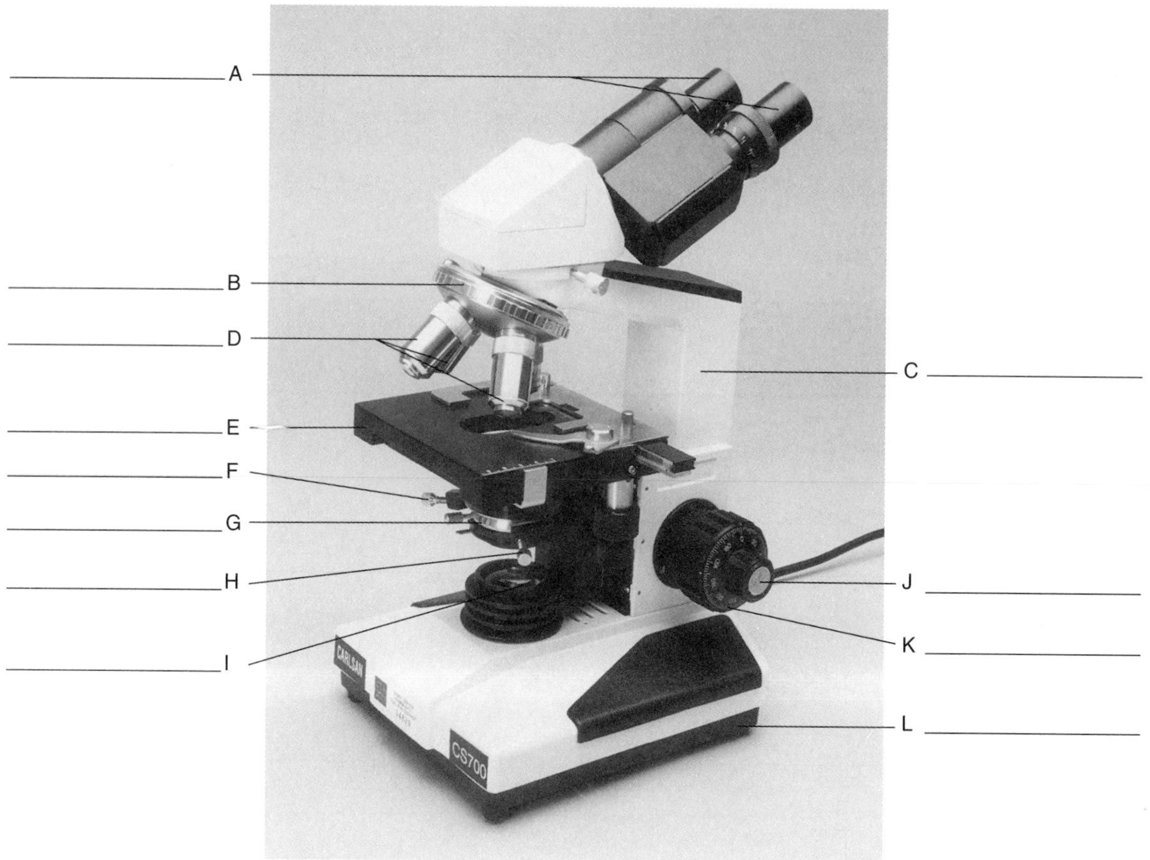

Part IV. Theory

1. List five reasons when it is absolutely required to wash your hands in the laboratory area.

   A. ______

   B. ______

   C. ______

   D. ______

   E. ______

2. Name three types of hazards in the lab setting:

   A. ______

   B. ______

   C. ______

3. Differentiate between qualitative and quantitative results. Give an example of each.

______

______

4. Name the four major divisions of the clinical lab.

   A. ______

   B. ______

   C. ______

   D. ______

5. Label each of the following according to its division.

   A. Hemoglobin ______

   B. Urine specific gravity ______

   C. Urine culture ______

   D. Blood glucose ______

   E. Throat culture ______

   F. White blood cell count ______

   G. Cholesterol ______

   H. Complete blood count ______

6. What is an MSDS?

______

______

______

7. What is the role of OSHA?

8. What is CLIA and what are the levels of laboratory testing?

9. List the items that must be present on the requisition form of a collected specimen.

Part V. Workplace Applications

1. On the thermometer drawings provided, mark the range of common laboratory temperatures for:
   a. Body and incubator temperature
   b. Room temperature
   c. Freezer temperature
   d. Refrigerator temperature

A

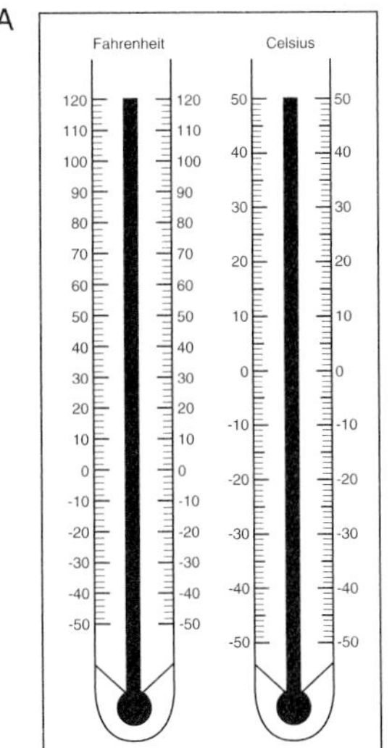
Fahrenheit
Celsius

B

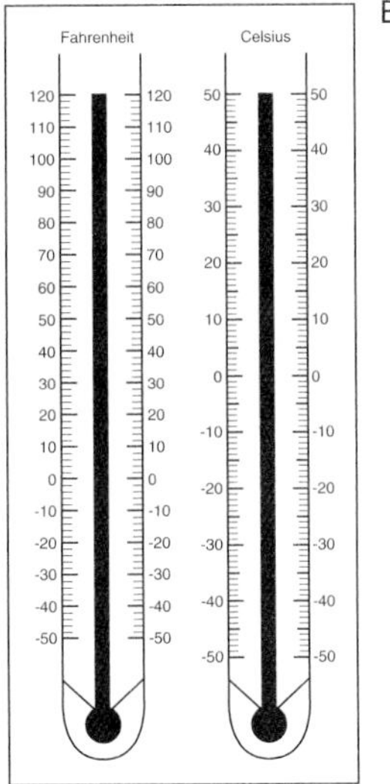
Fahrenheit
Celsius

C

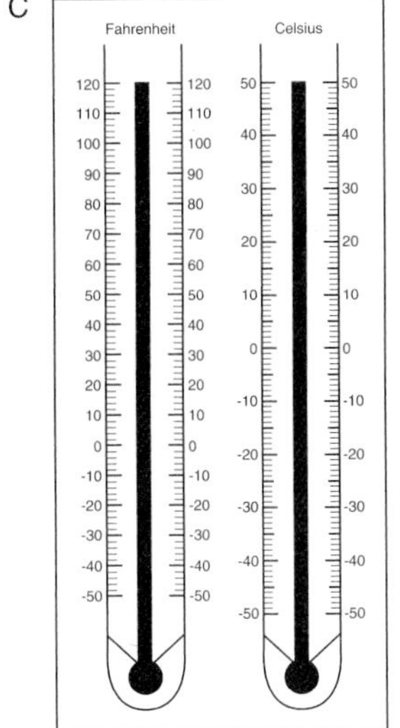
Fahrenheit
Celsius

D

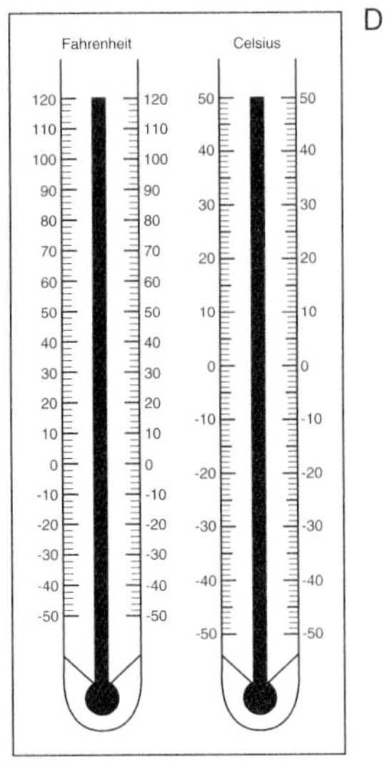
Fahrenheit
Celsius

2. Record the volume in milliliters for the two cylinders pictured.

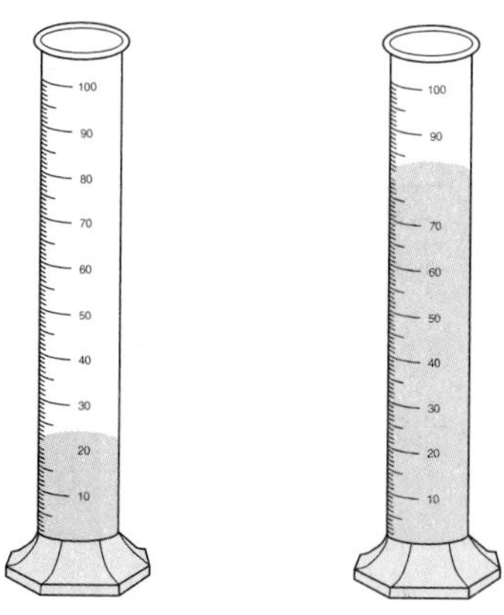

a. How much diluent do you have to add to a 1 ml sample to make a 1:10 dilution?

_______________ ml

b. How much diluent do you have to add to a 2 ml sample to make a 1:10 dilution?

_______________ ml

c. How much diluent do you have to add to a 1 ml sample to make a 1:20 dilution?

_______________ ml

d. How much diluent do you have to add to a 2 ml sample to make a 1:10 dilution?

_______________ ml

e. Your centrifuge starts to vibrate markedly while you are spinning a specimen. What should you check?

____

Part VI. Transdisciplinary Skills

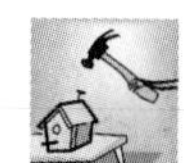

Directions: Proofread and make corrections to the following transcription.

4-14-20XX The patient arrived complaining of disuria and fever x 3 days. A urinalisis was performed. The microscopic results show presence of bacteria. CBC shows an elevated WBC.

Part VII. Certification Review

1. True or False: Mouth-pipetting is forbidden in the laboratory setting. ____

2. If the eyepiece of the microscope is 10x and the high power is 40x, what is the total magnification?

   ____

3. True or False: The coarse adjustment should always be used with the oil emersion lens. ____

4. Always carry the microscope by the ________________ with one hand under the

   ________________.

Chapter 48 Quiz

Name: ____

1. An ________________ is a portion of a well-mixed sample removed for testing.

2. A ______________ specimen is one in which blood vessels have ruptured.

3. MSDS stands for

   ____

   ____

4. When are laboratory assistants required to wash their hands?

   ____

   ____

5. What is the objective of quality control?

   ____

   ____

6. A simple lab test that can be performed at home is

   ____________________________ .

7. The FDA ensures quality of lab testing under what piece of legislation?

   ____

   ____

8. A ________________ lab test has numerical results.

9. A ________________ lab test has positive and negative results.

10. ________________________ is the government agency that deals with safety in the workplace.

CHAPTER 49

Assisting in the Analysis of Urine

Part I. Medical Terminology

Directions: Write the correct terms in the spaces provided.

1. ________________ Abnormal presence of a hemoglobin-like chemical of muscle tissue in urine, which is the result of muscle deterioration.
2. ________________ Essential amino acid found in milk, eggs, and other foods.
3. ________________ Decreased blood flow to a body part or organ, caused by constriction or plugging of the supplying artery.
4. ________________ ________________ Chemical reaction controlled by an enzyme.
5. ________________ white blood cells; leukocytes that have segmented nuclei; also known as polymorphonuclear neutrophils (PMNs) or segmented neutrophils.
6. ________________ Presence of glucose in the urine.
7. ________________ white blood cells; leukocytes that have unsegmented nuclei; monocytes and lymphocytes in particular.
8. ________________ Causing light to refract, thus creating a sharp boundary or image.
9. ________________ ________________ Level above which a substance cannot be reabsorbed by the renal tubules and is thus excreted in the urine.
10. ________________ Fluid that remains after a liquid is passed through a membranous filter.

Part II. Spelling

Phone-etics Game

Directions: Refer to the telephone keypad on p. 420 to spell out the missing words. Write the corresponding letters in the blanks provided.

The ________________ (7-4) is a measurement of the degree of acidity or alkalinity of the urine.

________________ (3-6-2-6) is the presence of small bubbles that persist for a long time after the specimen has been shaken; they must not be confused with any bubbles that rapidly disperse.

Normal urine ________________ (6-3-6-7) is said to be aromatic.

________________ (2-2-7-8-7) are formed when protein accumulates and precipitates in the kidney tubules and is washed into the urine.

1	ABC 2	DEF 3
GHI 4	JKL 5	MNO 6
PRS 7	TUV 8	WXY 9
*	0	#

Part III. Visual Aids

Directions: Identify the structures of the urinary system shown in the figure below.

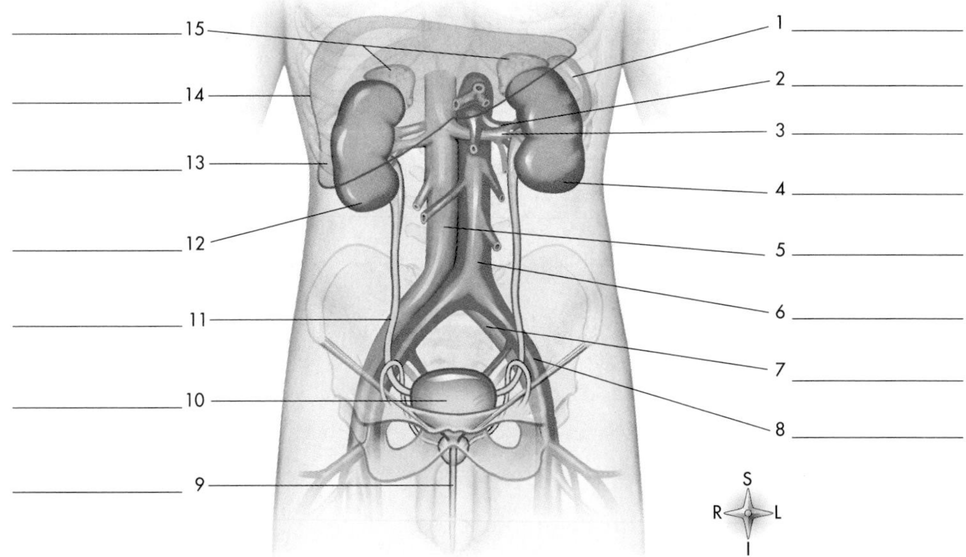

1. ______________________________
2. ______________________________
3. ______________________________
4. ______________________________
5. ______________________________
6. ______________________________
7. ______________________________
8. ______________________________
9. ______________________________
10. ______________________________
11. ______________________________
12. ______________________________
13. ______________________________
14. ______________________________
15. ______________________________

Directions: Label the structures of the kidney shown in the figure below.

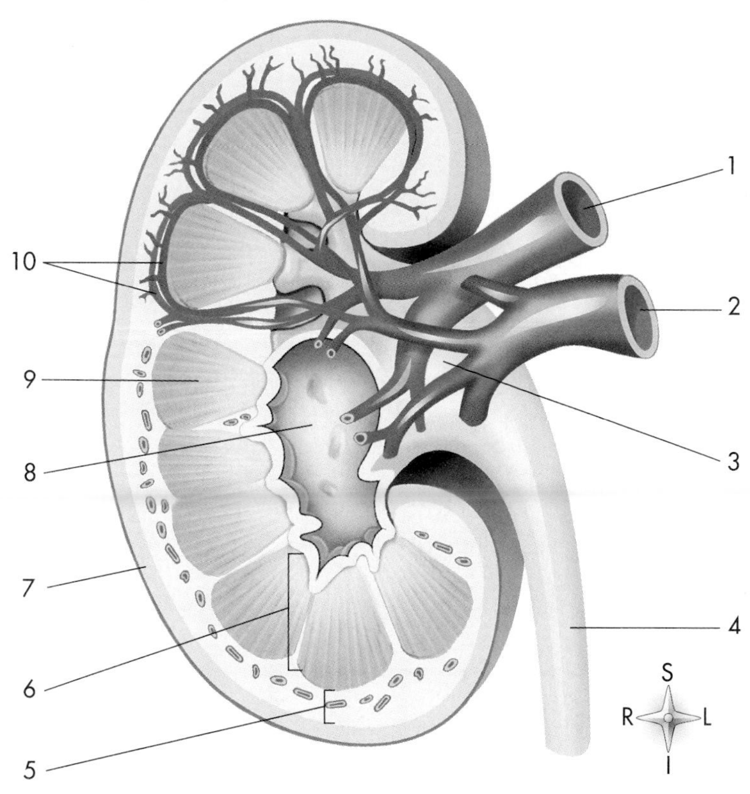

1. ______________________________
2. ______________________________

3. ____
4. ____
5. ____
6. ____
7. ____
8. ____
9. ____
10. ____

Part IV. Theory

A. List eight types of urine specimens.

1. ____
2. ____
3. ____
4. ____
5. ____
6. ____
7. ____
8. ____

B. Name three examinations in a routine urinalysis and give some examples of information determined from each examination.

1. ____
2. ____
3. ____

C. Describe a urinometer.

D. Describe a refractometer.

E. Differentiate between a Clinitest and a Acetest.

____

____

F. What is a sulfosalicylic acid test used for?

____

____

G. How does a urine pregnancy test work?

____

____

Part V. Workplace Applications

1. You are performing a microscopic examination of urine and you notice the blood cells shown in the figure below. What type are they?

   A. ______________________

   B. ______________________

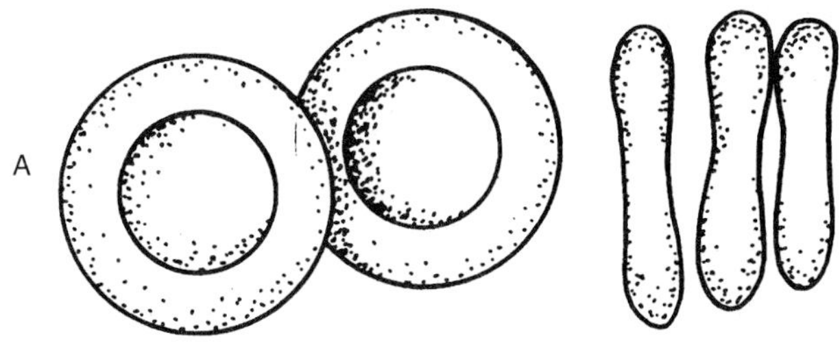

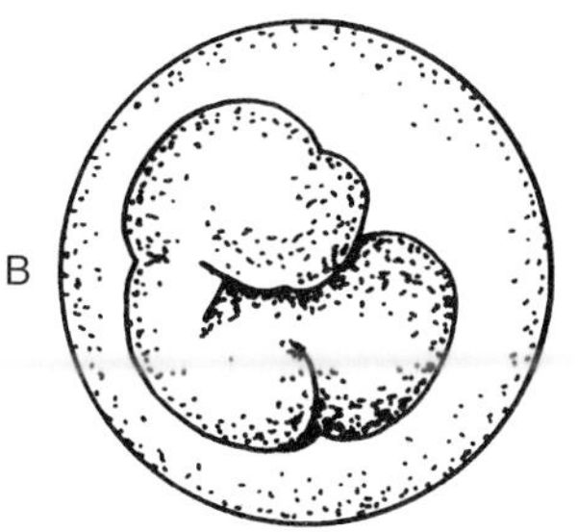

2. You are performing a microscopic examination of urine and you notice the pathogens shown in the figure below. What type are they?

   A. ______________________________

   B. ______________________________

   C. ______________________________

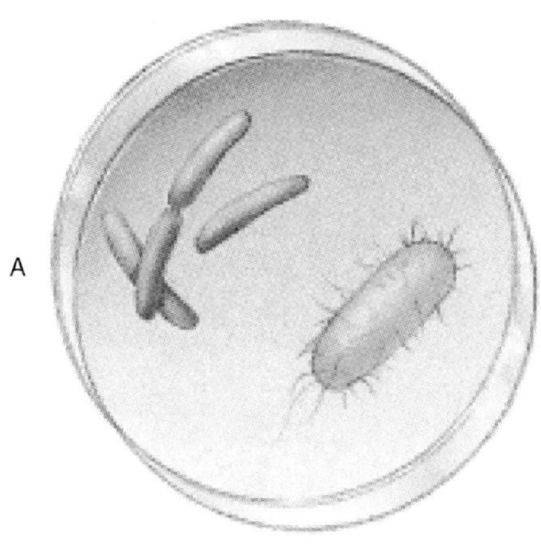

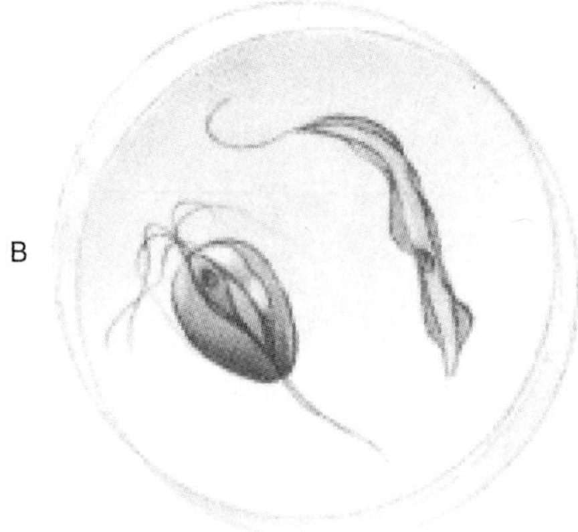

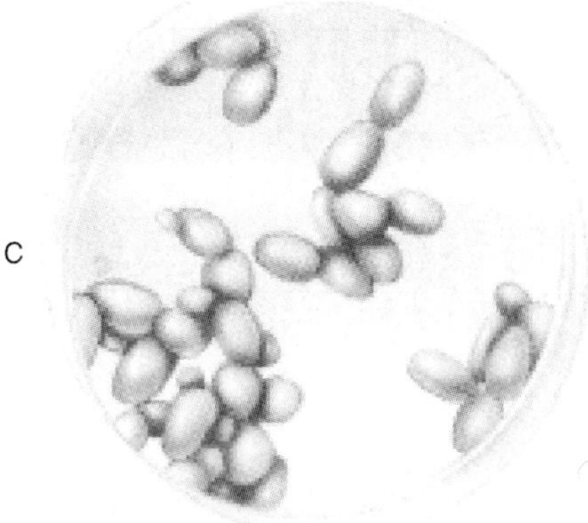

Part VI. Transdisciplinary Skills

Procedural Coding

You have looked up *urinalysis* in the *CPT* index, and you are confirming codes in the Pathology and Laboratory Section below. Answer the questions for these diagnostic studies.

Urinalysis

81000 Urinalysis by dipstick or tablet reagent for bilirubin, glucose, hemoglobin, ketones, leukocytes, nitrate, pH, protein, specific gravity, urobilinogen, any number of constituents: non-automated, with microscopy

81001 automated, with microscopy

81002 non-automated, without microscopy

81003 automated, without microscopy

1. What is the *CPT* code for a manual routine UA without microscopy? ________________
2. What code do you use for automated, without microscopy? ________________
3. What is the *CPT* manual routine UA with microscopy? ________________
4. An automated UA with a microscopic exam would need which *CPT* code? ________________

Part VII. Certification Review

Draw the following urine crystals.

1. Calcium oxalate (shaped like kites)
2. Triple phosphates (shaped like envelopes)

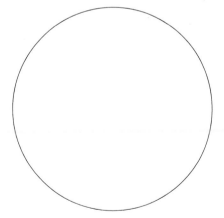

Chapter 49 Quiz

Name: ____

1. ____________ - to 50 cc of urine is needed for a routine urinalysis.

2. CCMS means ____________________ .

3. Bacteria in room temperature urine doubles every ____________ minutes.

4. Describe how to collect a 24-hour urine specimen.

   ____

   ____

5. Name four colors of urine.

   a. ______________________________

   b. ______________________________

   c. ______________________________

   d. ______________________________

6. Blood is filtered by the ____________ .

7. The functional unit of the kidney is the

   ______________________________ .

8. _______ ml of blood is filtered by the kidneys each minute.

9. Urine specimens should be labeled with: ______________________________

   ____

10. The dilution of urine is indicated by the

   ______________ ____________ .

CHAPTER 50

Assisting in Phlebotomy

Part I. Medical Terminology

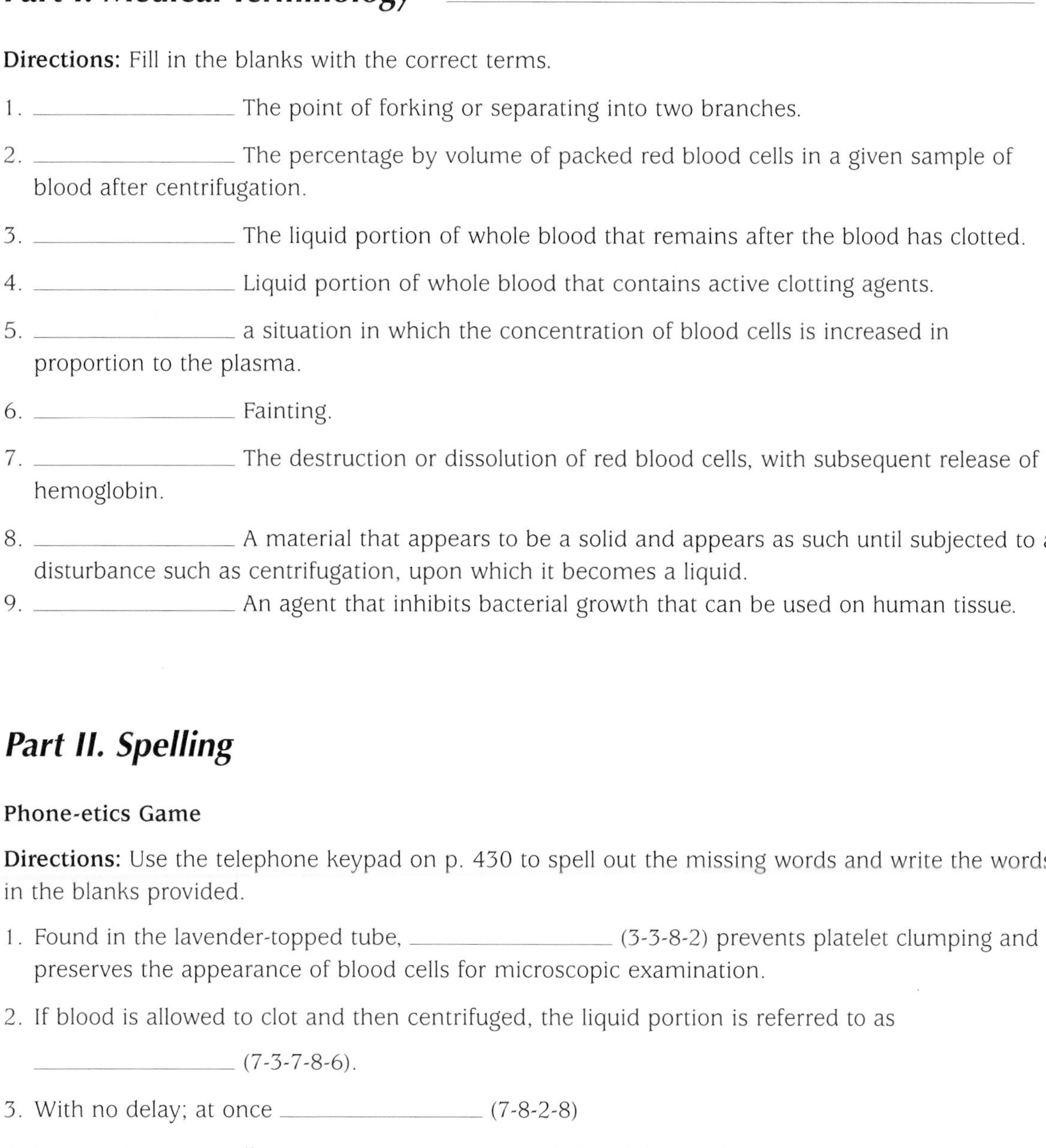

Directions: Fill in the blanks with the correct terms.

1. ________________ The point of forking or separating into two branches.
2. ________________ The percentage by volume of packed red blood cells in a given sample of blood after centrifugation.
3. ________________ The liquid portion of whole blood that remains after the blood has clotted.
4. ________________ Liquid portion of whole blood that contains active clotting agents.
5. ________________ a situation in which the concentration of blood cells is increased in proportion to the plasma.
6. ________________ Fainting.
7. ________________ The destruction or dissolution of red blood cells, with subsequent release of hemoglobin.
8. ________________ A material that appears to be a solid and appears as such until subjected to a disturbance such as centrifugation, upon which it becomes a liquid.
9. ________________ An agent that inhibits bacterial growth that can be used on human tissue.

Part II. Spelling

Phone-etics Game

Directions: Use the telephone keypad on p. 430 to spell out the missing words and write the words in the blanks provided.

1. Found in the lavender-topped tube, ________________ (3-3-8-2) prevents platelet clumping and preserves the appearance of blood cells for microscopic examination.
2. If blood is allowed to clot and then centrifuged, the liquid portion is referred to as ________________ (7-3-7-8-6).
3. With no delay; at once ________________ (7-8-2-8)
4. Some patients are allergic to ________________ (5-2-8-3-9) tourniquets.

1	ABC 2	DEF 3
GHI 4	JKL 5	MNO 6
PRS 7	TUV 8	WXY 9
*	0	#

Part III. Visual Aids

1. **Directions:** On the figure below, identify the parts of a Vacutainer (evacuated tube) system.

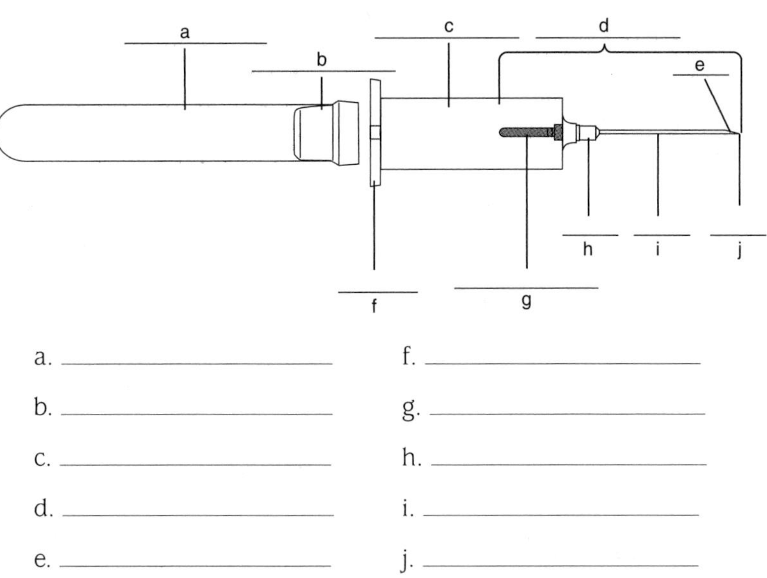

a. ______________________ f. ______________________

b. ______________________ g. ______________________

c. ______________________ h. ______________________

d. ______________________ i. ______________________

e. ______________________ j. ______________________

2. **Directions:** On the figure below, label the veins that are used for venipuncture:

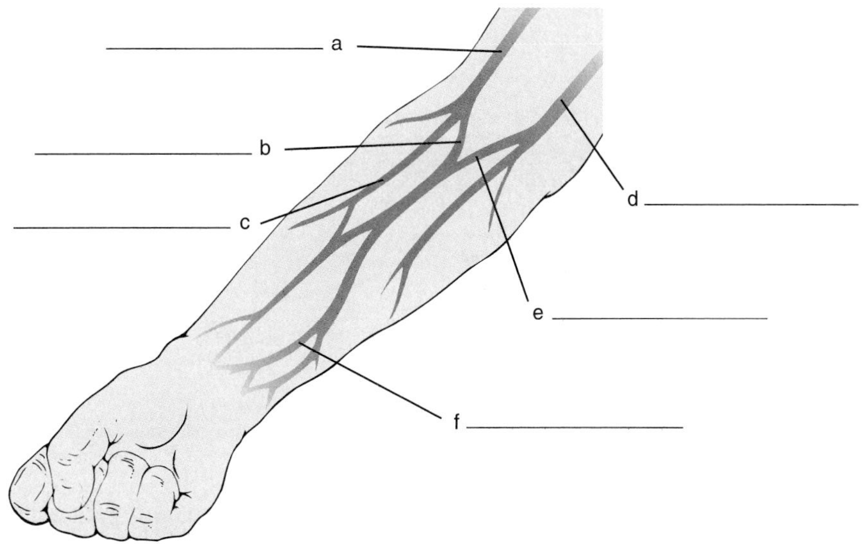

Part IV. Theory

A. **Directions:** List seven reasons that the laboratory may reject a specimen.

1. ______
2. ______
3. ______
4. ______
5. ______
6. ______
7. ______

B. The National Committee for Clinical Laboratory Standards has developed a set of standards outlining the order of draw for a multi-tube draw. The same order applies to the filling of tubes when the blood is collected in a syringe. A mnemonic device that is useful for remembering the order of the draw is **ST**OP, **R**ED **L**IGHT, **G**REEN **L**IGHT, **R**EADY, **G**O.

Directions: Use the mnemonic device and fill in the blanks.

1. ______ ______ tubes are collected first because they are sterile.
2. ______-topped tubes are second because they have no additive and thus nothing to transfer to another tube.
3. ______ blue-topped tubes are next because other anticoagulants might contaminate the sample that is collected for coagulation studies.
4. ______-topped tubes are next because heparin is less likely to interfere with EDTA than vice versa.
5. ______-topped tubes follow. EDTA binds with calcium, so this tube is drawn near the end.

6. ________________/________________ marble-topped tubes are next. They contain clot activator that could interfere with specimens if passed into another tube.

7. The ________________-topped tube is last because the contents can elevate electrolyte levels or damage cells if passed into another tube.

Part V. Workplace Applications

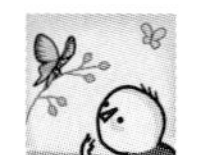

A. Identify the venipuncture supplies pictured below.

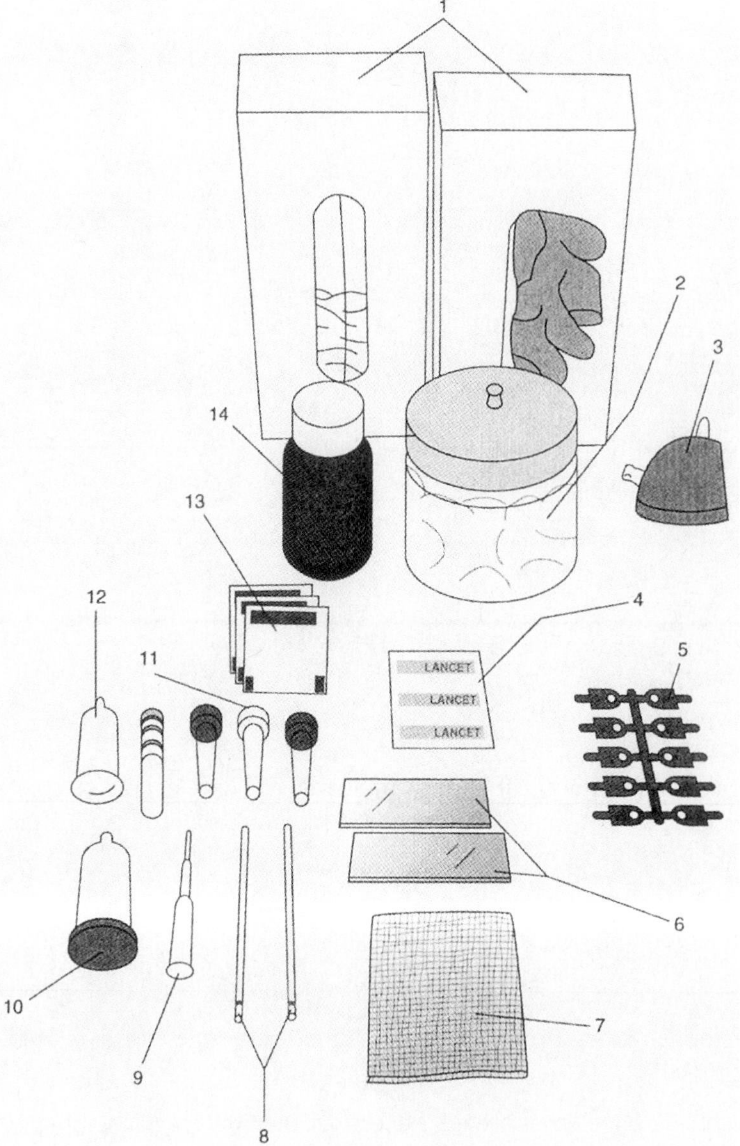

1. ______________________________
2. ______________________________
3. ______________________________
4. ______________________________
5. ______________________________
6. ______________________________
7. ______________________________
8. ______________________________
9. ______________________________
10. ______________________________
11. ______________________________
12. ______________________________
13. ______________________________
14. ______________________________

B. Capillary puncture may be warranted in:

1. ______________________________
2. ______________________________
3. ______________________________
4. ______________________________
5. ______________________________
6. ______________________________
7. ______________________________

Directions: Fill in the blanks.

C. ________________ tubes, also known as *microhematocrit tubes,* are small glass or plastic tubes, open on each end, that will hold a volume of 75 microliters.

D. Microcollection, or ________________, tubes hold up to 750 microliters of blood and are available with a variety of anticoagulants and additives.

E. For children younger than 1 year, dermal puncture is performed on the medial and lateral surfaces of the ________________ (bottom) of the heel.

F. True or False: After puncturing the dermis, it is important to wipe away the first drop of blood because this drop contains tissue fluid that could interfere with test results. _____

G. The most commonly used skin preparation is ________________% ________________ ________________, also known as *rubbing alcohol.*

H. If a blood culture is ordered, additional preparation is needed at the venipuncture site to eliminate contaminating bacteria. ________________-iodine solution (________________) is commonly used.

Chapter 50 Quiz

Name: ______________________________

1. What color tube has no additives and allows blood to clot?

   ____

2. Light blue tubes are used for ______________ testing.

3. Lavender tubes contain ________ .

4. Heparin tubes are __________ colored.

5. The major vein on the thumb side of the arm is the ____________ .

6. The practice of drawing blood is called

   ______________________ .

7. During venipuncture, blood is drawn from a ____________vein.

8. Bifurcation means:

   ____

   ____

9. Stat means:

   ____

   ____

10. Serum is:

    ____

    ____

CHAPTER 51

Assisting in the Analysis of Blood

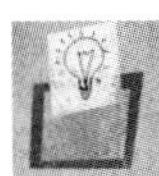

Part I. Medical Terminology

Matching:

1. ______ A condition marked by deficiency of red blood cells
2. ______ An apparatus consisting essentially of a compartment spun about a central axis to separate contained materials of different specific gravities, or to separate colloidal particles suspended in a liquid.
3. ______ Any of several complex proteins that are produced by cells and act as catalysts in specific biochemical reactions
4. ______ A substance, usually a peptide or steroid, produced by one tissue and conveyed by the bloodstream to another to effect physiological activity, such as growth or metabolism
5. ______ A substance produced by metabolism.
6. ______ An instrument for measuring the intensity of light, or, more especially, for comparing the relative intensities of different lights, or their relative illuminating power.
7. ______ A condition marked by an abnormally large number of red blood cells in the circulatory system
8. ______ An abnormal condition of pregnancy characterized by hypertension, edema, and protein in the urine
9. ______ Tests performed to assess the compatibility of blood to be transfused
10. ______ The major nitrogenous end product of protein metabolism and the chief nitrogenous component of the urine
11. ______ An enzyme that catalyzes the hydrolysis of urea to form ammonium carbonate

A. anemia
B. enzyme
C. urea
D. hormone
E. polycythemia vera
F. toxemia
G. metabolite
H. photometer
I. centrifuge
J. urease
K. type and cross match

Part II. Spell It Out

Phone-etics Game

Directions: Use the telephone keypad below to spell out the missing words. Write the corresponding words in the blanks provided.

1. The ________________ (2-2-2) is the most frequent laboratory procedure ordered on blood.
2. The ________________ (4-2-8) is a measurement of the percentage of packed red blood cells in a volume of blood.
3. The ________________ (4-4-2) determination is a rough measure of the oxygen-carrying capacity of the blood.
4. Increases in ________________ (7-2-2) are found in people with dehydration and polycythemia vera.
5. The ________________ (3-7-7) is a laboratory test that measures the rate at which erythrocytes gradually separate from plasma and settle to the bottom of a specially calibrated tube in an hour, and it is used as a general indication of inflammation.

1	ABC 2	DEF 3
GHI 4	JKL 5	MNO 6
PRS 7	TUV 8	WXY 9
*	0	#

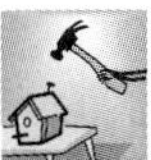

Part III. Visual Aids

A. **Directions:** Identify the blood cells shown in the figure below.

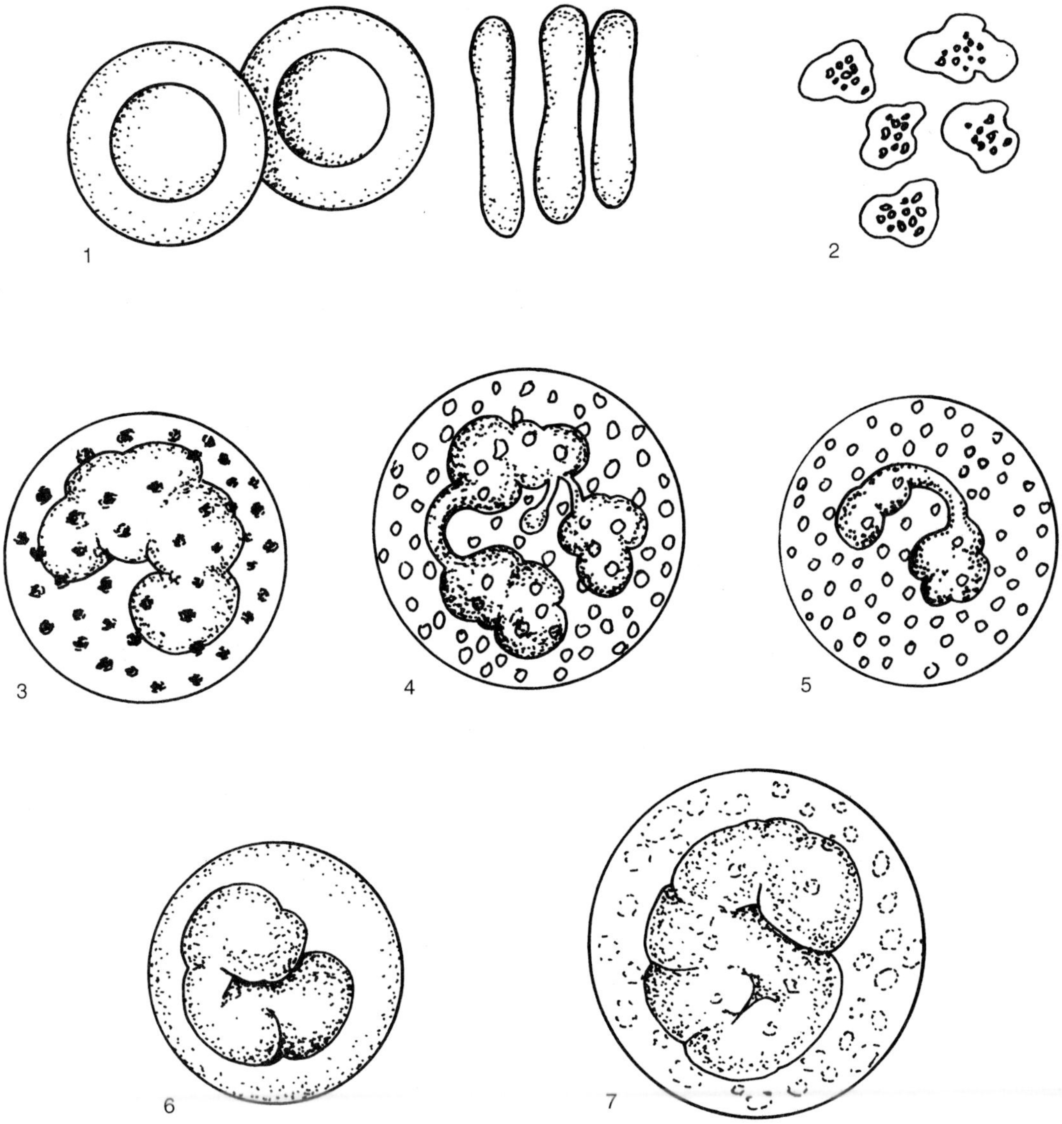

1. ______________________________
2. ______________________________
3. ______________________________
4. ______________________________
5. ______________________________
6. ______________________________
7. ______________________________

B. Practice counting manual differentials in the lab by using a Neubauer-type hemacytometer.

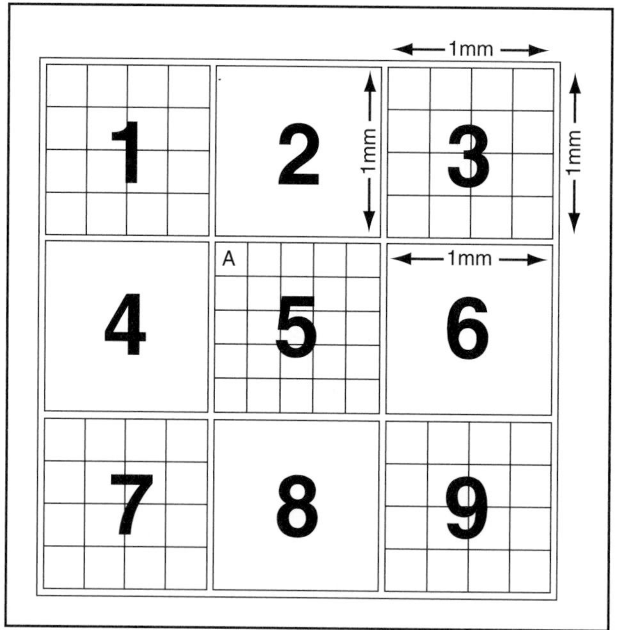

Part IV. Theory

Directions: Fill in the blanks.

A. Whole blood is composed of formed elements suspended in a clear yellow liquid portion called ________________. It makes up about 55% of the blood by volume. The remaining 45% consists of the formed cellular elements, which are the ________________ (red blood cells), ________________ (white blood cells), and ________________ (platelets).

B. ________________ actually carries the oxygen and carbon dioxide throughout the body. The life span of an erythrocyte is about ________________ days.

C. The granular leukocytes are called *polymorphonuclear leukocytes* and include the (hint "phils") ________________, ________________, and ________________.

D. The agranular leukocytes are the (hint "cytes") ________________ and ________________, both of which have clear cytoplasm and a solid nucleus.

E. ________________ are the smallest formed elements of the blood.

F. The platelets produce a substance that combines with ________________ ions in the blood to form ________________, which in turn converts the protein ________________ into thrombin in a complex series of reactions. Thrombin, an enzyme, converts fibrinogen, a protein substance, into ________________, an insoluble protein that forms an intricate network of minute thread-like structures called *fibrils* and causes the blood plasma to gel.

G. The ________________ test is also used to monitor the condition of patients who are taking warfarin (Coumadin).

H. Complete the following statements.

1. One person in ________________ is O positive.
2. One person in 15 is O ________________.
3. One person in ________________ is A positive.
4. One person in 16 is ________________ negative.
5. One person in 12 is B ________________.
6. One person in ________________ is B negative.
7. One person in 29 is ________________ positive.
8. One person in ________________ is AB negative.

I. List several commonly used blood chemistry tests.

1. ________________________________
2. ________________________________
3. ________________________________

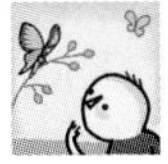

Part V. Workplace Applications

Directions: Identify the cells in the picture below. ________________

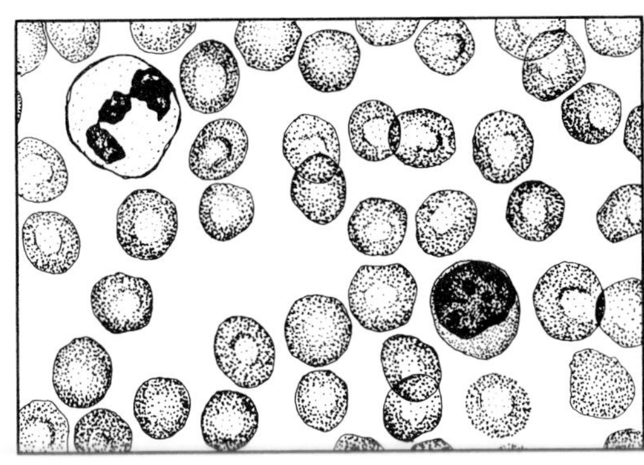

Part VI. Transdisciplinary Skills

Procedural Coding

You have looked up *blood count* in the *CPT* index, and you are confirming codes in the Pathology and Laboratory Section below. Answer the questions for the diagnostic studies.

Hematology and Coagulation

85007 Blood count, manual differential WBC count (includes RBC morphology and platelet estimation

85008 manual blood smear examination without differential parameters

85009 differential WBC count, buffy coat

85013 spun microhematocrit

85014 other than spun hematocrit

85015 hemoglobin

1. What is the *CPT* code for HCT? ________________
2. What code do you use for microhematocrit? ________________
3. What is the *CPT* code for Hgb? ________________
4. A CBC with manual diff would need which *CPT* code? ________________

Chapter 51 Quiz

Name: ____

1. Platelets are called ________________ .

2. A hemocytometer is used to

   ______________________________ .

3. Name three chemistry tests that are done in a doctor's office.

   a. ______________________________

   b. ______________________________

   c. ______________________________

4. ______________ is the study of poisons.

5. Describe buffy coat.

   ____

   ____

6. The ______________ section of the lab deals with the counting of blood cells.

7. The ___________ is the most frequently ordered blood test.

8. Fifty-five percent of whole blood is

   ______________________________.

9. WBCs are called ________________.

10. RBCs are called ________________.

CHAPTER 52

Assisting in Microbiology

Part I. Medical Terminology

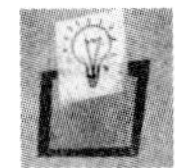

Directions: Fill in the blanks with the correct terms.

1. ________________ Pertaining to or originating in the hospital; said of an infection not present or incubating before admission to the hospital.
2. ________________ An agent that causes disease, especially a living microorganism such as a bacterium or fungus.
3. ________________ ________________ A bacterial or fungal culture that contains a single organism.
4. ________________ A differentiated structure within a cell, such as a mitochondrion, vacuole, or chloroplast, that performs a specific function.
5. ________________ One billionth (10^{-9}) of a meter.
6. ________________ An organism of microscopic or submicroscopic size.
7. ________________ A single-celled or multicellular organism in which each cell contains a distinct membrane-bound nucleus.
8. ________________ Requiring specialized media or growth factors to grow.
9. ________________ A small capsule-like sac that encloses certain organisms in their dormant or larval stage.
10. ________________ A sample, as of tissue, blood, or urine, used for analysis and diagnosis.
11. ________________ A unicellular organism that lacks a membrane-bound nucleus.
12. ________________ - ________________ ________________ ________________ A drug used to treat a broad range of infections.
13. ________________ ________________ Refers to conditions outside of a living body.
14. ________________ The process of removing pathogenic microorganisms or protecting against infection by such organisms.
15. ________________ The molecules needed for metabolism: carbohydrates, lipids, proteins, and nucleic acids.
16. ________________ ________________ The technique or process of keeping tissue alive and growing in a culture medium.
17. ________________ ________________ A drug that is used to treat infection.
18. ________________ A group of like or different atoms held together by chemical forces.

19. ________________ ________________ A medium used to keep an organism alive during transport to the laboratory.

20. ________________ Capable of living, developing, or germinating under favorable conditions.

21. ________________ ________________ A slide preparation in which a drop of liquid specimen or the like is covered with a coverslip and observed with a microscope.

Part II. Spell It Out

Phone-etics Game

Directions: Use the telephone keypad below to spell out the missing words. Write the words in the blanks provided.

1. Helminths go through the same life cycle as other worms. The adult worm lays eggs or ________________ (6-8-2).
2. Liquid media is called ________________ (2-7-6-8-4).
3. The addition of a powdered extract of seaweed to media is called ________________ (2-4-2-7).

1	ABC 2	DEF 3
GHI 4	JKL 5	MNO 6
PRS 7	TUV 8	WXY 9
*	0	#

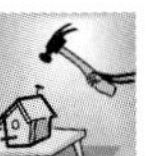

Part III. Visual Aids

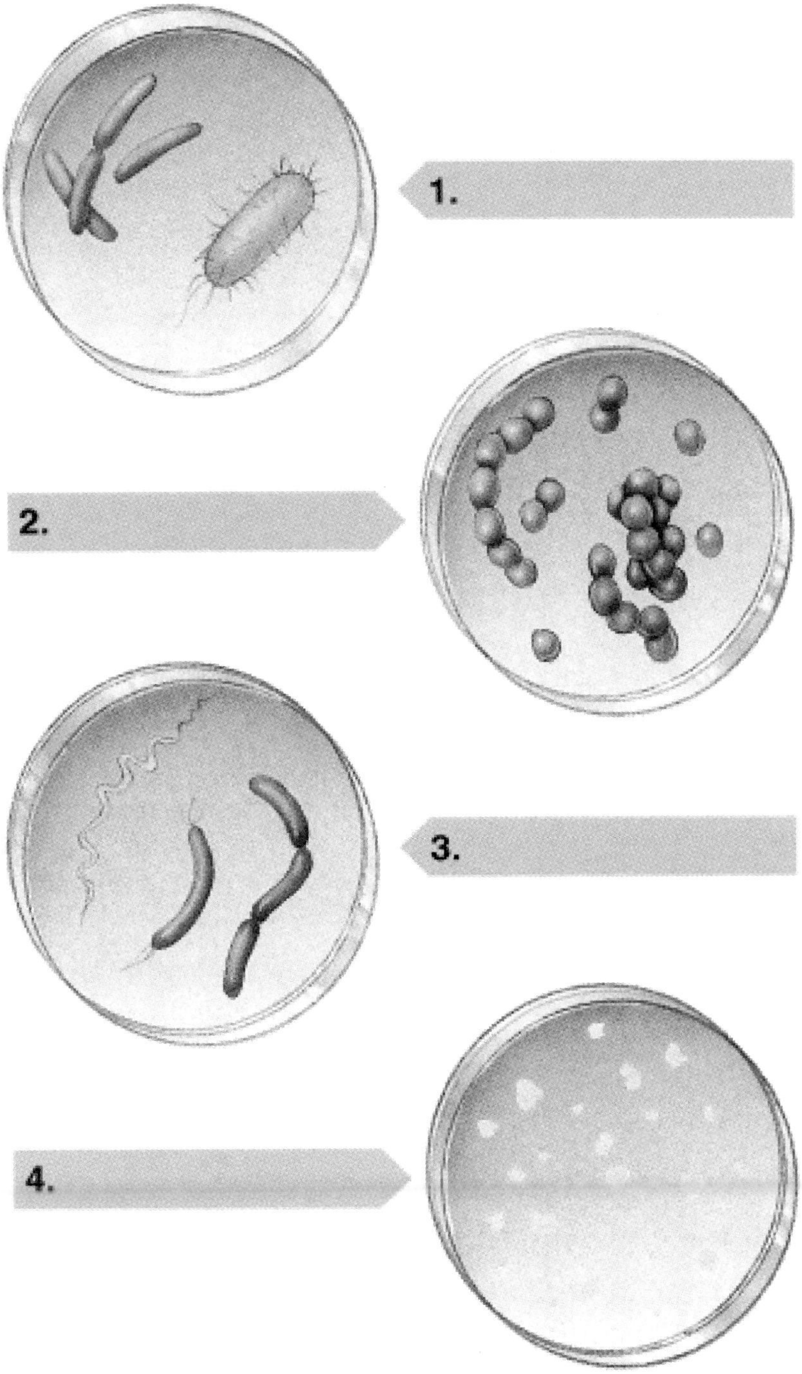

A. **Directions:** Identify the four shapes of bacteria shown in the figure above.

1. ____________________
2. ____________________
3. ____________________
4. ____________________

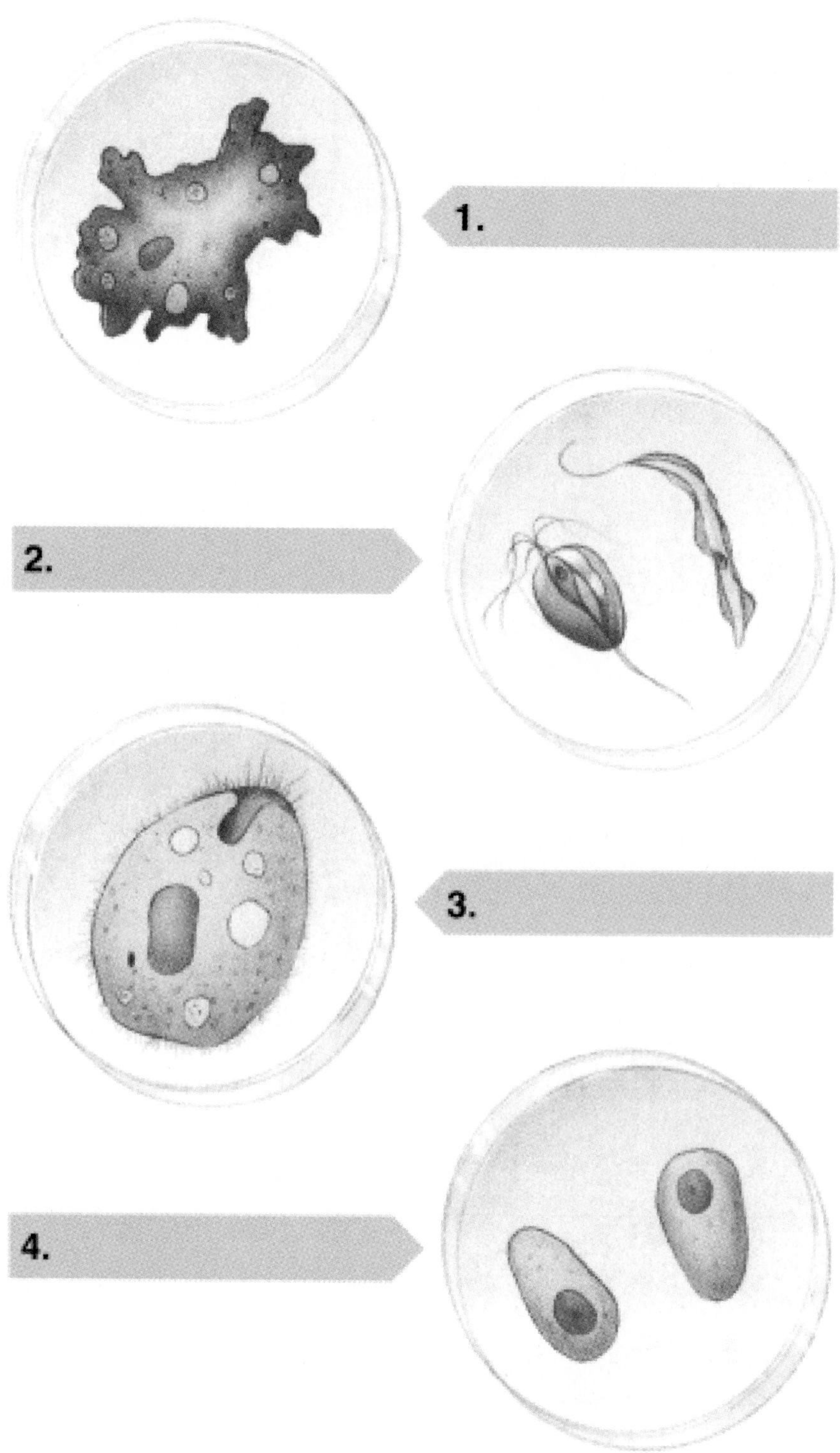

B. **Directions:** Identify the four types of disease-causing protozoa shown in the figure above.

1. ______________________________

2. ______________________________

3. ______________________________

4. ______________________________

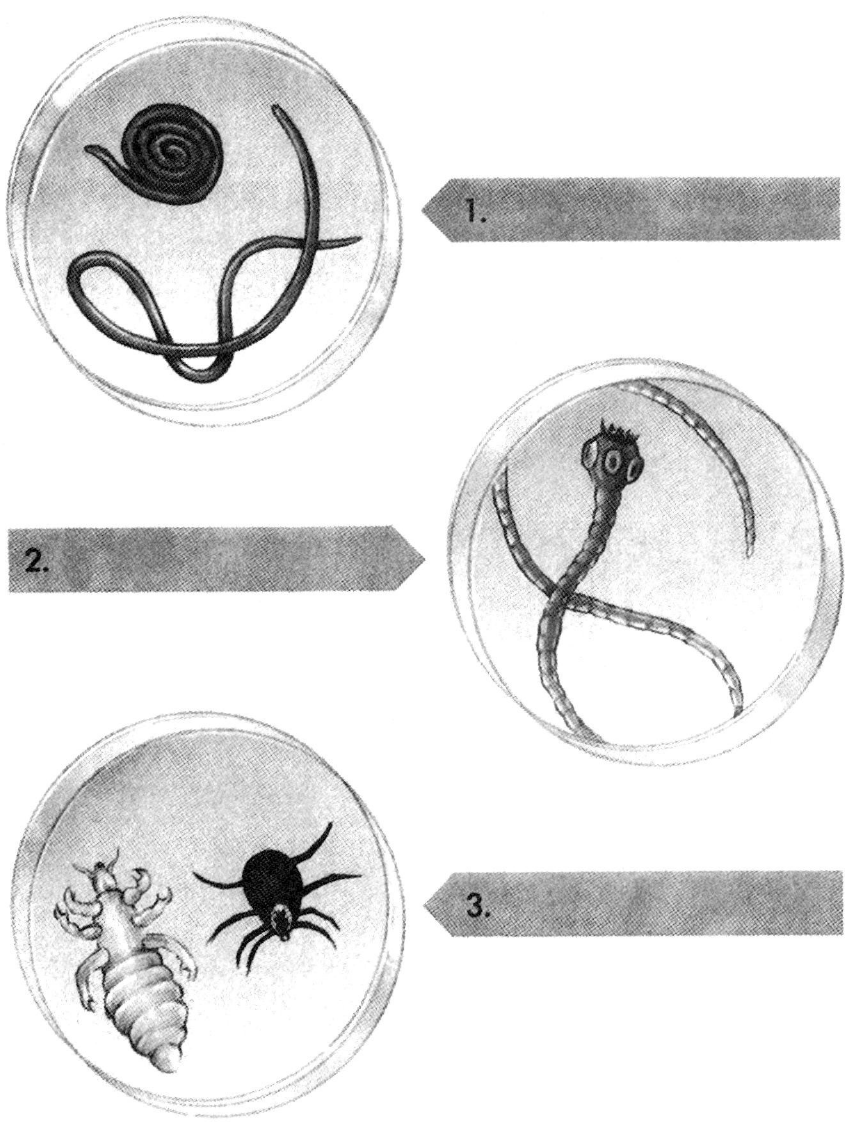

C. Identify the three pathogenic animals shown in the figure above.

1. ____

2. ____

3. ____

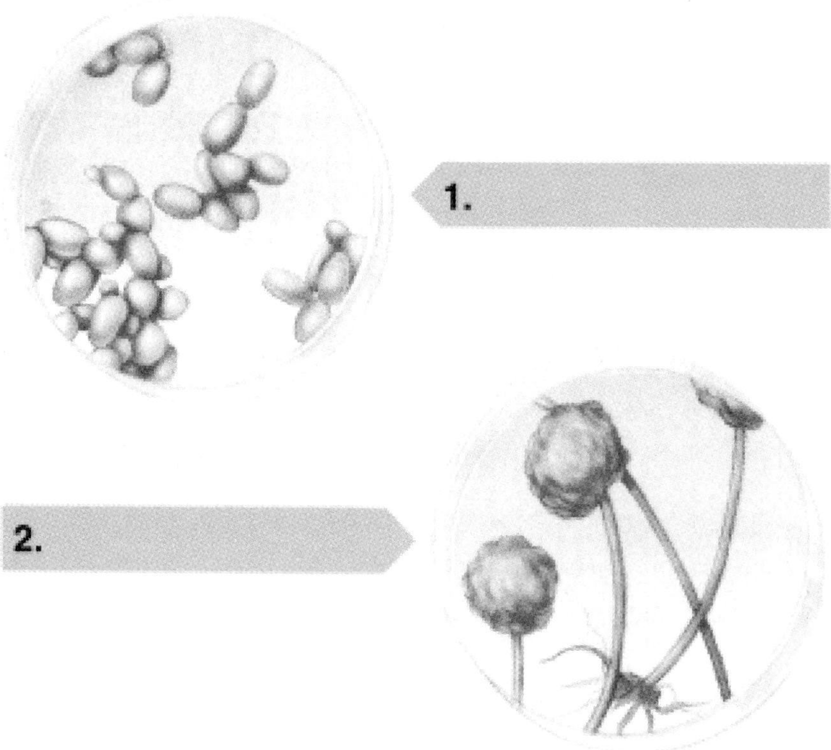

D. Identify the two fungi shown in the figure above.

1. ______________________________

2. ______________________________

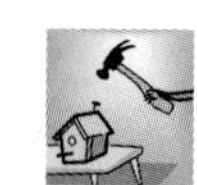

Part IV. Theory

A. Bacteria are also classified according to oxygen requirements. Those that require oxygen to live are called ______________; those that will die in the presence of oxygen are called ______________.

B. ______________ is the study of fungi and the diseases they cause.

C. ______________ are transmitted through contaminated feces, food, or drink and are present in moist environments and in bodies of water such as lakes and ponds.

D. Differentiate between Gram stain and acid fast stain.

____

____

____

____

E. Describe the four different classifications of media.

All-purpose or nutritive:

Selective:

Differential:

Enriched:

F. Complete the chart for transporting and processing of microbiology specimens.

Collection, Transport, and Processing of Specimens Commonly Submitted to the Physician's Office Laboratory

Specimen	Container	Patient Preparation	Special Instructions	Storage Before Processing
Blood		Disinfect venipuncture site with alcohol swab and Betadine.	Draw blood during febrile episodes; draw two sets from right and left arms.	
Body fluids (peritoneal, synovial. pleural, etc.)		Disinfect aspiration site with alcohol swab and Betadine.	Needle aspirations are preferable to swab collections.	
Eye			Moisten swab with Amie's or Stuart's medium before collection.	
Stool			Transport to lab within 24 hours if storing at 4°C.	

Specimen	Container	Patient Preparation	Special Instructions	Storage Before Processing
Rectal swab			Insert swav approx. 2.5 cm past anal sphincter.	
Gonorrhea culture		Wipe away exudate before culture; obtain culture with swab.	Do not refrigerate.	
Chlamydia culture		Urogenital swabs are preferred; epithelial cells, not exudate, must be obtained.	Transport immediately on ice to lab.	
Skin scraping (fungal culture)		Wipe skin with alcohol prep pad.	Scrape skin at leading edge of lesion.	
Sputum		Patient should rinse or gargle with mouthwash before collection.	Have patient collect from deep cough; do not collect saliva.	
Throat		Moisten swab with Stuart's or Amie's transport medium.	Swab pharynx and tonsils, not mouth, tongue, or teeth.	
Ova and parasites		A minimum of 3 specimens should be collected every other day for outpatients.	Wait 7 to 10 days if patient has been taking Pepto-Bismol, Kaopectate, or milk of magnesia.	
Urine		Instruct patient on clean-catch midstream collection.	Hold at 4°C and deliver to lab within 24 hours.	
Superficial wound		Wipe area with sterile saline solution or alcohol prep pad before collection.	Moisten swab with Amie's or Stuart's medium before collection.	
Deep wound or abscess		Wipe area with sterile saline solution or alcohol prep pad before collection.	Aspirate material, excise tissue,or insert swab deep into wound.	

Part V. Workplace Applications

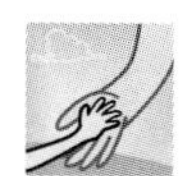

A. What two questions should the medical assistant ask himself or herself before collecting specimens for microbiological analysis?

____

____

B. Draw the pattern that you should make when you prepare a culture on an agar plate.

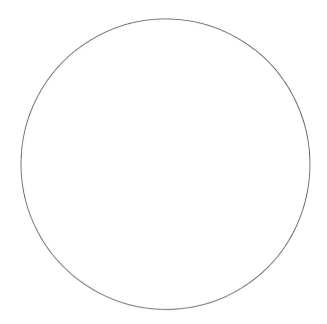

Part VI. Transdisciplinary Skills

Procedural Coding

You have looked up *culture* in the *CPT* Index, and you are confirming codes in the Pathology and Laboratory section below. Answer the questions for the diagnostic studies.

Microbiology

87040	Culture, bacterial; blood with isolation and presumptive identification of isolates (includes anaerobic)
87045	stool, with isolation and preliminary examination (e.g., KIA, LIA) *Salmonella* and *Shigella* species
87046	stool, additional pathogens (includes Campylobacter, Yersinia, Vibro, and E. coli), each plate
87070	any source, except urine, blood, stool

1. What is the *CPT* code for a stool culture for salmonella? ________________
2. What code do you use for a blood culture? ________________
3. What is the *CPT* code for a throat culture? ________________
4. A wound culture would need which *CPT* code? ________________
5. What is the *CPT* code for an extra stool culture for *Escherichia coli*? ________________

Chapter 52 Quiz

Name: ____

1. *S. pyogenes* needs to be cultured on

   ____________ ____________ .

2. The most common cause of UTIs is

   ______________________ .

3. Fungi are observed with what diagnostic prep?

   ____

   ____

4. Bacteria are identified by what characteristics?

   ____

   ____

5. What is the common name for *Enterobius vermicularis*?

   ____

   ____

6. Spherical bacteria are called

   ______________________ .

7. Rod-shaped bacteria are called

   ______________________ .

8. During a gram stain, ____________ is the decolorizing agent.

9. The organism that causes mononucleosis is ____________ ____________ .

10. An organism that causes disease is a

    ______________________ .

CHAPTER 53

Surgical Supplies and Instruments

Part I. Medical Terminology

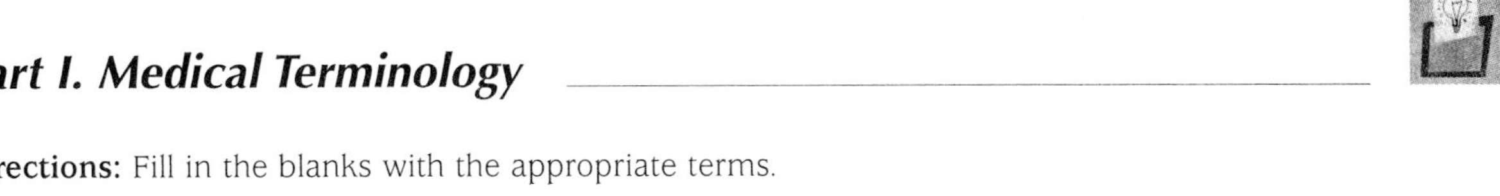

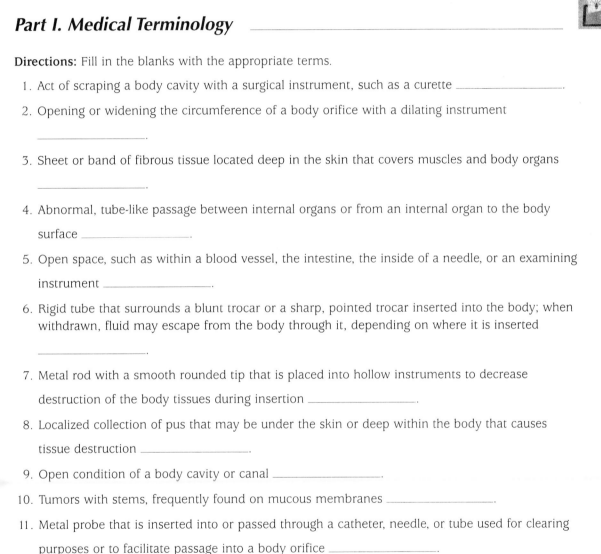

Directions: Fill in the blanks with the appropriate terms.

1. Act of scraping a body cavity with a surgical instrument, such as a curette ________________.
2. Opening or widening the circumference of a body orifice with a dilating instrument ________________.
3. Sheet or band of fibrous tissue located deep in the skin that covers muscles and body organs ________________.
4. Abnormal, tube-like passage between internal organs or from an internal organ to the body surface ________________.
5. Open space, such as within a blood vessel, the intestine, the inside of a needle, or an examining instrument ________________.
6. Rigid tube that surrounds a blunt trocar or a sharp, pointed trocar inserted into the body; when withdrawn, fluid may escape from the body through it, depending on where it is inserted ________________.
7. Metal rod with a smooth rounded tip that is placed into hollow instruments to decrease destruction of the body tissues during insertion ________________.
8. Localized collection of pus that may be under the skin or deep within the body that causes tissue destruction ________________.
9. Open condition of a body cavity or canal ________________.
10. Tumors with stems, frequently found on mucous membranes ________________.
11. Metal probe that is inserted into or passed through a catheter, needle, or tube used for clearing purposes or to facilitate passage into a body orifice ________________.
12. To cut or separate tissue with a cutting instrument or scissors ________________.

Part II.

A. List some of the features of a minor surgery room.

1. ______
2. ______
3. ______
4. ______
5. ______

B. List four surgical solutions.

1. ______
2. ______
3. ______
4. ______

C. List three local anesthetics.

1. ______
2. ______
3. ______

D. List two medications that help control bleeding.

1. ______
2. ______

E. List four groups of surgical instruments and give an example of each.

1. ______
2. ______
3. ______
4. ______

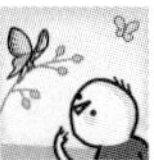

Part III. Visual Aids

1. **Directions:** Name the instruments pictured below.

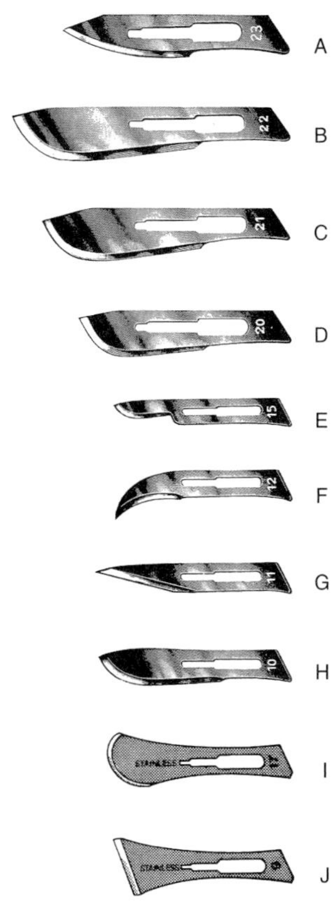

A. ______

B. ______

C. ______

D. ______

E. ______

F. ______

G. ______

H. ______

I. ______

J. ______

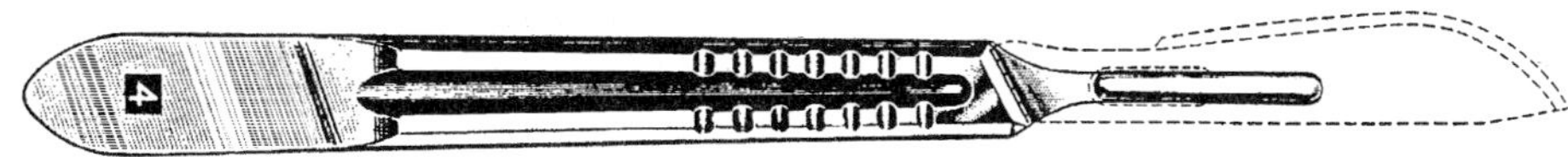

2. ______

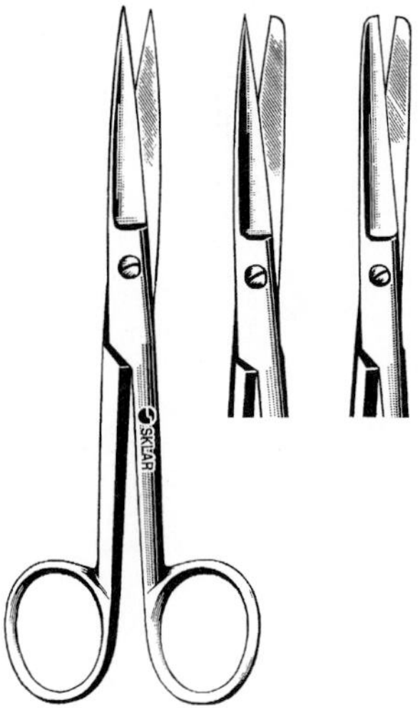

3. ______________________________

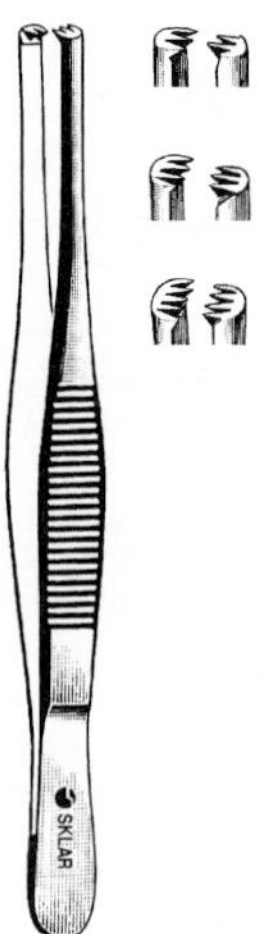

4. ______________________________

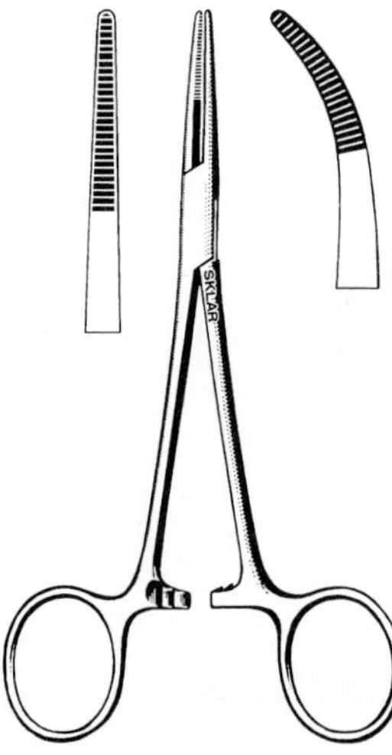

5. ______________________________

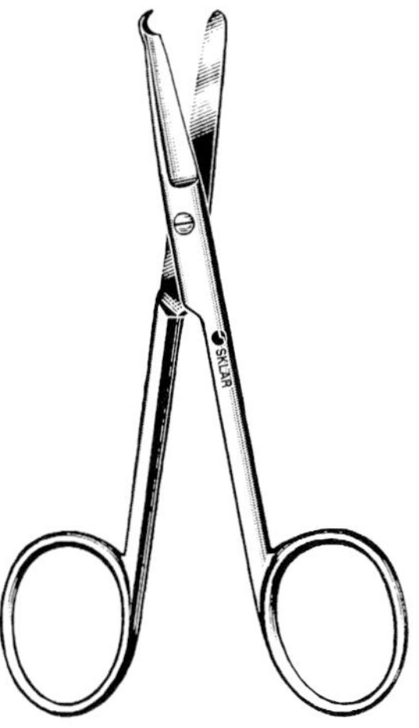

6. ______________________________

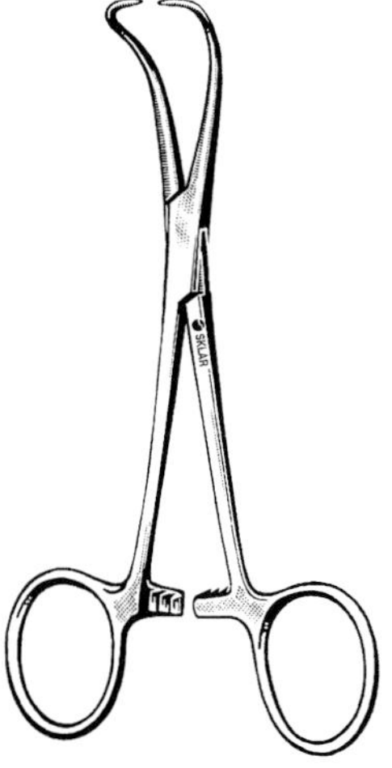

7. ______________________________

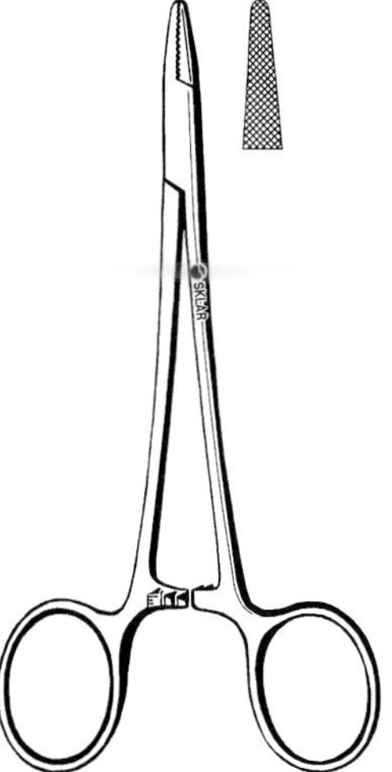

8. ______________________________

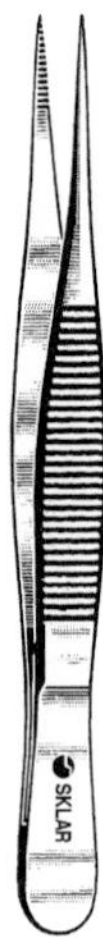

9. ______________________________

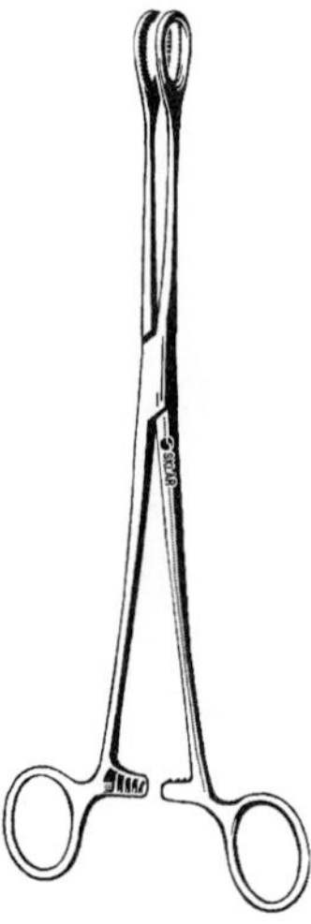

10. ______________________________

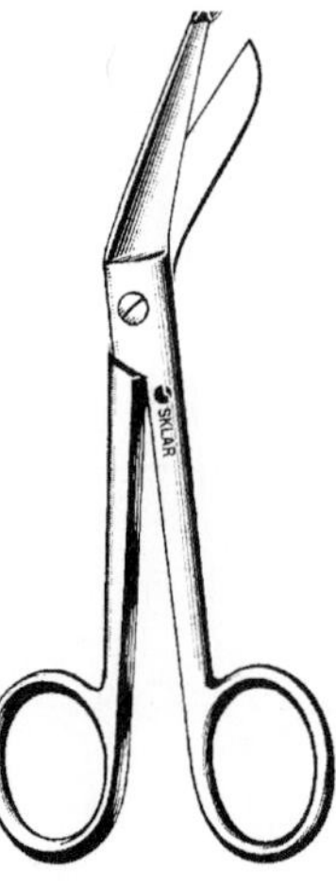

11. ______________________________

Part IV.

A. **Directions:** Indicate which statements are true (T) and which statements are false (F).

1. _____ Each instrument should always be unlocked before immersion in the chemical decontaminate to permit cleansing of the entire surface area.
2. _____ Instruments are always named after the person who designed them.
3. _____ Scissors have ratchets.
4. _____ *A mosquito* and *Kelly* are names of hemostats.

B. **Directions:** Match the following descriptions and instruments.

1. _____ Blade has beak or hook to slide under sutures.
2. _____ Jaws are shorter and look stronger than hemostat jaws.
3. _____ Design and construction vary; has fine tip for foreign object retrieval.
4. _____ Have very sharp hooks.
5. _____ Valves can be spread to facilitate viewing.
6. _____ Bandage scissors.
7. _____ Manufactured in different lengths; smooth-tipped; used to insert packing into or remove objects from nose and ear.

A. Bayonet forceps
B. Towel forceps (towel clamp)
C. Littauer stitch or suture scissors
D. Needle holders
E. Splinter forceps
F. Nasal specula
G. Probe tip is blunt

C. Search the Internet for surgical instruments. Review the names of instruments that you find on the Internet.

_______________ _______________
_______________ _______________
_______________ _______________
_______________ _______________
_______________ _______________

Chapter 53 Quiz

Name: ____

1. Metzenbaum, Mayo, and Iris are names of ______________________ .

2. Crile, Army-Navy, and Senn are ______________________ .

3. Allis, Bayonet, and Adson are ______________________ .

4. Hemostats are a type of forcep or ______________________ .

5. Normal physiologic sterile saline is ______________ %.

6. Local anesthetics have the ______________ suffix.

7. ______________ is the scraping of a body cavity with a surgical instrument.

8. An ________ is a metal rod with a smooth rounded tip that is placed in hollow instruments to prevent injury during insertion.

9. Betadine and HibiClens are examples of ______________________ .

10. Iodoform is used as a ____________ .

CHAPTER 54

Surgical Asepsis and Assisting with Surgical Procedures

Part I. Vocabulary

Directions: Match the following terms and definitions.

1. _____ Invasion of body tissues by microorganisms, which then proliferate and damage tissues
2. _____ Living organisms that can only be seen with a light microscope
3. _____ Disease-causing microorganisms
4. _____ Allowing a substance to pass or soak through
5. _____ Presence of pus-forming organisms in the blood
6. _____ Reducing the number of microorganisms to a relatively safe level
7. _____ Thick-walled dormant form of bacteria, very resistant to disinfection measures
8. _____ Complete destruction of all forms of microbial life
9. _____ Chemical agents that kill pathogens
10. _____ Having a rapid onset and severe symptoms
11. _____ Substance that kills microorganisms
12. _____ Being free from infection or infectious materials
13. _____ Persisting for a prolonged period
14. _____ Becoming unsterile by contact with any nonsterile material
15. _____ Pathologic process having a descriptive set of signs and symptoms
16. _____ Destruction of pathogens by physical or chemical means
17. _____ Swelling between layers of tissue

A. permeable
B. contamination
C. asepsis
D. disease
E. chronic
F. infection
G. antiseptic
H. edema
I. spores
J. pathogens
K. germicides
L. pyemia
M. acute
N. sterilization
O. disinfection
P. microorganisms
Q. sanitization

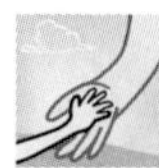

Directions: Rate yourself on the knowledge of the following procedures, with 1 being the lowest score and 5 being the highest score.

1. Demonstrate proper hand washing technique for surgical asepsis.	1	2	3	4	5
2. Clean and wrap instruments and equipment for autoclaving.	1	2	3	4	5
3. Load, run, and unload the autoclave properly.	1	2	3	4	5
4. Open a sterile pack to create a sterile field.	1	2	3	4	5
5. Open and add the contents of a sterile pack to a sterile field.	1	2	3	4	5
6. Transfer sterile instruments.	1	2	3	4	5
7. Assist with a minor surgical procedure.	1	2	3	4	5
8. Assist with suturing.	1	2	3	4	5
9. Remove sutures.	1	2	3	4	5
10. Properly apply dressing and bandage to surgical site.	1	2	3	4	5

Part III. ______________________________

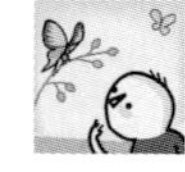

Directions: Fill in the blanks.

1. The physician must have the patient's written, ________________ consent before doing any surgical procedure. To sign an informed consent form, permitting the physician to legally perform the surgery, the patient must understand ________________ procedure will be done, ________________ it should be done, the potential ________________ and ________________ of the surgery, alternative treatments (including no treatment), and the possible risks of any alternative treatment. This legal requirement is not simply met by having the patient ________________ the operative permit. A ________________ must occur during which the physician provides the patient or the patient's legal representative with enough information to decide whether to proceed with the proposed surgical treatment. After this discussion, the patient either ________________ or ________________ to consent to the surgery.
   The patient then signs or refuses to sign the consent form. If the patient signs with an *X*, the medical assistant should write "patient's mark" beside the *X*, and in addition, have a ________________ ________________ witness the signature. The discussion must be fully ________________ in the patient's medical record. A copy of the ________________ form must also be included in the patient's record. Treatment may not exceed the scope of the permit.
   NOTE: The patient must not be under the influence of any ________________ medication at the time he or she is signing the consent form. This condition must ________________ be violated.

Part IV. ______

A. List five reasons a postoperative patient should call the office.

1. ______
2. ______
3. ______
4. ______
5. ______

B. **Directions:** Indicate which statements are true (T) and which statements are false (F).

1. ____ Air currents carry bacteria, so body motions over a sterile field and talking should be kept to a minimum.
2. ____ Infection can cause death in some circumstances.
3. ____ A sterile field can get wet.
4. ____ Sterile team members should always face each other.
5. ____ You should always keep the sterile field in your view.
6. ____ You should never turn your back on a sterile field or wander away from it.
7. ____ When autoclaving, you should place a gauze sponge around the tips of sharp instruments to prevent them from piercing the wrapping material.
8. ____ Nonsterile persons should never reach over a sterile field.
9. ____ All hinged instruments are wrapped in the closed position to allow full steam penetration of the joint.
10. ____ When using sterilizing bags, you should insert the grasping end of the instruments first.

Chapter 54 Quiz

Name: ____

1. Using electrocautery requires the patient to be connected to a ______________ .

2. True or False: Laser surgery requires sterile water to be available. __________

3. Endoscopes are either rigid or _______ .

4. Cryosurgery is __________ the tissue.

5. ____________ consent is required before any surgical procedure.

6. Name three types of sterilization.
   a. ______________________________
   b. ______________________________
   c. ______________________________

7. A machine that uses steam and pressure to kill pathogens and spores is an ____________________________ .

8. What is the purpose of autoclave tape?
   ____
   ____

9. What should be written on the outside of instruments after they are wrapped?
   ____
   ____

10. Sterile supplies expire after ___________ days to ___________ months depending on the packaging.

CHAPTER 55

Career Development and Life Skills

Part I. Vocabulary

Directions: Match the following terms and definitions.

1. _____ To give an expert judgment of the value or merit of; in this chapter, the evaluation of work performance.
2. _____ A return offer made by one who has rejected an offer or job.
3. _____ A failure to pay financial debts, especially a student loan.
4. _____ A postponement, especially of repayment of a student loan.
5. _____ Expressing sincerity and honest feeling.
6. _____ Not tolerable or bearable.
7. _____ To imitate or practice.
8. _____ The exchange of information or services among individuals, groups, or institutions; in this chapter, it involves meeting and getting to know individuals in the same or similar career fields and sharing information about available opportunities.
9. _____ Having a clear decisive relevance to the matter in hand.
10. _____ To read and mark corrections.
11. _____ Something produced by a cause or necessarily following from a set of conditions.
12. _____ To correct by removing errors.
13. _____ Having or marked by keen insight and ability to penetrate deeply and thoroughly.
14. _____ Marked by compact, precise expression without wasted words.
15. _____ A condensed statement or outline.
16. _____ The work in which a person is regularly employed.

A. succinct
B. counteroffer
C. synopsis
D. appraisals
E. rectify
F. proofread
G. intolerable
H. default
I. pertinent
J. ramification
K. networking
L. vocation
M. subtle
N. genuineness
O. mock
P. deferment

Part II. ____

A. **Directions:** List nine methods of job searching.

1. ____
2. ____
3. ____
4. ____
5. ____
6. ____
7. ____
8. ____
9. ____

B. **Directions:** Complete the job application that is included in this workbook. Use factual information. Remember: Neatness counts.

C. **Directions:** Prepare a draft resume using the blank pages included in this chapter.

DIAMONTE
HOSPITAL

APPLICATION FOR EMPLOYMENT

This application is not a contract. It is intended to provide information for evaluating your suitability for employment. Please read each question carefully and give an honest and complete answer. Qualified applicants receive consideration for employment without unlawful discrimination because of sex, religion, race, color, national origin, age, disability, or other classification protected by law. Applications will remain active for three months.

PLEASE TYPE OR PRINT ALL INFORMATION

Date: ____________

Position(s) applying for: ____________

How did you learn about us? ☐ Walk-in ☐ Friend ☐ Relative ☐ Job hotline ☐ Employee ☐ Other
☐ Advertisement (Please state name of publication) ____________ Referred by: ____________

Name: ____________
Last *First* *Middle initial*

Mailing address: ____________
City *State* *Zip code*

Phone: (___) ____________ (___) ____________ Social Security #: ____________
Home *Message*

If related to anyone in our employ, state name and department: ____________

If you have been employed under another name, please list here: ____________

Are you under 18 years of age? ☐ Yes ☐ No

Are you currently employed? ☐ Yes ☐ No

May we contact your present employer? ☐ Yes ☐ No

Do you have legal rights to work in this country?
(Proof of legal rights to work in this country will be required upon employment) ☐ Yes ☐ No

Have you ever been employed with us before? ☐ Yes ☐ No *If "yes," give date(s):* ____________

Are you available to work: ☐ Full-time ☐ Part-time ☐ Shift work ☐ Temporary

Are you available to work overtime if required? ☐ Yes ☐ No

How flexible are you in accepting varying scheduled hours? ☐ Very flexible ☐ Somewhat flexible
☐ Need set schedule

Minimum salary desired: ____________

Have you ever been discharged from a job or forced to resign? ☐ Yes ☐ No
Explain: ____________

Have you ever been convicted of a felony?
If "yes," please explain: ☐ Yes ☐ No
Criminal convictions are not an absolute bar to employment but will be considered with respect to the specific requirements of the job for which you are applying. ____________

EDUCATION

High school: ______________________ High school graduate/GED: ☐Yes ☐No
______________________ Date: __________

College: ______________________ Graduated: ☐Yes ☐No
Major/field(s) of study: ______________________ Degree: __________
Date: __________

College: ______________________ Graduated: ☐Yes ☐No
Major/field(s) of study: ______________________ Degree: __________
Date: __________

Technical, business, or correspondence school: ______________________ Graduated: ☐Yes ☐No
Major/field(s) of study: ______________________ Degree: __________
Date: __________

Describe any specialized training, apprenticeship, and skills such as computer, office equipment, etc. ______________________

LICENSES AND CERTIFICATIONS

Type of license(s)/certification(s): ______________________ Expiration date: __________
Type of license(s)/certification(s): ______________________ Expiration date: __________
Type of license(s)/certification(s): ______________________ Expiration date: __________
Verified by: __________
Date: __________

REFERENCES

(Give name, address, and telephone number of three references that you have known for at least one year who are not related to you.)

Name: ______________________ Phone: __________ Years acquainted: ______
Address: ______________________ Business: __________

Name: ______________________ Phone: __________ Years acquainted: ______
Address: ______________________ Business: __________

Name: ______________________ Phone: __________ Years acquainted: ______
Address: ______________________ Business: __________

EMPLOYMENT EXPERIENCE

(Please list all employment experience, with most recent employment first. If more space is needed, please use the Additional Employment form.)

Employer: ____________________ Duties and skills performed: ____________________
Address: ____________________
Phone number(s) ____________________
Job title: ____________________
Supervisor's name/title: ____________________
Reason for leaving: ____________________
Salary received: ____________________ *hourly / weekly / monthly*
Employed from: ____________ to ____________
month / year *month / year*

Employer: ____________________ Duties and skills performed: ____________________
Address: ____________________
Phone number(s) ____________________
Job title: ____________________
Supervisor's name/title: ____________________
Reason for leaving: ____________________
Salary received: ____________________ *hourly / weekly / monthly*
Employed from: ____________ to ____________
month / year *month / year*

Employer: ____________________ Duties and skills performed: ____________________
Address: ____________________
Phone number(s) ____________________
Job title: ____________________
Supervisor's name/title: ____________________
Reason for leaving: ____________________
Salary received: ____________________ *hourly / weekly / monthly*
Employed from: ____________ to ____________
month / year *month / year*

Do you expect any of the employers listed above to give you a poor reference? ☐ *Yes* ☐ *No*
If yes, explain: ____________________

APPLICANT'S STATEMENT

I hereby certify that the statements and information provided are true, and I understand that any false statements or omissions are cause for termination. I agree to submit to a drug test and physical following any conditional offer of employment, and I grant permission to Diamonte Hospital to investigate my criminal history, education, prior employment history, and references, and hereby release all persons or agencies from all liability or any damage for issuing this information.

I understand that this application is current for only **three months**. At the end of that time, if I do not hear from Diamonte Hospital and still wish to be considered for employment, it will be necessary to update my application.

_______________________________ _______________________

Signature of Applicant *Date*

____

Print Name

DIAMONTE HOSPITAL

Draft Resumé

Draft Resumé

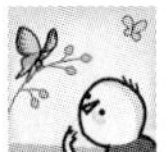

Part III.

Directions: Evaluate Teresa O'Sullivan's cover letter. Describe what you like about the letter and make notes of additional information that you would include in your own cover letter.

Theresa O'Sullivan
233 Wentworth Street, San Diego, CA 92100
Telephone (619) 222-3333

June 15, 20xx

Arthur M. Blackburn, MD
2200 Broadway
Any Town, US 98765

Dear Doctor Blackburn:

In a few weeks, I will complete my formal training in medical assisting with an Associate in Science degree from Ola Vista Community College.

The medical assisting program at Ola Vista includes theory and practical application in both administrative and clinical skills. My six-week supervised externship gave me additional practical experience in two specialty practices.

While studying at Ola Vista, I also worked part-time for a physician in family practice, while maintaining a 3.5 grade point average. My experience as Dr. Madden's employee is outlined on the enclosed resumé. I have enjoyed my work in Dr. Madden's office and am now seeking full-time employment.

If you will require a replacement or addition to your staff in the near future, may I be considered as an applicant? I will follow up with a telephone call within a week.

Sincerely yours,

Theresa O'Sullivan

Enc. Resumé

Part IV.

A. **Directions:** Set some realistic goals for your career in medical assisting by answering the following questions.

1. Where am I today?

2. Where will I be in five years?

3. Where will I be in ten years?

4. What additional skills do I need to get where I want to be?

B. **Directions:** Plan a budget for yourself using your actual living expenses.

The Guideline Budget

MONTHLY INCOME	AMOUNT
Net Income	
Spouse Net Income	
Child Support	
Other Income	

MONTHLY EXPENSES	AMOUNT
Rent	
Gas	
Electric	
Home/Renters Insurance	
Water/Sewage	
Trash	
Home Telephone	
Cell Telephone	
Pager	
Cable TV/Satellite	
Internet/DSL	
Child Care	
Lawn Care	
Clothing	
Food-Home	
Food-Work or School	
Food-Eating Out	
Laundry/Dry Cleaning	
Medical Expenses	
Dental Expenses	
Life Insurance	
Medical Insurance	
Dental Insurance	
Eyeglasses	
Prescriptions	
Automobile Payment	
Automobile Insurance	
Repairs	
Gas/Oil	
Furniture	
Beauty/Barber Shop	
Pet Expenses	
Student Loan	
Others Loans	
Credit Cards	
Church/charities	
Birthdays	
Anniversaries	
Christmas	
Vacation Planning	
Entertainment	

Chapter 55 Quiz

Name: ____

1. A fact sheet that summarizes an applicant's qualifications, education, and experience is called a ____________ .

2. True or False: Salary expectation should be clearly stated in the resume.

   ____

3. Name two of the most effective ways of job searching.

   a. ______________________________

   b. ______________________________

4. True or False: It is illegal for someone to ask about number of children, religion, and marital status during an interview.

   ____

5. Name the four phases of a job interview.

   a. ______________________________

   b. ______________________________

   c. ______________________________

   d. ______________________________

6. Name three traditional job search techniques.

   a. ______________________________

   b. ______________________________

   c. ______________________________

7. What is the purpose of a cover letter for a resume?

   ____

   ____

8. When writing career objectives, what should you ask yourself?

   ____

   ____

9. List three things that employers want.

   a. ______________________________

   b. ______________________________

   c. ______________________________

10. Describe three types of skills that could be included on a resume.

    a. ______________________________

    b. ______________________________

    c. ______________________________

PROCEDURE CHECKLISTS

Student Name ______________________ Date ____________ Score ____________

Procedure 9-1 Answering the Telephone

Task: To answer the phone in a professional manner, respond to a request for action, and accurately record a message.

Equipment and Supplies:
- Telephone
- Message pad
- Pen or pencil
- Appointment book
- Script for conversation

Standards: Complete the procedure and all critical steps in ____________ minutes with a minimum score of ____________ % within three attempts.

Scoring: Divide points earned by total possible points. Failure to perform a critical step that is indicated with an asterisk (*), will result in an unsatisfactory overall score.

Time began ____________ **Time ended** ____________

Steps	Possible Points	First Attempt	Second Attempt	Third Attempt
1. Answer the phone after the first ring and before the third ring, speaking directly into the transmitter, with the mouthpiece 1 inch from the mouth.	20			
2. Speak distinctly with a pleasant tone and expression, at a moderate rate, and with sufficient volume. Remember to smile.	10			
3. Identify yourself and the office.*	20			
4. Verify the identity of the caller.	10			
5. Provide the caller with the requested information or service, if possible.	10			
6. Take a message for further action, if required.	20			
7. Terminate the call in a pleasant manner and replace the receiver gently.	10			

Documentation in the Medical Record

____

____

____

____

Comments:

Total Points Earned ________ Divided by ________ Total Possible Points = ________ % Score

Instructor's Signature ______________________

Student Name ______________________ Date ____________ Score ____________

Procedure 9-2 Taking a Message

Task: To take an accurate telephone message and follow up on the requests made by the caller.

Equipment and Supplies:
- Telephone
- Message pad
- Pen or pencil
- Notepad

Standards: Complete the procedure and all critical steps in ____________ minutes with a minimum score of ____________ % within three attempts.

Scoring: Divide points earned by total possible points. Failure to perform a critical step that is indicated with an asterisk (*), will result in an unsatisfactory overall score.

Time began ____________ **Time ended** ____________

Steps	**Possible Points**	**First Attempt**	**Second Attempt**	**Third Attempt**
1. Answer the telephone using the guidelines in Procedure 9-1, Answering the Telephone.	**10**			
2. Using a message pad or notepad, take the phone message, obtaining the following information: a. the name of the person to whom the call is directed b. the name of the person calling c. the caller's daytime and/or telephone number d. the reason for the call e. the action to be taken f. the date and time of the call g. the initials of the person taking the call	**20**			
3. Repeat the information back to the caller after the message is recorded on the message pad.	**10**			
4. Provide the caller with an approximation of the time and date that he or she will be called back, if possible.	**10**			
5. End the call and wait for the caller to hang up first.	**10**			
6. Deliver the phone message to the appropriate person. Separate trays or slots for each staff member are helpful.	**10**			
7. Follow up on important messages.	**10**			

Steps	Possible Points	First Attempt	Second Attempt	Third Attempt
8. Keep old message books for future reference. Carbonless copies will allow the facility to keep a permanent record of phone messages.	10			
9. File pertinent phone messages in the patient's chart.	10			

Comments:

Total Points Earned ________ Divided by ________ Total Possible Points = ________ % Score

Instructor's Signature ____________________

Student Name ______________________ Date ____________ Score ____________

Procedure 9-3 Calling Pharmacy with New or Refill Prescription Orders

Task: To call in an accurate prescription to the pharmacy for a patient in the most efficient manner.

Equipment and Supplies:
- Prescription
- Notepad
- Patient chart
- Telephone

Standards: Complete the procedure and all critical steps in ____________ minutes with a minimum score of ____________ % within three attempts.

Scoring: Divide points earned by total possible points. Failure to perform a critical step that is indicated with an asterisk (*), will result in an unsatisfactory overall score.

Time began ____________ **Time ended** ____________

Steps	**Possible Points**	**First Attempt**	**Second Attempt**	**Third Attempt**
1. Receive the call from the patient requesting a prescription, using appropriate telephone technique.	**10**			
2. Obtain the following information from the patient: a. patient's name b. telephone number where he or she can be reached c. patient's symptoms and current condition d. history of this condition e. treatments the patient has tried f. pharmacy name and telephone number	**20**			
3. Write the prescription in the patient's chart that the physician wishes the patient to have. Be very careful to transcribe the information correctly. Read it back to the physician.	**10**			
4. If the prescription is a refill, give the physician the patient's chart with the message requesting a refill attached, along with the information in procedure step two as listed above.	**10**			
5. Note the comments that the physician writes in the chart. If the prescription is written or a refill is approved, call the patient's pharmacy and ask to speak to a member of the pharmacy staff.	**10**			
6. Ask the pharmacy staff member to repeat the prescription back to you.	**10**			

Steps	Possible Points	First Attempt	Second Attempt	Third Attempt
7. Note the date and time that the prescription was called to the pharmacy in the chart.	**10**			
8. Call the patient to notify him or her that the prescription has been called in. Provide any information regarding the prescription doses, frequency, etc. that is requested by the physician. Tell the patient when to return to the office, if necessary. Ask the patient to write this information down.	**20**			

Comments:

Total Points Earned ________ Divided by ________ Total Possible Points = ________ % Score

Instructor's Signature ____________________

Student Name ______________________ Date ____________ Score ____________

Procedure 10-1 Preparing and Maintaining the Appointment Book

Task: To establish the matrix of the appointment page, arrange appointments for one day, and enter information.

Equipment and Supplies:
- Page from appointment book
- Office policy for office hours and doctors' availability
- Clerical supplies
- Calendar
- Description of patients to be scheduled

Standards: Complete the procedure and all critical steps in ____________ minutes with a minimum score of ____________ % within three attempts.

Scoring: Divide points earned by total possible points. Failure to perform a critical step that is indicated with an asterisk (*), will result in an unsatisfactory overall score.

Time began ____________ **Time ended** ____________

Steps	Possible Points	First Attempt	Second Attempt	Third Attempt
1. Identify each patient's complaint.	15			
2. Establish the matrix of the appointment page for the day.	15			
3. Consult guidelines to determine the length of time necessary for each patient.	15			
4. Allot appointment time according to the complaint and facilities available.*	25			
5. Enter information in the appointment book. NOTE: A telephone number must follow the patient's name. If the patient is new, add the letters NP (new patient) after his or her name.	15			
6. Allow buffer time in the morning and afternoon.	15			

Comments:

Total Points Earned ________ Divided by ________ Total Possible Points = ________ % Score

Instructor's Signature ________________________

Student Name ________________ Date ________ Score ________

Procedure 10-2 Scheduling a New Patient

Task: To schedule a new patient for a first office visit.

Equipment and Supplies:
- Appointment book
- Scheduling guidelines
- Appointment card
- Telephone

Standards: Complete the procedure and all critical steps in ________ minutes with a minimum score of ________ % within three attempts.

Scoring: Divide points earned by total possible points. Failure to perform a critical step that is indicated with an asterisk (*), will result in an unsatisfactory overall score.

Time began ________ **Time ended** ________

Steps	Possible Points	First Attempt	Second Attempt	Third Attempt
1. Obtain the patient's full name, birth date, address, and telephone number. NOTE: Verify the spelling of the name.	10			
2. Determine whether the patient was referred by another physician.	10			
3. Determine the patient's chief complaint and when the first symptoms occurred.*	20			
4. Search the appointment book for the first suitable appointment time and an alternate time.	10			
5. Offer the patient a choice of these dates and times.	10			
6. Enter the mutually agreed-upon time in the appointment book, followed by the patient's telephone number. NOTE: Indicate that the patient is new by adding the letters NP.	15			
7. If new patients are expected to pay at the time of the visit, explain this financial arrangement when the appointment is made.	10			
8. Offer travel directions for reaching the office and parking instructions.	5			
9. Repeat the day, and time of the appointment before saying good-bye to the patient.	10			

Comments:

Total Points Earned ________ Divided by ________ Total Possible Points = ________ % Score

Instructor's Signature ______________________

Student Name ______________________ Date ____________ Score ____________

Procedure 10-3 Scheduling Outpatient Admissions and Procedures

Task: To schedule a patient for an outpatient diagnostic test ordered by a physician within the time frame needed by the physician, confirm the appointment with the patient, and issue all required instructions.

Equipment and Supplies:
- Diagnostic test order from physician
- Name, address, and telephone number of diagnostic facility
- Patient chart
- Test preparation instructions
- Telephone

Standards: Complete the procedure and all critical steps in ____________ minutes with a minimum score of ____________ % within three attempts.

Scoring: Divide points earned by total possible points. Failure to perform a critical step that is indicated with an asterisk (*), will result in an unsatisfactory overall score.

Time began ____________ **Time ended** ____________

Steps	Possible Points	First Attempt	Second Attempt	Third Attempt
1. Obtain an oral or written order from the physician for the exact procedure to be performed.	10			
2. Determine the patient's availability.	10			
3. Telephone the diagnostic facility. • Order the specific test needed. • Establish the date and time. • Give the name, age, address, and telephone number of the patient. • Determine any special instructions for the patient. • Notify the facility of any urgency for test results.	25			
4. Notify the patient of the arrangements, including: • Name, address, and telephone number of the diagnostic facility. • Date and time to report for the test. • Instructions concerning preparation for the test (e.g., eating restrictions, fluids, medications, enemas). • Ask the patient to repeat the instructions.	25			
5. Note arrangements on the patient's chart below.	20			
6. Place reminder in a "tickler" file or on a desk calendar.	10			

Documentation in the Medical Record

____

____

____

____

Comments:

Total Points Earned ________ Divided by ________ Total Possible Points = ________ % Score

Instructor's Signature ____________________

Student Name ______________________ Date ____________ Score ____________

Procedure 10-4 Scheduling Inpatient Admissions

Task: To schedule a patient for inpatient admission within the time frame needed by physician, confirm with the patient, and issue all required instructions.

Equipment and Supplies:
- Admissions orders from physician
- Name, address, and telephone number of inpatient facility
- Patient demographic information
- Patient chart
- Any preparation instructions for the patient
- Telephone
- Admission packet for the patient

Standards: Complete the procedure and all critical steps in ____________ minutes with a minimum score of ____________ % within three attempts.

Scoring: Divide points earned by total possible points. Failure to perform a critical step that is indicated with an asterisk (*), will result in an unsatisfactory overall score.

Time began ____________ **Time ended** ____________

Steps	Possible Points	First Attempt	Second Attempt	Third Attempt
1. Obtain an oral or written order from the physician for the admission.	10			
2. Precertify the admission with the patient's insurance company, if necessary.	20			
3. Determine the physician and patient availability if the admission is not an emergency.	10			
4. Telephone the diagnostic facility and schedule the admission. • Order any specific tests needed. • Provide the patient's admitting diagnosis. • Establish the date and time. • Convey the patient's room preferences. • Give the name, age, address, and telephone number of the patient. • Provide the demographic information for the patient, including insurance policy numbers and addresses for filing claims. • Determine any special instructions for the patient. • Notify the facility of any urgency for test results.	20			

Steps	Possible Points	First Attempt	Second Attempt	Third Attempt
5. Notify the patient of the arrangements, including: • Name, address, and telephone number of the facility. • Date and time to report for admission. • Instructions concerning preparation for any procedures, if necessary (e.g., eating restrictions, fluids, medications, enemas) • Tell what preadmission testing will be necessary, if any. • Ask the patient to repeat the instructions.	**20**			
6. Note arrangements and the admission on the patient's chart.	**10**			
7. Place reminder on the physician's tickler or desk calendar, if needed. Be sure the information is listed on the office schedule. If the physician keeps a list of all inpatients, add the patient's name to that list.	**10**			

Comments:

Total Points Earned ________ Divided by ________ Total Possible Points = ________ % Score

Instructor's Signature ____________________

Student Name ______________________ Date __________ Score __________

Procedure 10-5 Scheduling Inpatient Surgical Procedures

Task: To schedule a patient for inpatient surgery within the time frame needed by physician, confirm with the patient, and issue all required instructions.

Equipment and Supplies:
- Orders from physician
- Name, address, and telephone number of inpatient facility
- Patient demographic information
- Patient chart
- Any preparation instructions for the patient
- Telephone

Standards: Complete the procedure and all critical steps in __________ minutes with a minimum score of __________ % within three attempts.

Scoring: Divide points earned by total possible points. Failure to perform a critical step that is indicated with an asterisk (*), will result in an unsatisfactory overall score.

Time began __________ **Time ended** __________

Steps	Possible Points	First Attempt	Second Attempt	Third Attempt
1. Obtain an oral or written order from the physician for the admission.	10			
2. Precertify the admission with the patient's insurance company, if necessary.	10			
3. Determine the physician availability if the surgery is not an emergency. Another physician may be the surgeon. If this is the case, the surgery will need to be coordinated with his or her office as well.	10			
4. Telephone the hospital surgical department and schedule the procedure. • Order any specific tests needed. • Provide the patient's admitting diagnosis. • Establish the date and time. • Give the name, age, address, and telephone number of the patient. • Provide the demographic information for the patient, including insurance policy numbers and addresses for filing claims. • Determine any special instructions for the patient. • Notify the facility of any urgency for the surgery.	20			

Steps	Possible Points	First Attempt	Second Attempt	Third Attempt
5. Notify the patient of the arrangements, if the patient is not already admitted to the hospital. Include: • Name, address, and telephone number of the facility. • Date and time to report for admission. • Instructions concerning preparation for any procedures, if necessary (e.g., eating restrictions, fluids, medications, enemas) • Tell what preadmission testing will be necessary, if any. • Ask the patient to repeat the instructions.	**20**			
6. The physician should review the consent form with the patient. Have the patient sign a consent for the surgical procedure. Keep the original consent in the patient's chart and give a copy to the patient.	**10**			
7. Note arrangements on the patient's chart.	**10**			
8. Place reminder on the physician's tickler or desk calendar, if needed. Be sure the information is listed on the office schedule. If the physician keeps a list of all inpatients, add the patient's name to that list. Follow up with the hospital after the procedure regarding the patient's condition as required by the physician.	**10**			

Comments:

Total Points Earned ________ Divided by ________ Total Possible Points = ________ % Score

Instructor's Signature ____________________

Student Name ______________ Date __________ Score __________

Procedure 11-1 Preparing Charts for Scheduled Patients

Task: To prepare patient charts for the daily appointment schedule and have them ready for the physician before the patients' arrival.

Equipment and Supplies:
- Appointment schedule for current date
- Patient files
- Clerical supplies (e.g., pen, tape, stapler)

Standards: Complete the procedure and all critical steps in ______________ minutes with a minimum score of ______________ % within three attempts.

Scoring: Divide points earned by total possible points. Failure to perform a critical step that is indicated with an asterisk (*), will result in an unsatisfactory overall score.

Time began ______________ **Time ended** ______________

Steps	Possible Points	First Attempt	Second Attempt	Third Attempt
1. Review the appointment schedule.	10			
2. Identify full name of each scheduled patient.	10			
3. Pull patients' charts for files, checking each patient's name on your list as each is pulled.*	10			
4. Review each chart to insure that: • All information has been correctly entered. • Any previously ordered tests have been performed and the results mounted permanently in the chart. • The results have been entered on the chart. • Replenish forms inside the chart, such as progress notes, etc.	40			
5. Annotate the appointment list with any special concerns.	10			
6. Arrange the charts sequentially according to each patient's appointment.	10			
7. Place the charts in the appropriate examination room or other specified location.	10			

Comments:

Total Points Earned ________ Divided by ________ Total Possible Points = ________ % Score

Instructor's Signature ______________________

Student Name ________________ Date ________ Score ________

Procedure 11-2 Registering a New Patient

Task: To complete a registration form for a new patient with information for credit and insurance claims, and to inform and orient the patient to the facility.

Equipment and Supplies:
- Registration form
- Clerical supplies (pen, clipboard)
- Private conference area

Standards: Complete the procedure and all critical steps in ________ minutes with a minimum score of ________ % within three attempts.

Scoring: Divide points earned by total possible points. Failure to perform a critical step that is indicated with an asterisk (*), will result in an unsatisfactory overall score.

Time began ________ **Time ended** ________

Steps	**Possible Points**	**First Attempt**	**Second Attempt**	**Third Attempt**
1. Determine whether the patient is new.	10			
2. Obtain and record the necessary information: • Full name, birth date, name of spouse (if married) • Home address, telephone number (include ZIP and area codes) • Occupation, name of employer, business address, telephone number • Social Security number and driver's license number, if any • Name of referring physician, if any • Name and address of person responsible for payment • Method of payment • Health insurance information (photocopy both sides of insurance ID card) • Name of primary carrier • Type of coverage • Group policy number • Subscriber number • Assignment of benefits, if required	50			
3. Review the enter form and confirm patient eligibility for insurance coverage.	10			
4. Determine that required referrals have been received, if applicable.	10			
5. Explain medical and financial procedures to patients.*	10			
6. Collect copays or balance payment charges.	10			

Comments:

Total Points Earned ________ Divided by ________ Total Possible Points = ________ % Score

Instructor's Signature ______________________

Student Name ________________ Date ________ Score ________

Procedure 12-1 Composing Business Correspondence

Task: To compose a letter that will convey information in an accurate and concise manner, which is easy to comprehend by the reader.

Equipment and Supplies:
- Computer or word processor
- Word processing software
- Draft paper
- Letterhead
- Printer
- Pen or pencil
- Highlighter
- Envelope
- Correspondence to be answered
- Other pertinent information needed to compose a letter
- Electronic or hard cover dictionary and thesaurus
- Writer's handbook
- Portfolio

Standards: Complete the procedure and all critical steps in ________ minutes with a minimum score of ________ % within three attempts.

Scoring: Divide points earned by total possible points. Failure to perform a critical step that is indicated with an asterisk (*), will result in an unsatisfactory overall score.

Time began ________ **Time ended** ________

Steps	Possible Points	First Attempt	Second Attempt	Third Attempt
1. Read through any correspondence to be answered and highlight the specific questions that should be addressed.	10			
2. Make any necessary notes on the letter or a copy of the letter. A scrap sheet of paper may be used.	10			
3. Prepare a draft of the letter and save it in the computer or word processor, using good grammatical skills.	10			
4. Proofread a printed copy of the letter, using proofreader's marks to make corrections.	10			
5. Make any necessary corrections.	10			
6. Allow the physician or other interested party to proofread the letter, if the medical assistant is not the person whose signature will appear at the bottom.	10			

Steps	Possible Points	First Attempt	Second Attempt	Third Attempt
7. Make any final changes, then print the letter on stationery. Allow the person whose name appears at the bottom to sign the letter.	20			
8. Address the envelope using OCR guidelines and place the letter and any supporting documents inside.	10			
9. Mail the letter using correct postage.	10			

Comments:

Total Points Earned ________ Divided by ________ Total Possible Points = ________ % Score

Instructor's Signature ____________________

Student Name ______________________ Date ____________ Score ____________

Procedure 12-2 Proofreading Written Correspondence

Task: To compose a clearly written, grammatically correct business letter, which is easily understandable by the reader, and to eliminate spelling errors.

Equipment and Supplies:
- Stationary
- Computer or typewriter
- Correspondence to be answered or notes

Standards: Complete the procedure and all critical steps in ____________ minutes with a minimum score of ____________ % within three attempts.

Scoring: Divide points earned by total possible points. Failure to perform a critical step that is indicated with an asterisk (*), will result in an unsatisfactory overall score.

Time began ____________ **Time ended** ____________

Steps	Possible Points	First Attempt	Second Attempt	Third Attempt
1. Place the stationary into the printer or typewriter.	10			
2. Scan through the letter to be answered or the notes about the correspondence to be written and highlight any questions that should be answered or points to be made.	10			
3. Write the letter using grammatical guidelines.	10			
4. Print a draft copy of the letter. Read it carefully and highlight changes to be made or note any additions to be made. Use proofreaders' marks.	20			
5. Revise the letter using the notes.	10			
6. Read the letter once again on the screen. Complete a spell and grammatical check if those tools are available on the computer.	10			
7. Print a final draft. Read the letter word-for-word and check once again for errors.	10			
8. Have another person proofread especially important correspondence.	10			
9. Complete the final preparations for mailing the letter. Address the letter using guidelines for OCR and fast processing at the post office.	10			

Comments:

Total Points Earned ________ Divided by ________ Total Possible Points = ________ % Score

Instructor's Signature ________________________

Student Name ________________ Date ________ Score ________

Procedure 12-3 Preparing a FAX for Transmission

Task: To send a FAX from the medical office and assure that it arrives at its destination in a confidential manner.

Equipment and Supplies:
- FAX machine
- FAX cover sheet
- Correspondence to be sent

Standards: Complete the procedure and all critical steps in ________ minutes with a minimum score of ________ % within three attempts.

Scoring: Divide points earned by total possible points. Failure to perform a critical step that is indicated with an asterisk (*), will result in an unsatisfactory overall score.

Time began ________ **Time ended** ________

Steps	Possible Points	First Attempt	Second Attempt	Third Attempt
1. Fill out a FAX cover sheet. Include the name of the person sending the FAX, and the person's phone number. List the name of the person to receive the FAX and the FAX number where the document is being sent. Use cover sheets that contain a confidentiality statement.	20			
2. Note the number of pages that are being sent, including the cover page.	20			
3. Turn the last page upside down and write the fax number on the top of the document. Many machines require the documents to be in place prior to starting the fax. This allows the user to see the number without having to memorize it and make an error.	20			
4. Follow the instructions for individual FAX machines.	20			
5. Be sure the machine is set to provide a verification that the fax went through. Print the verification and attach it to the fax. Verify the arrival of critical FAX documents on the phone. File the fax and verification sheet in the appropriate location.	20			

Comments:

Total Points Earned ________ Divided by ________ Total Possible Points = ________ % Score

Instructor's Signature ______________________

Student Name ______________________ Date ____________ Score ____________

Procedure 12-4 Opening the Daily Mail

Task: To sort through the mail that arrives in the medical office on a daily basis in an efficient way.

Equipment and Supplies:
- Computer or word processor
- Letterhead stationary
- Pen or pencil
- Highlighter
- Staple remover
- Paper clips
- Letter opener
- Date stamp
- Draft paper
- Stapler
- Transparent tape

Standards: Complete the procedure and all critical steps in ____________ minutes with a minimum score of ____________ % within three attempts.

Scoring: Divide points earned by total possible points. Failure to perform a critical step that is indicated with an asterisk (*), will result in an unsatisfactory overall score.

Time began ____________ **Time ended** ____________

Steps	Possible Points	First Attempt	Second Attempt	Third Attempt
1. Sort the mail according to importance and urgency: • Physician's personal mail • Ordinary First Class mail • Checks from patients • Periodicals and newspapers • All other pieces, including drug samples	10			
2. Open the mail neatly and in an organized manner.	10			
3. Stack the envelopes so that they are all facing in the same direction.	10			
4. Pick up the top one and tap the envelope so that when you open it you will not cut the contents.	10			
5. Open all envelopes along the top edge for easiest removal of contents.	10			
6. Remove the contents of each envelope and hold the envelope to the light to see that nothing remains inside.	10			
7. Make a note of the postmark when this is important.	10			

Steps	Possible Points	First Attempt	Second Attempt	Third Attempt
8. Discard the envelope after you have checked to see that there is a return address on the message contained inside. Some offices make it a policy to attach the envelope to each piece of correspondence until it has received attention.	**10**			
9. Date stamp the letter and attach any enclosures.	**10**			
10. If there is an enclosure notation at the bottom of the letter, check to be certain that the enclosure was included. Should it be missing, indicate this on the notation by writing the word ***no*** and circling it.	**10**			

Comments:

Total Points Earned ________ Divided by ________ Total Possible Points = ________ % Score

Instructor's Signature ______________________

Student Name ______________________ Date ____________ Score ________

Procedure 12-5 Addressing Outgoing Mail Using U.S. Post Office OCR Guidelines

Task: To correctly address business correspondence so that the mail arrives and is processed by the U.S. Post Office as efficiently as possible.

Equipment and Supplies
- Envelopes
- Computer or typewriter
- Correspondence

Standards: Complete the procedure and all critical steps in ____________ minutes with a minimum score of ____________ % within three attempts.

Scoring: Divide points earned by total possible points. Failure to perform a critical step that is indicated with an asterisk (*), will result in an unsatisfactory overall score.

Time began ____________ **Time ended** ____________

Steps	Possible Points	First Attempt	Second Attempt	Third Attempt
1. Place the envelope into the printer or typewriter.	10			
2. Enter the word processing program, such as Microsoft Word, and check the "Tools" section for envelopes. If this is not available in the word processing program, or a typewriter is being used, judge the area on the envelope that can be read by the optical character reader (OCR). The address block should start no higher than $2\frac{3}{4}$ inches from the bottom. Leave a bottom margin of at least 5/8 inch and left and right margins of at least 1 inch. Nothing should be written or printed below the address block or to the right of it.	20			
3. Use dark type on a light background, no script or italics, and capitalize everything in the address.	10			
4. Type the address in block format, using only approved abbreviations and eliminating all punctuation.*	20			
5. Type the city, state, and zip code on the last line of the address.	10			
6. No line should have more than 27 total characters, including spaces.	10			

Steps	Possible Points	First Attempt	Second Attempt	Third Attempt
7. Leave a 5/8″ by 4¾″ space blank in the bottom right corner of the envelope.	10			
8. Mail addressed to other countries includes the city and postal code on the third line, and the name of the country on a fourth line.	10			

Comments:

Total Points Earned ________ Divided by ________ Total Possible Points = ________ % Score

Instructor's Signature ____________________

Student Name ______________________ Date ____________ Score ________

Procedure 13-1 Initiating a Medical File for a New Patient

Task: To initiate a medical file for a new patient that will contain all the personal data necessary for a complete medical record and any other information required by the agency.

Equipment and Supplies:
- Computer or typewriter
- Clerical supplies
- Information on filing system
- Registration form
- File Folder
- Label
- ID card for numeric system
- Cross-reference card
- Financial card
- Routing slip or encounter form
- Private conference area

Standards: Complete the procedure and all critical steps in ____________ minutes with a minimum score of ____________ % within three attempts.

Scoring: Divide points earned by total possible points. Failure to perform a critical step that is indicated with an asterisk (*), will result in an unsatisfactory overall score.

Time began ____________ **Time ended** ____________

Steps	Possible Points	First Attempt	Second Attempt	Third Attempt
1. Determine that the patient is new to the office.	10			
2. Obtain and record the required personal data.	10			
3. Type the information onto the patient history form.	10			
4. Review entire form.	10			
5. Select label and file folder for the record.	10			
6. Type the caption on the label and apply to folder	10			
7. For numeric filing, prepare a cross-reference.	10			
8. Prepare the financial card or enter into a computerized ledger.	10			
9. Place the patient's history and other required forms in the folder.	10			
10. Clip an encounter form or routing slip on the outside of the folder	10			

Comments:

Total Points Earned ________ Divided by ________ Total Possible Points = ________ % Score

Instructor's Signature ________________________

Student Name ______________ Date ______________ Score ______________

Procedure 13-2 Preparing an Informed Consent for Treatment Form

Task: To adequately and completely inform the patient regarding the treatment or procedure that he or she is to receive, and provide legal protection for the facility and the provider.

Equipment and Supplies:
- Pen
- Consent form

Standards: Complete the procedure and all critical steps in ______________ minutes with a minimum score of ______________ % within three attempts.

Scoring: Divide points earned by total possible points. Failure to perform a critical step that is indicated with an asterisk (*), will result in an unsatisfactory overall score.

Time began ______________ **Time ended** ______________

Steps	Possible Points	First Attempt	Second Attempt	Third Attempt
1. After the physician provides the details of the procedure to be done, prepare the consent form. Be sure that the form addresses the following: a. the nature of the procedure or treatment b. the risks and/or benefits of the procedure or treatment c. any reasonable alternatives to the procedure or treatment d. the risks and/or benefits of each alternative e. the risks and/or benefits of not performing the procedure or treatment	**20**			
2. Personalize the form with the patient's name and any other demographic information that the form lists.	**10**			
3. Deliver the form to the physician for use as the patient is counseled about the procedure.	**10**			
4. Witness the signature of the patient on the form, if necessary. The physician will usually sign the form as well.	**10**			
5. Provide a copy of the consent form to the patient.	**10**			
6. Place the consent form in the patient's chart. The facility where the procedure is to be performed may require a copy.	**10**			

Steps	Possible Points	First Attempt	Second Attempt	Third Attempt
7. Ask the patient if he or she has any questions about the procedure. Refer questions that the medical assistant cannot or should not answer to the physician. Be sure that all of the questions expressed by the patient are answered.	**20**			
8. Provide information regarding the date and time for the procedure to the patient.	**10**			

Comments:

Total Points Earned ________ Divided by ________ Total Possible Points = ________ % Score

Instructor's Signature ______________________

Student Name ______________ Date ______________ Score ______________

Procedure 13-3 Adding Supplementary Items to Established Patient Files

Task: To initiate a medical file for a new patient that will contain all the personal data necessary for a complete medical record and any other information required by the agency.

Equipment and Supplies:
- Computer or typewriter
- Clerical supplies, sorter, stapler
- Information on filing system
- Mending tape
- Patient file folders
- Assorted correspondence and reports
- File stamp and a pen

Standards: Complete the procedure and all critical steps in ______________ minutes with a minimum score of ______________ % within three attempts.

Scoring: Divide points earned by total possible points. Failure to perform a critical step that is indicated with an asterisk (*), will result in an unsatisfactory overall score.

Time began ______________ **Time ended** ______________

Steps	Possible Points	First Attempt	Second Attempt	Third Attempt
1. Group all papers according to patients' names.*	20			
2. Remove and pins or paper clips.	10			
3. Mend and damaged or torn records.	10			
4. Attach any small items to standard-sized paper.	10			
5. Staple any related papers together.	10			
6. Place your initials or FILE stamp in the upper left corner.	10			
7. Code the document by underlining or writing the patient's name in the upper right corner.	10			
8. Continue steps 2-7 until all documents have been conditioned, released, indexed, and coded.	10			
9. Place all documents in the sorter in filing sequence.	10			

Comments:

Total Points Earned ________ Divided by ________ Total Possible Points = ________ % Score

Instructor's Signature ____________________

Student Name ______________________ Date ______________ Score ______________

Procedure 13-4 Preparing a Record Release Form

Task: To provide a legal document to another provider or healthcare facility that indicates the patient's consent to the release of his or her medical records.

Equipment and Supplies:
- Medical record release form
- Pen
- Envelope

Standards: Complete the procedure and all critical steps in ______________ minutes with a minimum score of ______________ % within three attempts.

Scoring: Divide points earned by total possible points. Failure to perform a critical step that is indicated with an asterisk (*), will result in an unsatisfactory overall score.

Time began ______________ **Time ended** ______________

Steps	Possible Points	First Attempt	Second Attempt	Third Attempt
1. Explain to the patient that a medical record release form will be necessary to obtain records from another provider. If the patient is having records sent to another provider, a release will also be required.	20			
2. Review the record release form with the patient and ask if the form is understood or if there are any questions about the form.	20			
3. Have the patient sign the form in the space indicated. If other demographic information is required, such as a social security number or other names used, complete that information as well.	20			
4. Make a copy of the form for the file and then mail it to the appropriate facility. Note the date that the form was sent. Provide a copy to the patient if requested.	20			
5. Follow-up to assure that the requested records actually arrived.	20			

Comments:

Total Points Earned ________ Divided by ________ Total Possible Points = ________ % Score

Instructor's Signature ________________________

Student Name ________________ Date ________ Score ________

Procedure 13-5 Transcribing a Machine-Dictated Letter Using a Computer or Word Processor

Task: To transcribe a machine-dictated letter into a mailable document without error or detectable corrections, using a computer or word processor.

Equipment and Supplies:
- Word processor, computer, or typewriter
- Transcribing machine
- Stationary
- Reference manual

Standards: Complete the procedure and all critical steps in ________ minutes with a minimum score of ________ % within three attempts.

Scoring: Divide points earned by total possible points. Failure to perform a critical step that is indicated with an asterisk (*), will result in an unsatisfactory overall score.

Time began ________ **Time ended** ________

Steps	**Possible Points**	**First Attempt**	**Second Attempt**	**Third Attempt**
1. Assemble supplies.	**10**			
2. Set up the format for selected letter style.	**20**			
3. Keyboard the text while listening to the dictation.	**20**			
4. Edit the letter on the monitor.	**20**			
5. Execute a spell check.	**20**			
6. Direct the document to a printer.	**10**			

Comments:

Total Points Earned ________ Divided by ________ Total Possible Points = ________ % Score

Instructor's Signature ________________

Student Name ______________________ Date ____________ Score ________

Procedure 13-6 Filing Medical Records and Documents Using the Alphabetical System

Task: To file records efficiently using an alphabetical system and assure that the records can be easily and quickly retrieved.

Equipment and Supplies:
- Medical records
- Physical filing equipment
- Cart to carry records, if needed
- Alphabetic file guide
- Staple remover
- Stapler
- Paper clips

Standards: Complete the procedure and all critical steps in ____________ minutes with a minimum score of ____________ % within three attempts.

Scoring: Divide points earned by total possible points. Failure to perform a critical step that is indicated with an asterisk (*), will result in an unsatisfactory overall score.

Time began ____________ **Time ended** ____________

Steps	**Possible Points**	**First Attempt**	**Second Attempt**	**Third Attempt**
1. Using alphabetical guidelines, place the records to be filed in alphabetical order. If a stack of documents is to be filed, place them in alphabetical order inside an alphabetic file guide or sorter. Use rules for filing documents alphabetically.	20			
2. Go to the filing storage equipment (shelves, cabinets, or drawers) and locate the spot in the alphabet for the first file.	20			
3. Place the file in the cabinet or drawer in correct alphabetical order.	20			
4. If adding a document to a file, place it on top, so that the most recent information is seen first. This puts the information in the file in reverse chronological order.	20			
5. Securely fasten documents to the chart. Do not just drop the documents inside the chart. Refile the chart in its proper place.	20			

Comments:

Total Points Earned ________ Divided by ________ Total Possible Points = ________ % Score

Instructor's Signature ______________________

Student Name ______________________ Date ____________ Score ____________

Procedure 13-7 Filing Medical Records and Documents Using the Numeric System

Task: To file records efficiently using a numeric system and assure that the records can be easily and quickly retrieved.

Equipment and Supplies:
- Medical records
- Physical filing equipment
- Cart to carry records, if needed
- Numeric file guide
- Staple remover
- Stapler
- Paper clips

Standards: Complete the procedure and all critical steps in ____________ minutes with a minimum score of ____________ % within three attempts.

Scoring: Divide points earned by total possible points. Failure to perform a critical step that is indicated with an asterisk (*), will result in an unsatisfactory overall score.

Time began ____________ **Time ended** ____________

Steps	Possible Points	First Attempt	Second Attempt	Third Attempt
1. Using numeric guidelines, place the records to be filed in numeric order. If a stack of documents is to be filed, write the chart number on the document. Use rules for filing documents alphabetically.	20			
2. Go to the filing storage equipment (shelves, cabinets, or drawers) and locate the numeric spot for the first file.	20			
3. Place the file in the cabinet or drawer in correct numeric order.	20			
4. If adding a document to a file, place it on top, so that the most recent information is seen first. This puts the information in the file in reverse chronological order.	20			
5. Securely fasten documents to the chart. Do not just drop the documents inside the chart.	20			

Comments:

Total Points Earned ________ Divided by ________ Total Possible Points = ________ % Score

Instructor's Signature ______________________

Student Name ______________ Date ______________ Score ______________

Procedure 13-8 Color Coding Patient Charts

Task: To color code patient charts using the agecy's established coding system to effectively facilitate filing and finding.

Equipment and Supplies:
- 20 Patient charts
- Information on filing system
- 20 file folders
- Full range of color labels

Standards: Complete the procedure and all critical steps in ______________ minutes with a minimum score of ______________ % within three attempts.

Scoring: Divide points earned by total possible points. Failure to perform a critical step that is indicated with an asterisk (*), will result in an unsatisfactory overall score.

Time began ______________ **Time ended** ______________

Steps	**Possible Points**	**First Attempt**	**Second Attempt**	**Third Attempt**
1. Assemble patient charts.	10			
2. Arrange charts in indexing order.	15			
3. Pick up the first chart and note the second letter of the surname.	15			
4. Chose a folder and/or caption label of the appropriate color.	15			
5. Type the patients' name on label in indexing order and apply to folder tab.	15			
6. Repeat steps 4 and 5 until all charts have been coded.	15			
7. Check any group for any isolated color.	15			

Comments:

Total Points Earned ______________ Divided by ______________ Total Possible Points = ______________ % Score

Instructor's Signature ______________

Student Name ______________________ Date __________ Score __________

Procedure 14-1 Explaining Professional Fees

Task: To explain the physician's fees so that the patient understands his or her obligations and rights for privacy.

Equipment and Supplies:
- Patient's statement
- Copy of physician's fee schedule
- Quiet, private area with the patient feels free to ask questions

Standards: Complete the procedure and all critical steps in __________ minutes with a minimum score of __________ % within three attempts.

Scoring: Divide points earned by total possible points. Failure to perform a critical step that is indicated with an asterisk (*), will result in an unsatisfactory overall score.

Time began __________ **Time ended** __________

Steps	Possible Points	First Attempt	Second Attempt	Third Attempt
1. Determine that the patient has the correct bill.	10			
2. Examine the bill for possible errors.	15			
3. Refer to the fee schedule for services rendered.	15			
4. Explain itemized billing: • Date of each service • Type of service rendered • Fee	15			
5. Display a professional attitude toward the patient.	15			
6. Determine whether the patient has specific concerns that may hinder payment.	15			
7. Make appropriate arrangements for a discussion between the physician and patient if further explanation is necessary for resolution of the problem.	15			

Comments:

Total Points Earned __________ Divided by __________ Total Possible Points = __________ % Score

Instructor's Signature ______________________

Student Name ______________________ Date ____________ Score ________

Procedure 14-2 Posting Service Charges and Payments Using Pegboard

Task: To post one day's charges and payments and computer the daily bookkeeping cycle using a pegboard.

Equipment and Supplies:
- Patient's statement
- Calculator
- Pen
- Daysheet
- Carbon
- Receipts
- Ledger cards
- Balances from previous day

Standards: Complete the procedure and all critical steps in ____________ minutes with a minimum score of ____________ % within three attempts.

Scoring: Divide points earned by total possible points. Failure to perform a critical step that is indicated with an asterisk (*), will result in an unsatisfactory overall score.

Time began ____________ **Time ended** ____________

Steps	**Possible Points**	**First Attempt**	**Second Attempt**	**Third Attempt**
1. Prepare the board: • Place a new daysheet on the board. • Cover daysheet with carbon. • Place bank of receipts over the pegs, aligning the top receipt with the first open writing line on the daysheet.	5			
2. Carry forward balances from the previous day.	5			
3. Pull ledger cards for patient being seen today.	5			
4. Insert the ledger card under the first receipt, aligning the first available writing line of the card with the carbonized strip on the receipt.	5			
5. Enter the patientís name, the date, receipt number, and any existing balance from the ledger card.	5			
6. Detach the charge slip from the receipt and clip it to the patientís chart.	5			
7. Accept the returned charge slip at the end of the visit.	5			
8. Enter the appropriate fee from the fee schedule.	5			

Steps	Possible Points	First Attempt	Second Attempt	Third Attempt
9. Locate the receipt on the board with a number matching the charge slip.	5			
10. Reinsert the patientís ledger card under the receipt.	5			
11. Write the service code number and fee on the receipt.	5			
12. Accept the patient's payment and record the amount of payment and the new balance.	5			
13. Give the completed receipt to the patient.	5			
14. Follow your agency's procedure for refilling the ledger card.	5			
15. Repeat step 4 to 14 for each service of the day.	10			
16. Total all columns of the daysheet at the end of the day.	5			
17. Write preliminary totals in pencil.	5			
18. Complete proof of totals and enter totals in ink.	5			
19 Enter figures for accounts receivable control.	5			

Comments:

Total Points Earned ________ Divided by ________ Total Possible Points = ________ % Score

Instructor's Signature ________________

Student Name ______________________ Date ______________ Score __________

Procedure 14-3 Making Credit Arrangements with a Patient

Task: To assist the patient in paying for services by making mutually beneficial credit arrangements according to established office policy.

Equipment and Supplies:
- Patient's ledger
- Calendar
- Truth in lending form
- Assignment of benefits form
- Patient's insurance form
- Private area for interview

Standards: Complete the procedure and all critical steps in ______________ minutes with a minimum score of ______________ % within three attempts.

Scoring: Divide points earned by total possible points. Failure to perform a critical step that is indicated with an asterisk (*), will result in an unsatisfactory overall score.

Time began ______________ **Time ended** ______________

Steps	**Possible Points**	**First Attempt**	**Second Attempt**	**Third Attempt**
1. Answer all questions about credit thoroughly and kindly.	**10**			
2. Inform the patient of the office policy regarding credit: • Payment at the time of first visit • Payment by bank card • Credit application	**20**			
3. Have the patient complete the credit application.	**10**			
4. Check the completed credit application.	**10**			
5. Discuss with the patient the possible arrangements and ask the patient to decide which of those arrangements is most suitable.	**10**			
6. Prepare the truth in lending form and have the patient sign it if the agreement requires more than four installments.	**10**			
7. Have the patient execute an assignment of insurance benefits.	**10**			
8. Make a copy of the patient's insurance ID and have the patient's sign a consent for release of the information to the insurance company.	**10**			
9. Keep credit information confidential.	**10**			

Comments:

Total Points Earned ________ Divided by ________ Total Possible Points = ________ % Score

Instructor's Signature ________________________

Student Name ________________ Date ________ Score ________

Procedure 14-4 Preparing Monthly Billing Statements

Task: To Process monthly statements and evaluate accounts for collection procedures in accordance with the agency's credit policy.

Equipment and Supplies:
- Typewriter or computer
- Patient accounts
- Agency's credit policy
- Statement forms

Standards: Complete the procedure and all critical steps in ________ minutes with a minimum score of ________ % within three attempts.

Scoring: Divide points earned by total possible points. Failure to perform a critical step that is indicated with an asterisk (*), will result in an unsatisfactory overall score.

Time began ________ **Time ended** ________

Steps	**Possible Points**	**First Attempt**	**Second Attempt**	**Third Attempt**
1. Assemble all accounts that have outstanding balances.	**20**			
2. Separate accounts that need special attention in accordance with the agency's credit policy.	**20**			
3. Prepare routine statements, including • Date the statement is prepared • Name and address of the person responsible for payment • Name of the patient, if different from the person responsible for payment • Itemization of dates, services, and charges for the month • Any unpaid balance carried forward (may or may not be itemized, depending on office policy)	**20**			
4. Determine the action to be taken on accounts separated in step 2.	**20**			
5. Make a note of the necessary action on the ledger card (telephone call, collection letter series, small claims court, or assignment of collection agency).	**20**			

Comments:

Total Points Earned ________ Divided by ________ Total Possible Points = ________ % Score

Instructor's Signature ______________________

Student Name ______________________ Date ______________ Score ______________

Procedure 14-5 Aging Accounts Receivable

Task: To determine the age of accounts and decide what collection activity is needed.

Equipment and Supplies
- Patient ledger cards with a balance due
- Pen
- Computer
- Calculator

Standards: Complete the procedure and all critical steps in ______________ minutes with a minimum score of ______________ % within three attempts.

Scoring: Divide points earned by total possible points. Failure to perform a critical step that is indicated with an asterisk (*), will result in an unsatisfactory overall score.

Time began ______________ **Time ended** ______________

Steps	Possible Points	First Attempt	Second Attempt	Third Attempt
1. Prompt the computer to compile a report on the age of accounts receivable. Many programs will have this report option that can be easily accessed.	10			
2. Divide the accounts into categories as listed below: • 0 to 30 days old • 30 to 60 days old • 60 to 90 days old • 90 to 120 days old • over 120 days old	20			
3. If the computer program does not perform this function, manually pull all ledger cards that have a balance due and divide them into the categories as listed above.	10			
4. Examine the accounts to see which are awaiting an insurance payment. Action need not be taken if an insurance payment is expected and is not long overdue. Return those ledgers to the ledger tray.	10			
5. Follow the office procedure for collections on the accounts left. Collection reminder stickers may be placed on the statements sent to the patient, or a collection letter may be sent. Be sure that the stickers are inside the envelope, not on the outside.	10			

Steps	Possible Points	First Attempt	Second Attempt	Third Attempt
6. Call patients whose accounts are over 90 days old. Attempt to make payment arrangements with the patient.	10			
7. Send a collection letter to patients whose accounts are over 120 days old, if indicated, to encourage the patient to pay the account. If it is the office policy, mention that the account is in danger of being sent to a collection agency.	10			
8. Add the total accounts receivable for each category and arrive at a figure outstanding for each. The physician may wish to have a report weekly or monthly on these figures.	10			
9. Note any arrangements made with patients regarding payment of the accounts in the chart and/or on the ledger. Send a follow-up letter to remind the patients of their payment agreements.	10			

Comments:

Total Points Earned ________ Divided by ________ Total Possible Points = ________ % Score

Instructor's Signature ____________________

Student Name ____________ Date ____________ Score ____________

Procedure 15-1 Assigning ICD-9-CM Codes

Task: To assign the proper ICD-9-CM code based on a medical documentation for auditing and billing purposes.

Equipment and Supplies:
- Patient medical record
- Current ICD-9-CM code book
- Medical dictionary

Standards: Complete the procedure and all critical steps in ____________ minutes with a minimum score of ____________ % within three attempts.

Scoring: Divide points earned by total possible points. Failure to perform a critical step that is indicated with an asterisk (*), will result in an unsatisfactory overall score.

Time began ____________ **Time ended** ____________

Steps	**Possible Points**	**First Attempt**	**Second Attempt**	**Third Attempt**
1. Identify the key term in the diagnostic statement.	20			
2. Locate the diagnosis in the alphabetic index.	10			
3. Read and understand footnotes. NOTE: This includes any symbols, instructions, or cross-references.	10			
4. Locate the diagnosis in the Tabular List.	10			
5. Read and understand the inclusions and exclusions.	10			
6. Make certain you include 4th and 5th digits where available.	10			
7. Assign the code. NOTE: All diagnosis elements need to be identified. Double-check the code to insure an accurate transfer to the patient form.	30			

Comments:

Total Points Earned ________ Divided by ________ Total Possible Points = ________ % Score

Instructor's Signature ______________________

Student Name ______________________ Date ____________ Score ________

Procedure 16-1 Assigning CPT Codes

Task: To assign the proper CPT codes based on medical documentation for auditing and billing purposes.

Equipment and Supplies:
- Patient medical record
- Current CPT code book
- Medical dictionary

Standards: Complete the procedure and all critical steps in ____________ minutes with a minimum score of ____________ % within three attempts.

Scoring: Divide points earned by total possible points. Failure to perform a critical step that is indicated with an asterisk (*), will result in an unsatisfactory overall score.

Time began ____________ **Time ended** ____________

Steps	Possible Points	First Attempt	Second Attempt	Third Attempt
1. Identify if the patient is new or established. NOTE: An office (or outpatient) visit for the evaluation and management of a new patient requires these three key components: • A detailed history • A detailed examination • Medical decision-making of low complexity	10			
2. Indicate where the patient is being seen.	10			
3. Determine whether the visit is a consultation.	10			
4. Determine whether the visit is due to illness or is a preventative medical service.	10			
5. Determine the level of history.	10			
6. Determine the level of examination.	10			
7. Determine the level of medical decision making.	10			
8. Assign the most accurate CPT code.	30			

Comments:

Total Points Earned ________ Divided by ________ Total Possible Points = ________ % Score

Instructor's Signature ______________________

Student Name ______________________ Date ____________ Score ________

Procedure 17-1 Completing the Insurance Claim Form

Task: To accurately complete a CMS-1500 (formerly HCFA-1500) claim form.

Equipment and Supplies:
- Patient information form
- Photocopy of patient's insurance ID card
- Encounter Form
- Patient record
- Patient's ledger
- CMS-1500 form
- Typewriter or computer

Standards: Complete the procedure and all critical steps in ____________ minutes with a minimum score of ____________ % within three attempts.

Scoring: Divide points earned by total possible points. Failure to perform a critical step that is indicated with an asterisk (*), will result in an unsatisfactory overall score.

Time began ____________ **Time ended** ____________

Steps	Possible Points	First Attempt	Second Attempt	Third Attempt
Patient/Insured Section				
Block 1 Check the type of health insurance coverage applicable to the claim.	2			
Block 1a Enter the patient's insurance identification number or Medicare ID number exactly as it appears on his/her insurance card.	2			
Block 2 Enter the patient's last name, first name and middle initial following OCR guidelines.	2			
Block 3 Enter the patient's birth date in MM DD YYYY format, and enter an "x" in the appropriate box for gender.	2			
Block 4 For commercial and Blue Cross/Blue Shield claims, enter "SAME" if patient and insured (policy-holder) are the same person. If the insured's name is different from the patient, enter the last name, first name, and middle initial in this block. If there is insurance primary to Medicare, list the name of the insured here. If Medicare is primary, leave blank. For CHAMPUS/TRICARE, enter the "sponsor's" name.	2			
Block 5 Enter the patient's street address on the first line, city and state on the second line, and the zip code and telephone number on the third line. Remember to use all capital letters and no punctuation.	2			

Steps	Possible Points	First Attempt	Second Attempt	Third Attempt
Block 6 Check the appropriate box for the patient's relationship to insured. If Medicare is primary, leave blank.	2			
Block 7 Enter the insured's address and telephone number, unless the insured and the patient are the same, in which case enter "SAME." Complete this item only when Blocks 4 and 11 are completed. For Medicare and Medicaid, leave blank.	2			
Block 8 Check the appropriate box for the patient's marital status and whether employed or a student.	2			
Block 9 (Required if 11d is marked "yes".) If the patient has other medical insurance coverage, and he/she is not the insured, enter the insured's name, and complete boxes 9a through 9d. If there is no other insurance, leave 9a through 9d blank and proceed to Block 10.	2			
Block 9a Enter the policy or group number of the insured's secondary insurance coverage. If the secondary policy is Medigap, enter the policy and/or group number preceded by **MEDIGAP.**	2			
Block 9b Enter the insured's birth date in MM DD YYYY format, and enter an "x" in the appropriate gender box.	2			
Block 9c Enter the name of the insured's employer or school, if applicable. Leave blank if a Medigap PayerID is entered in item 9d. Otherwise, enter the claims processing address of the Medigap insurer.	2			
Block 9d Enter the name of the secondary insurance plan or program. If the secondary insurer is a Medigap policy, enter the 9-digit PayerID number of the Medigap insurer. If there is no PayerID number, enter the Medigap insurance program or plan name.	2			
Block 10 Check the appropriate boxes in this section to identify whether the patient's condition was related to either his/her employment, auto accident, or other accident.	2			
Block 10a Check "no" unless the illness, accident, or injury was the result of employment or occurred on the job or in the process of performing one's job.	2			
Block 10b Check "no" unless the claim is due to an injury resulting from an automobile accident. In the case of an auto accident, enter the two-letter state code where the accident occurred.	2			

Steps	Possible Points	First Attempt	Second Attempt	Third Attempt
Block 10c Enter an "x" in the appropriate box.	2			
Block 10d This block is usually reserved for Medicaid as secondary payor claims. In some states, this block is used only if the patient is entitled to Medicaid. If this is the case, enter the patient's Medicaid number preceded by MCD. For Medicare, leave blank. Some third party payors want the word "attachment(s)" entered into this field if there are attachments included with the claim.	2			
Block 11 For commercial carriers, enter the group policy name/number from the patient's card. For BC/BS and Medicaid, leave blank. For insurance primary to Medicare, enter the insured's policy or group number. If Medicare is primary, the word "NONE" must appear in this block. By doing so indicates that Medicare is primary.	2			
NOTE: For a claim to be considered for Medicare Secondary Payer, a copy of the primary payer's explanation of benefits (EOB) must be included with the claim form.	2			
Block 11a Enter the insured's birth date and sex if different from Block 3. For Medicare and Medicaid, leave blank.	2			
Block 11b Enter the employer's name if applicable. On Medicare claims, if there is a second policy and the insured's status is retired, enter the date of retirement preceded by the word "RETIRED."	2			
Block 11c Enter the 9-digit Payer ID number of the primary insurer. If no such number exists, enter the complete name of the primary payer's program or plan name.	2			
Block 11d Check "no" if patient is covered by only one insurance policy. If the answer is "yes," give the name of the company and any other information available in Block 9. For Medicare and Medicaid, leave blank.	2			
Block 12 The patient or authorized person must sign and date this item unless a signature is on file. If this is the case, the words "SIGNATURE ON FILE" should be entered here. Leave blank on Medicaid claims.	2			
Block 13 The patient or authorized person should sign and date this item if he or she agrees that benefits are to be paid directly to the provider. For Medicare supplements and cross-over claims, "SIGNATURE ON FILE" must also appear in this block. For Medicaid, leave blank.	2			

Steps	Possible Points	First Attempt	Second Attempt	Third Attempt
Physician/Supplier Information				
Block 14 Enter the date of the first symptom of the current illness, injury, or pregnancy in this block if one is documented in the chart notes or the date of the last menstrual cycle if the claim is related to pregnancy.	2			
Block 15 Enter the date the patient was first treated for this condition. Leave blank for Medicare claims.	2			
Block 16 Enter date(s) patient unable to work in current occupation if it is a workers' compensation claim. Not required for most other carriers.	2			
Block 17 Enter the name of the referring (or ordering) physician, if applicable.	2			
Block 17a Enter the UPIN/NPI number of the referring/ordering physician listed in Block 17.	2			
Block 18 If the claim is for a related hospital stay, enter the dates of hospital admission and discharge. If the patient has not been discharged, leave the "to" box blank.	2			
Block 19 This block is usually left blank. Some private payors insert the word "attachment(s)" when specific documentation accompanies the claim.	2			
Block 20 If laboratory procedures are listed on the claim in Block 24, and these services were performed in the provider's facility, the "NO" box in is checked with an "x" or left blank. If lab work shown on the claim was done by an outside lab and billed to the provider, check the "YES" box, and enter the total amount of the charges. Leave this block blank if no lab tests were done.	2			
Block 21 Enter the patient's diagnosis(es) using ICD-9-CM code number(s), listing the primary diagnosis first. Up to four codes (in priority order) can be entered in Block 21.	2			
Block 22 Required only for replacement claims for Medicaid. Enter the appropriate 3-digit replacement code followed by the 17-digit transaction control number of the most current incorrectly paid claim.	2			
Block 23 For private and commercial carriers and Medicaid, enter the 10-digit prior authorization number for those procedures requiring prior approval assigned by the peer review organization (PRO). Consult the specific guidelines for the payor to whom the claim is being submitted.	2			

Steps	Possible Points	First Attempt	Second Attempt	Third Attempt
Block 24a The first date of service for the charge on this line should be placed in the "From" column. When a claim is for more than one day of the same service on a line item, the days must be in consecutive order. The last date of service is required in the "To" column. Enter the month, day, and year (in the MM DD YYYY format) for each procedure, service, or supply. When "from" and "to" dates are shown for a series of identical services, enter the number of days or units in 24G.	2			
Block 24b Enter the appropriate place of service code.	2			
Block 24c Enter the appropriate type of service code. NOTE: For private payors and Medicare, leave blank. All others, refer to specific guidelines.	2			
Block 24d Enter the procedure, service, or supply code using appropriate 5-digit CPT or HCPCS procedure code. Enter a two-position modifier when applicable.	2			
Block 24e Link the procedure/service code back to the diagnosis code in Block 21 by indicating the applicable number of the diagnosis code (1, 2, 3 or 4) to that line's procedure code.	2			
Block 24f Enter the charge for each listed procedure, supply, and /or service.	2			
Block 24g Enter the number of days or units. If only one service is performed, enter the number 1.	2			
Block 24h Leave blank for all claims with the exception of certain Medicaid claims.	2			
Block 24i For certain carriers, enter an "X" or "E" as appropriate if documentation indicates a medical emergency existed. Leave blank for Medicare claims.	2			
Block 24j For commercial claims, BC/BS, Medicare, Medicaid, and TRICARE, leave blank. (Refer to specific third-payor guidelines.)	2			
Block 24k Enter the five-digit number that has been assigned when the provider was approved by the third-party payor. For Medicare, it is referred to as the "billing number." Blue Cross-Blue Shield and Medicaid have their own numbers. This is not the same of the UPIN number.	2			
Block 25 Enter the provider's nine-digit Federal tax identification number and check the appropriate box in this field; or, in the case of an unincorporated practice or sole proprietorship, enter the provider's social security number.	2			

Steps	Possible Points	First Attempt	Second Attempt	Third Attempt
Block 26 Enter the patient's account number as assigned by the supplier's accounting system, if available. If you are submitting the claim electronically, you are required to provide a patient account number.	2			
Block 27 Check the appropriate block to indicate whether the provider accepts assignment of benefits. If the supplier is a *participating provider* (PAR), assignment must be accepted for all covered charges. For nonPAR provider's, this can be left blank. For Medicaid, check "YES."	2			
Block 28 Total column 24f and enter the total charges in this field.	2			
Block 29 Enter the total amount, if any, that has been paid by the patient. Leave blank if no payment has been made.	2			
Block 30 Used when there is a secondary insurance. Enter the balance owing as indicated on the explanation of benefits (EOB).	2			
Block 31 Enter the signature of the provider, or his/her representative and his or her initials, and the date the form was signed. The signature may be typed, stamped, or handwritten; however, the characters should not fall outside of the block.	2			
Block 32 Enter the name and address of the facility where the services were performed if other than patient's home or physician's office. For Medicare, enter the name and address of the facility regardless of where services were provided.	2			
Block 33 Enter the provider's billing name, address, zip code, and telephone number. Also, enter the billing number (from Block 24k). Enter the Group NPI number, if the provider is a member of a group practice. Refer to specific third-payor guidelines.	2			

Comments:

Total Points Earned ________ Divided by ________ Total Possible Points = ________ % Score

Instructor's Signature ______________________

Student Name ______________________ Date ______________ Score ______________

Procedure 18-1 Obtaining a Managed Care Precertification

Task: Using the information in the case study, obtain precertification from a patient's HMO for requested services/procedures.

Equipment and Supplies:
- Patient record
- Precertification form
- Patient's insurance information
- Telephone/FAX machine
- Pen/Pencil

Standards: Complete the procedure and all critical steps in ______________ minutes with a minimum score of ______________ % within three attempts.

Scoring: Divide points earned by total possible points. Failure to perform a critical step that is indicated with an asterisk (*), will result in an unsatisfactory overall score.

Time began ______________ **Time ended** ______________

Steps	Possible Points	First Attempt	Second Attempt	Third Attempt
1. Assemble the necessary documents and equipment.	20			
2. Examine the patient record, and determine the service/procedure for which preauthorization is being requested, including the specialist's name and phone number, and the reason for the request.	20			
3. Complete the referral form, providing all pertinent information requested.	20			
4. Proofread the completed form to ascertain accuracy.	20			
5. Role play the act of faxing the completed form to the patient's insurance carrier. Place a copy of the completed form in the patient's medical record.	20			

Documentation in the Medical Record

___

___

___

___

Comments:

Total Points Earned ________ Divided by ________ Total Possible Points = ________ % Score

Instructor's Signature ____________________

Student Name ________________ Date ________ Score ________

Procedure 18-2 Obtaining a Managed Care Referral

Task: Using the information in the case study, accurately complete a referral form for the managed care patient.

Equipment and Supplies:
- Patient record
- Referral form
- Patient's insurance information
- Pen/Pencil

Standards: Complete the procedure and all critical steps in ________ minutes with a minimum score of ________ % within three attempts.

Scoring: Divide points earned by total possible points. Failure to perform a critical step that is indicated with an asterisk (*), will result in an unsatisfactory overall score.

Time began ________ **Time ended** ________

Steps	Possible Points	First Attempt	Second Attempt	Third Attempt
1. Assemble the necessary documents and equipment.	20			
2. Examine the patient record, and determine the service for which the patient is to be referred, including the specialist's name and phone number, and the reason for the referral.	20			
3. Role plan with a partner the act of telephoning the patient's insurance carrier.	20			
4. Complete the referral form, providing all information requested.	20			
5. Proofread the completed form to ascertain accuracy. Place a copy of the completed form in the patient's medical record.	20			

Documentation in the Medical Record

____

____

____

____

Comments:

Total Points Earned ________ Divided by ________ Total Possible Points = ________ % Score

Instructor's Signature ______________________

Student Name ______________________ Date ____________ Score ____________

Procedure 19-1 Writing Checks in Payment of Bills

Task: To correctly write checks for payment of bills.

Equipment and Supplies:
- Checkbook
- Bills to be paid

Standards: Complete the procedure and all critical steps in ______________ minutes with a minimum score of ______________ % within three attempts.

Scoring: Divide points earned by total possible points. Failure to perform a critical step that is indicated with an asterisk (*), will result in an unsatisfactory overall score.

Time began ______________ **Time ended** ______________

Steps	**Possible Points**	**First Attempt**	**Second Attempt**	**Third Attempt**
1. Locate bill to be paid. Fill out stub first.	**10**			
2. Complete check and stub with pen or typewriter.	**10**			
3. Date the check.	**10**			
4. Write the Payee on the appropriate line.	**10**			
5. Leave no space before the name and follow with three dashes. Omit personal titles.	**10**			
6. Enter amount correctly and in a manner that prevents alteration.*	**20**			
7. Verify amount with check stub.	**20**			
8. Make a notation on the bill that is being paid. Include date and check number. File.	**10**			

Comments:

Total Points Earned ________ Divided by ________ Total Possible Points = ________ % Score

Instructor's Signature ______________________

Student Name ______________________ Date ____________ Score ____________

Procedure 19-2 Preparing a Bank Deposit

Task: To prepare a bank deposit for the day's receipts and complete appropriate office records related to the deposit.

Equipment and Supplies:
- Currency
- Six checks for deposit
- Deposit slip
- Endorsement stamp (optional)
- Typewriter
- Envelope

Standards: Complete the procedure and all critical steps in ____________ minutes with a minimum score of ____________ % within three attempts.

Scoring: Divide points earned by total possible points. Failure to perform a critical step that is indicated with an asterisk (*), will result in an unsatisfactory overall score.

Time began ____________ **Time ended** ____________

Steps	**Possible Points**	**First Attempt**	**Second Attempt**	**Third Attempt**
1. Organize currency.	10			
2. Total the currency and record the amount on the deposit slip.	10			
3. Place restrictive endorsement on checks.*	20			
4. List each check separately on the deposit slip by ABA number or patient last name.	20			
5. Total the amount of currency and checks and enter on deposit slip.	10			
6. Enter the amount of the deposit in the checkbook.	10			
7. Keep a copy of the deposit slip for office records.	10			
8. Place currency, checks, and deposit in envelope for transport to bank.	10			

Comments:

Total Points Earned ________ Divided by ________ Total Possible Points = ________ % Score

Instructor's Signature ______________________

Student Name ______________________ Date ____________ Score ____________

Procedure 19-3 Reconciling a Bank Statement

Task: To reconcile a bank statement with checking account.

Equipment and Supplies:
- Ending balance of previous statement
- Current bank statement
- Cancelled checks for current month
- Checkbook stubs
- Calculator
- Pen

Standards: Complete the procedure and all critical steps in ____________ minutes with a minimum score of ____________ % within three attempts.

Scoring: Divide points earned by total possible points. Failure to perform a critical step that is indicated with an asterisk (*), will result in an unsatisfactory overall score.

Time began ____________ **Time ended** ____________

Steps	**Possible Points**	**First Attempt**	**Second Attempt**	**Third Attempt**
1. Compare opening balance of the new statement with the closing balance of previous statement.	**10**			
2. Compare canceled checks with items on statement.	**10**			
3. Arrange checks in numerical order and compare to stubs.	**10**			
4. Place a checkmark on the matching stub.	**10**			
5. List and total outstanding checks.	**10**			
6. Verify that all previous outstanding checks have cleared.	**10**			
7. Subtract the total of outstanding checks from the statement balance.*	**10**			
8. Add to the total in Step 7 any deposits made but not included in statement balance.	**10**			
9. Total any bank charges that appear on the bank statement and subtract them from the check-book balance.	**10**			
10. If the checkbook and statement do not agree, match bank statement entries with the check-book entries.	**10**			

Comments:

Total Points Earned ________ Divided by ________ Total Possible Points = ________ % Score

Instructor's Signature ________________________

Student Name ______________ Date ______________ Score ______________

Procedure 20-1 Making Travel Arrangements

Task: To make travel arrangements for the physician or another staff member.

Equipment and Supplies:
- Travel plan
- Telephone
- Telephone directory
- Typewriter or computer
- Typing paper

Standards: Complete the procedure and all critical steps in ______________ minutes with a minimum score of ______________ % within three attempts.

Scoring: Divide points earned by total possible points. Failure to perform a critical step that is indicated with an asterisk (*), will result in an unsatisfactory overall score.

Time began ______________ **Time ended** ______________

Steps	Possible Points	First Attempt	Second Attempt	Third Attempt
1. Verify the dates of the planned trip. • Desired date and time of departure • Desired date and time of return • Preferred mode of transportation • Number in party • Preferred lodging and price range • Preferred ticketing method (electronic or paper)	**20**			
2. Telephone a trusted travel agency to arrange for transportation and lodging reservations.	**10**			
3. Arrange for traveler's checks, if desired.	**10**			
4. Pick up tickets/e-receipts or arrange for delivery	**10**			
5. Check tickets to confirm conformance with the travel plan	**10**			
6. Check to see that hotel and air reservations are confirmed.	**10**			
7. Prepare an itinerary, including all the necessary information • Date and time of departure • Flight numbers or identifying information of other modes of travel • Mode of transportation to hotel(s) • Name, address, and telephone number of hotel(s), with confirmation numbers if available • Name, address, and telephone number of travel agency • Date and time of return	**10**			

Steps	Possible Points	First Attempt	Second Attempt	Third Attempt
8. Place one copy of itinerary in the office file.	**10**			
9. Give several copies of the itinerary to the traveler.	**10**			

Comments:

Total Points Earned ________ Divided by ________ Total Possible Points = ________ % Score

Instructor's Signature ____________________

Student Name ______________ Date ______________ Score ______________

Procedure 20-2 Arranging a Group Meeting

Task: To plan and execute a productive meeting that will result in achieved goals.

Equipment and Supplies:
- Meeting room
- Agenda
- Visual aids and equipment
- Handouts
- Stopwatch or clock
- Computer or word processor
- Paper
- List of items for the agenda

Standards: Complete the procedure and all critical steps in ______________ minutes with a minimum score of ______________ % within three attempts.

Scoring: Divide points earned by total possible points. Failure to perform a critical step that is indicated with an asterisk (*), will result in an unsatisfactory overall score.

Time began ______________ **Time ended** ______________

Steps	Possible Points	First Attempt	Second Attempt	Third Attempt
1. Determine the purpose of the meeting and draft a list of the items to be discussed. Include the desired results of the meeting.	10			
2. Determine where the meeting will be held, the time and date of the meeting, and the individuals who should attend.	10			
3. Send a memo, email, or letter to the individuals who should attend the meeting at least ten days in advance, if possible. Send a copy to any supervisors who should be kept informed about the issues to be raised in the meeting.	10			
4. Be sure that the notice includes the following information: a. date b. time c. place d. directions, if not in a common meeting room or away from the office e. speakers and/or meeting topics f. cost and registration information, if applicable g. list of items individuals should bring to the meeting	10			
5. Finalize the list of items to discuss and place them in priority order.	10			

Steps	Possible Points	First Attempt	Second Attempt	Third Attempt
6. Delegate any tasks that others can accomplish and follow-up to be sure that they fulfill their duties prior to the meeting.	10			
7. Assign a staff member the task of keeping notes and keeping time during the meeting.	10			
8. Make a list of all items that need to be taken to the meeting, including equipment such as microphones, projectors, screens, computers, disks containing presentations, etc.	10			
9. Compile the final agenda for the meeting.	10			
10. On the meeting day, transport all items needed to the meeting room. Begin and end the meeting on time. Stay on track and follow the agenda.	10			

Comments:

Total Points Earned ________ Divided by ________ Total Possible Points = ________ % Score

Instructor's Signature ____________________

Student Name ______________________ Date ____________ Score ____________

Procedure 23-1 Accounting for Petty Cash

Task: To establish a petty cash fund, maintain an accurate record of expenditures for 1 month, and replenish the fund as necessary.

Equipment and Supplies:
- Form for petty cash fund
- Pad of vouchers
- Disbursement journal
- Two checks
- List of petty cash expenditures

Standards: Complete the procedure and all critical steps in ____________ minutes with a minimum score of ____________ % within three attempts.

Scoring: Divide points earned by total possible points. Failure to perform a critical step that is indicated with an asterisk (*), will result in an unsatisfactory overall score.

Time began ____________ **Time ended** ____________

Steps	**Possible Points**	**First Attempt**	**Second Attempt**	**Third Attempt**
1. Determine the amount needed in the petty cash fund.	**10**			
2. Write a check in the determined amount.	**10**			
3. Record the beginning balance in the petty cash fund.	**10**			
4. Post the amount to miscellaneous on the disbursement record.	**10**			
5. Prepare a petty cash voucher for each amount withdrawn from the fund.	**10**			
6. Record each voucher in the petty cash record and enter the new balance.	**10**			
7. Write a check to replenish the fund as necessary. NOTE: The total of the vouchers plus the fund balance must equal the beginning amount.	**10**			
8. Total the expense columns and post to the appropriate accounts in the disbursement record.	**10**			
9. Record the amount added to the fund.	**10**			
10. Record the new balance in the petty cash fund.	**10**			

Documentation in the Medical Record

____

____

____

____

Comments:

Total Points Earned ________ Divided by ________ Total Possible Points = ________ % Score

Instructor's Signature ____________________

Student Name ______________________ Date ____________ Score ____________

Procedure 23-2 Processing an Employee Payroll

Task: To process payroll and compensate employees, making deductions accurately.

Equipment and Supplies:
- Checkbook
- Computer and payroll software, if applicable
- Pen
- Tax withholding tables
- Federal employers tax guide

Standards: Complete the procedure and all critical steps in ____________ minutes with a minimum score of ____________ % within three attempts.

Scoring: Divide points earned by total possible points. Failure to perform a critical step that is indicated with an asterisk (*), will result in an unsatisfactory overall score.

Time began ____________ **Time ended** ____________

Steps	Possible Points	First Attempt	Second Attempt	Third Attempt
1. Be sure that all information has been collected on the employees, including a copy of the social security card, a W-4 form, and an I-9 form.	20			
2. Review the time cards for all employees. Determine if any employees need counseling due to late arrivals or habitual absences.	20			
3. Figure the salary or hourly wages that are due the employee for the period worked.	20			
4. Figure the deductions that must be taken from the paycheck. This usually includes, but is not limited to: • Federal, state, and local taxes • Social security withholdings • Medicare withholdings • Other deductions, such as insurance, savings, etc. • Donations to organizations, such as the United Way	20			
5. Write the check for the balance due the employee. Most software programs can print the checks and explanations of deductions.	20			

Comments:

Total Points Earned ________ Divided by ________ Total Possible Points = ________ % Score

Instructor's Signature ______________________

Student Name ______________________ Date ____________ Score ____________

Procedure 23-3 Establishing and Maintaining a Supply Inventory and Ordering System

Task: To establish an inventory of all expendable supplies in the physician's office and follow an efficient plan of order control using a card system.

Equipment and Supplies:
- File box
- Inventory and order control cards
- List of supplies on hand
- Metal tabs
- Reorder tabs
- Pen or pencil

Standards: Complete the procedure and all critical steps in ____________ minutes with a minimum score of ____________ % within three attempts.

Scoring: Divide points earned by total possible points. Failure to perform a critical step that is indicated with an asterisk (*), will result in an unsatisfactory overall score.

Time began ____________ **Time ended** ____________

Steps	**Possible Points**	**First Attempt**	**Second Attempt**	**Third Attempt**
1. Write the name of each item on a separate card.	**10**			
2. Write the amount of each item on hand in the space provided.	**10**			
3. Place a reorder tag at the point where the supply should be replenished.	**20**			
4. Place a metal tab over the *order* section of the card.	**20**			
5. When the order has been placed, note the date and quantity ordered and move the table to the *on order* section of the card.	**20**			
6. Then the order is received, note the date and quantity in the appropriate column, remove the tab, and refile the card. NOTE: If the order is only partially filled, let the tab remain until the order is complete.	**20**			

Comments:

Total Points Earned ________ Divided by ________ Total Possible Points = ________ % Score

Instructor's Signature ____________________

Student Name ______________________ Date ____________ Score ________

Procedure 23-4 Preparing a Purchase Order

Task: To prepare an accurate purchase order for supplies or equipment.

Equipment and Supplies:
- List of current inventory
- Purchase order
- Pen
- Phone
- Fax machine

Standards: Complete the procedure and all critical steps in ____________ minutes with a minimum score of ____________ % within three attempts.

Scoring: Divide points earned by total possible points. Failure to perform a critical step that is indicated with an asterisk (*), will result in an unsatisfactory overall score.

Time began ____________ **Time ended** ____________

Steps	Possible Points	First Attempt	Second Attempt	Third Attempt
1. Review the current inventory and determine what items need to be ordered.	**10**			
2. Complete the purchase order accurately, filling in all applicable spaces and blanks with the information requested.	**15**			
3. List the items to be ordered, including quantity, item numbers, size, color, price, and extended price. Be sure that all applicable information is included.	**15**			
4. Provide the physician's signature, DEA certificate, and medical license where needed.	**15**			
5. Call in, fax, mail, or submit the order electronically to the vendor. Keep a copy for your records. Keep any verification provided that the order was received.	**15**			
6. Note on the inventory which items are on order.	**15**			
7. Keep a copy of the order in the appropriate place in the office filing system.	**15**			

Comments:

Total Points Earned ________ Divided by ________ Total Possible Points = ________ % Score

Instructor's Signature ______________________

Student Name ______________________ Date ____________ Score ____________

Procedure 24-1 Performing Medical Aseptic Hand Washing

Task: To minimize the number of pathogens on your hands, thus reducing the risk of pathogenic transmission.

Equipment and Supplies:
- Sink with running water
- Anti-microbial liquid soap in a dispenser (bar soap is not acceptable)
- Nail brush or orange stick
- Paper towels in a dispenser
- Water-based antimicrobial lotion

Standards: Complete the procedure and all critical steps in ____________ minutes with a minimum score of ____________ % within three attempts.

Scoring: Divide points earned by total possible points. Failure to perform a critical step that is indicated with an asterisk (*), will result in an unsatisfactory overall score.

Time began ____________ **Time ended** ____________

Steps	**Possible Points**	**First Attempt**	**Second Attempt**	**Third Attempt**
1. Remove all jewelry except your wristwatch, which should be pulled up above your wrist or removed, and a plain gold wedding ring.	10			
2. Turn on the faucet and regulate the water temperature to lukewarm.	10			
3. Allow your hands to become wet, apply soap, and lather using a circular motion with friction while holding your fingertips downward. Rub well between your fingers.	10			
4. Rinse well, holding your hands so that the water flows from your wrists downward to your fingertips.	10			
5. Wet your hands again and repeat the scrubbing procedure using vigorous, circular motion over wrists and hands for at least 1 to 2 minutes.	10			
6. Rinse your hands a second time, keeping fingers lower than your wrists.	10			
7. Dry your hands with paper towels. Do not touch the paper towel dispenser as you are obtaining towels.	10			
8. If faucets are not foot operated, turn off the water faucet with the paper towel.*	10			

Steps	Possible Points	First Attempt	Second Attempt	Third Attempt
9. After completion of drying your hands and turning off faucets (if necessary) place used towels into waste container	**10**			
10. Apply a water-based antibacterial hand lotion to prevent chapped or dry skin.	**10**			

Comments:

Total Points Earned ________ Divided by ________ Total Possible Points = ________ % Score

Instructor's Signature ______________________

Student Name ______________________ Date __________ Score __________

Procedure 24-2 Sanitization of Instruments

Task: To remove all contaminated matter from instruments in preparation for disinfection or sterilization.

Equipment and Supplies:
- Sink with hot running water
- Sanitizing agent or low-sudsing soap with enzymatic action
- Utility gloves
- Brush
- Towels
- Appropriate waste container

Standards: Complete the procedure and all critical steps in __________ minutes with a minimum score of __________ % within three attempts.

Scoring: Divide points earned by total possible points. Failure to perform a critical step that is indicated with an asterisk (*), will result in an unsatisfactory overall score.

Time began __________ **Time ended** __________

Steps	**Possible Points**	**First Attempt**	**Second Attempt**	**Third Attempt**
1. Put on utility gloves.*	**20**			
2. Separate sharp instruments from other instruments to be sanitized.	**10**			
3. Rinse the instruments under cold running water.	**10**			
4. Open hinged instruments and scrub all grooves, crevices, and serrations with a brush.*	**20**			
5. Rinse well with hot water.	**10**			
6. Towel dry all instruments thoroughly.	**10**			
7. Remove utility gloves and wash hands thoroughly.	**10**			
8. Place sanitized instruments in designated area for disinfection or sterilization.	**10**			

Comments:

Total Points Earned ________ Divided by ________ Total Possible Points = ________ % Score

Instructor's Signature ______________________

Student Name ______________ Date ______________ Score ______________

Procedure 24-3 Removing Contaminated Latex Gloves

Task: To minimize pathogen exposure by aseptically removing and discarding contaminated gloves.

Equipment and Supplies:
- Latex examination gloves
- Biohazard waste container

Standards: Complete the procedure and all critical steps in ______________ minutes with a minimum score of ______________ % within three attempts.

Scoring: Divide points earned by total possible points. Failure to perform a critical step that is indicated with an asterisk (*), will result in an unsatisfactory overall score.

Time began ______________ **Time ended** ______________

Steps	Possible Points	First Attempt	Second Attempt	Third Attempt
1. With the dominant hand, grasp the glove of the opposite hand near the palm and begin removing the first glove. Arms should be extended from the body and hands pointed down.	20			
2. Pull the glove inside out until you reach the fingers, holding the contaminated glove in the dominant gloved hand.	20			
3. Insert the thumb of the non-gloved hand inside the cuff of the remaining contaminated glove.	20			
4. Pull the glove down the hand inside out over the contaminated glove being held leaving the contaminated side of both gloves on the inside.	20			
5. Properly dispose of the inside out contaminated gloves in a biohazard waste container. Perform a medical aseptic hand wash as described in Procedure 24-1.	20			

Documentation in the Medical Record

____

____

____

____

Comments:

Total Points Earned ________ Divided by ________ Total Possible Points = ________ % Score

Instructor's Signature ____________________

Student Name ________________ Date ________ Score ________

Procedure 25-1 Obtaining a Medical History

Task: To obtain an acceptable written background from the patient to help the physician determine the cause and effects of the present illness. This includes the chief complaint (CC), present illness (PI), past history (PH). family history (FH), and social history (SH).

Equipment and Supplies:
- A history form
- Two pens, a red pen for recording patient allergies and a black pen to meet legal documentation guidelines
- A quiet, private area

Standards: Complete the procedure and all critical steps in ________ minutes with a minimum score of ________ % within three attempts.

Scoring: Divide points earned by total possible points. Failure to perform a critical step that is indicated with an asterisk (*), will result in an unsatisfactory overall score.

Time began ________ **Time ended** ________

Steps	**Possible Points**	**First Attempt**	**Second Attempt**	**Third Attempt**
1. Greet and identify the patient in a pleasant manner. Introduce yourself and explain your role.	**10**			
2. Take patient to a quiet, private area for the interview and explain to the patient why the information is needed.	**10**			
3. Complete the history form by utilizing therapeutic communication techniques. Make sure that all medical terminology is adequately explained. A self-history may have been mailed to the patient before the visit. If so, review the self-history for completeness.	**10**			
4. Speak in a pleasant, distinct manner, remembering to keep eye contact with your patient.	**10**			
5. Record the following statistical information on the patient information form: • Patient's full name, including middle initial • Address, including apartment number and ZIP code • Marital status • Sex (gender) • Age and date of birth • Telephone number for home and work • Insurance information if not already available • Employer's name, address, telephone number	**10**			

Steps	Possible Points	First Attempt	Second Attempt	Third Attempt
6. Record the following medical history on the patient history (PH) form: Chief complaint Present illness Past history Family history Social history	10			
7. Ask about allergies to drugs and any other substances, and record any allergies in red ink on every page of the history form, on the front of the chart, and on each progress note page. Some practices apply allergy alert labels to the front of each chart.	10			
8. Record all information legibly and neatly, and spell words correctly. Print rather than write in longhand. Do not erase, scribble or use white-out. If you make an error, draw a single line through the error, write error above it, add the correction, and initial and date the entry.	10			
9. Thank the patient for cooperating, and direct him or her back to the reception area.	10			
10. Review the record for errors before you pass it to the physician. Use the information on the record to complete the patient's chart. Keep the information confidential.	10			

Documentation:

Your patient's CC is dizziness for 2 weeks. She denies headaches, history (Hx) of ear infections, or Hx of hypertension. Her BP is 172/94, T – 97.6, P – 88, R – 22. Document pertinent patient findings using the SOAPE method.

S: ______

O: ______

A: ______

P: ______

E: ______

Total Points Earned ______ Divided by ______ Total Possible Points = ______ % Score

Instructor's Signature ______

Student Name ______________________ Date ____________ Score ________

Procedure 27-1 Determining Fat-Fold Measurement

Task: To accurately determine and record a measurement of body fat.

Equipment and Supplies:
- Fat-fold body calipers
- Pencil and paper

Standards: Complete the procedure and all critical steps in ____________ minutes with a minimum score of ____________ % within three attempts.

Scoring: Divide points earned by total possible points. Failure to perform a critical step that is indicated with an asterisk (*), will result in an unsatisfactory overall score.

Time began ____________ **Time ended** ____________

Steps	Possible Points	First Attempt	Second Attempt	Third Attempt
1. Read the directions for the caliper before you begin.	5			
2. Gather the equipment and supplies needed to complete the procedure and wash hands.	5			
3. Identify the patient.	5			
4. Explain the procedure to the patient.	5			
5. Using the triceps of the upper arm, grasp the skinfold with thumb and index finger. Make sure that the fold is in a parallel angle by keeping the thumb and index finger in line with one another. Be sure you do not grasp muscle tissue or pinch too tightly.	5			
6. Place calipers over the fold and measure.	10			
7. Record the measurement.	10			
8. Grasp the subscapular region located beneath the shoulder blade and obtain your second measurement.	10			
9. Record the measurement.	5			
10. Using the suprailiac area located posteriorly and immediately superior to the fanning of the hip bone, obtain your third measurement.	10			
11. Record the measurement.	5			

Steps	Possible Points	First Attempt	Second Attempt	Third Attempt
12. Determine total percent of body fat using Table 27-4.	10			
13. Record the calculations in the patient's medical record.	5			
14. Disinfect equipment and return to its proper place.	5			
15. Wash your hands.	5			

Documentation in the Medical Record

Comments:

Total Points Earned ________ Divided by ________ Total Possible Points = ________ % Score

Instructor's Signature ____________________

Student Name ______________________ Date ____________ Score ________

Procedure 27-2 Teaching the Patient to Read Food Labels

Task: To accurately explain the nutritional labeling of food products to the patient.

Equipment and Supplies:
- One each of four bars: Snickers, Twix, Healthy Choice, Fat Free Fruit Bar
- Pencil and Paper

Standards: Complete the procedure and all critical steps in ____________ minutes with a minimum score of ____________ % within three attempts.

Scoring: Divide points earned by total possible points. Failure to perform a critical step that is indicated with an asterisk (*), will result in an unsatisfactory overall score.

Time began ____________ **Time ended** ____________

Steps	Possible Points	First Attempt	Second Attempt	Third Attempt
1. Explain what you are going to talk about to the patient. Be sure to include reasons why food labels are a valuable source of nutritional information in diet planning.	10			
2. Using the labels on each bar, point out the nutritional information according to the guidelines in the text.	10			
3. Give the patient pencil and paper to write down the serving size of each type of candy bar.	10			
4. Together compare similarities and differences.	10			
5. Next have the patient write down the total caloric amount for each product serving.	10			
6. Compare similarities and differences.	10			
7. Write down the percentage of total, saturated, and unsaturated fats.	10			
8. Compare similarities and differences.	10			
9. Together analyze the nutritional level of each.	10			
10. Discuss any new information that was learned and ask the patient if he or she will use this information when shopping and how it will be implemented into nutritional planning.	10			

Comments:

Total Points Earned ________ Divided by ________ Total Possible Points = ________ % Score

Instructor's Signature ______________________

Student Name ______________________ Date ____________ Score ____________

Procedure 28-1 Obtaining an Oral Temperature Using a Digital Thermometer

Task: To accurately determine and record a patient's temperature using a digital thermometer.

Equipment and Supplies:
- Digital thermometer
- Probe covers
- Biohazard waste container

Standards: Complete the procedure and all critical steps in ____________ minutes with a minimum score of ____________ % within three attempts.

Scoring: Divide points earned by total possible points. Failure to perform a critical step that is indicated with an asterisk (*), will result in an unsatisfactory overall score.

Time began ____________ **Time ended** ____________

Steps	Possible Points	First Attempt	Second Attempt	Third Attempt
1. Wash hands and assemble equipment and supplies.*	10			
2. Identify your patient and explain the procedure. Be sure that the patient has not eaten, drunk fluids, smoked, or exercised for 30 minutes before taking the temperature.*	20			
3. Prepare the probe for use as described in package directions. Make sure probe covers are *always* used.	10			
4. Place the probe under the patient's tongue, and instruct the patient to close the mouth tightly. Assist the patient by holding the probe end.	10			
5. When the "beep" is heard, remove the probe from the patient's mouth and immediately eject the probe cover into the appropriate waste container.	10			
6. Note the reading in the LED window of the processing unit you are holding.	10			
7. Record the reading on the patient's medical record as T = 97.7°.	20			
8. Wash hands and disinfect equipment as indicated.	10			

Documentation in the Medical Record

____

____

____

____

Comments:

Total Points Earned ________ Divided by ________ Total Possible Points = ________ % Score

Instructor's Signature ____________________

Student Name ________________ Date ________ Score ________

Procedure 28-2 Obtaining an Aural Temperature Using the Tympanic Thermometer

Task: To accurately determine and record a patient's temperature using the tympanic thermometer.

Equipment and Supplies:
- Tympanic thermometer
- Disposable probe covers
- Biohazard waste container

Standards: Complete the procedure and all critical steps in ________ minutes with a minimum score of ________ % within three attempts.

Scoring: Divide points earned by total possible points. Failure to perform a critical step that is indicated with an asterisk (*), will result in an unsatisfactory overall score.

Time began ________ **Time ended** ________

Steps	Possible Points	First Attempt	Second Attempt	Third Attempt
1. Wash hands.	10			
2. Gather the necessary equipment and supplies.	10			
3. Identify your patient and explain the procedure.	10			
4. Place disposable probe cover on probe.	10			
5. Follow the package directions to start the thermometer.	10			
6. Insert the probe into the ear canal far enough to seal the opening. Do not apply pressure.	10			
7. Press the button on the probe as directed. The temperature will be on the display screen in 1 to 2 seconds.	10			
8. Remove the probe, note the reading, and discard the probe cover without touching it.	10			
9. Wash your hands and disinfect the equipment if indicated.	10			
10. Record temperature results as T = 98.6° (T) on the patient's medical record.	10			

Documentation in the Medical Record

____

____

____

____

Comments:

Total Points Earned ________ Divided by ________ Total Possible Points = ________ % Score

Instructor's Signature ____________________

Student Name ______________________ Date ____________ Score ____________

Procedure 28-3 Obtaining an Axillary Temperature

Task: To accurately determine and record a patient's temperature using the axillary method.

Equipment and Supplies:
- Digital unit
- Thermometer sheath or probe cover
- Supply of tissues
- Biohazard waste container

Standards: Complete the procedure and all critical steps in ____________ minutes with a minimum score of ____________ % within three attempts.

Scoring: Divide points earned by total possible points. Failure to perform a critical step that is indicated with an asterisk (*), will result in an unsatisfactory overall score.

Time began ____________ **Time ended** ____________

Steps	Possible Points	First Attempt	Second Attempt	Third Attempt
1. Wash your hands.	10			
2. Gather equipment and supplies.	5			
3. Introduce yourself, identify your patient, and explain the procedure.	10			
4. Prepare thermometer or digital unit in same manner as done for oral usage.	10			
5. Remove clothing and gown patient as needed to access axillary region.	5			
6. Pat the patient's axillary area dry if needed.	10			
7. Cover the thermometer or probe and place the tip into the center of the armpit, pointing the stem to the upper chest, making sure the thermometer is touching only skin, not clothing.	10			
8. Instruct the patient to hold the arm snugly across the chest or abdomen until the thermometer beeps.	10			
9. Remove the thermometer, note the digital reading, and dispose of the cover in the biohazard waste container.	10			
10. Disinfect the thermometer if indicated and Wash hands.	10			
11. Record the axillary temperature on the patient's medical record, for example, T = 97.6° (A)	10			

Documentation in the Medical Record

____

____

____

____

Comments:

Total Points Earned ________ Divided by ________ Total Possible Points = ________ % Score

Instructor's Signature ______________________

Student Name ______________________ Date ____________ Score ________

Procedure 28-4 Obtaining Rectal Temperature

Task: To accurately determine and record a patient's temperature using the rectal method.

Equipment and Supplies:
- Digital thermometer for rectal use
- Thermometer sheath or probe cover
- Lubricant
- A supply of tissues
- Nonsterile gloves
- Biohazard waste container

Standards: Complete the procedure and all critical steps in ____________ minutes with a minimum score of ____________ % within three attempts.

Scoring: Divide points earned by total possible points. Failure to perform a critical step that is indicated with an asterisk (*), will result in an unsatisfactory overall score.

Time began ____________ **Time ended** ____________

Steps	Possible Points	First Attempt	Second Attempt	Third Attempt
1. Wash your hands.	10			
2. Introduce yourself, identify your patient, and explain the procedure.	5			
3. Remove patient clothing from waist down and drape as needed.	5			
4. Place adult patient in Sims' position.	5			
5. Prepare thermometer using a sheath or probe cover on the red probe in the digital unit.	10			
6. Put on gloves.*	10			
7. Lubricate the probe tip and insert into the rectum past the sphincter.*	10			
8. Hold the thermometer in place until a beep is heard.	10			
9. Remove the thermometer and note the reading on the LED window. Offer tissues to patient.	5			
10. Remove the sheath or probe cover as well as your gloves and discard into appropriate biohazard waste container.	15			
11. Wash hands.*	10			

Steps	Possible Points	First Attempt	Second Attempt	Third Attempt
12. Assist patient with positioning and dressing as needed.	5			
13. Record temperature with (R) which indicates a rectal temperature for example, T = 99.6° (R).	10			

Documentation in the Medical Record

___

___

___

___

Comments:

Total Points Earned ______ Divided by ______ Total Possible Points = ______ % Score

Instructor's Signature ______________

Student Name ________________ Date ________ Score ________

Procedure 28-5 Obtaining an Apical Pulse

Task: To assess the patient's apical heart rate.

Equipment and Supplies:
- A watch with a second hand
- Stethoscope
- Alcohol wipes
- Patient gown

Standards: Complete the procedure and all critical steps in ________ minutes with a minimum score of ________ % within three attempts.

Scoring: Divide points earned by total possible points. Failure to perform a critical step that is indicated with an asterisk (*), will result in an unsatisfactory overall score.

Time began ________ **Time ended** ________

Steps	Possible Points	First Attempt	Second Attempt	Third Attempt
1. Wash your hands and clean stethoscope earpieces with alcohol swabs.	10			
2. Introduce yourself, identify your patient, and explain the procedure.	10			
3. Assist patient in disrobing from waist up and provide patient gown open to the front.	10			
4. Patient should be either sitting or in supine position.	10			
5. Place the stethoscope just below the left nipple in the intercostal space between the 5th and 6th ribs.	10			
6. Listen carefully for the heartbeat.	10			
7. Count the pulse for one full minute.* Note any irregularities in rhythm and volume.	10			
8. Assist the patient to sit up and dress.	10			
9. Wash hands.	10			
10. Record the pulse in the patient chart as AP (e.g., AP = 96) and record any arrhythmias.	10			

Documentation in the Medical Record

____

____

____

____

Comments:

Total Points Earned ________ Divided by ________ Total Possible Points = ________ % Score

Instructor's Signature ____________________

Student Name _______________ Date _______ Score _______

Procedure 28-6 Assessing the Patient's Pulse

Task: To determine and record a patient's pulse rate, rhythm, volume, and elasticity.

Equipment and Supplies:
- A watch with a second hand

Standards: Complete the procedure and all critical steps in _______ minutes with a minimum score of _______ % within three attempts.

Scoring: Divide points earned by total possible points. Failure to perform a critical step that is indicated with an asterisk (*), will result in an unsatisfactory overall score.

Time began _______ **Time ended** _______

Steps	Possible Points	First Attempt	Second Attempt	Third Attempt
1. Wash your hands.	10			
2. Introduce yourself, identify your patient, and explain the procedure.	10			
3. Place the patient's arm in a relaxed position, palm downward.	10			
4. Gently grasp the palm side of the patient's wrist with your first three fingertips approximately 1 inch above the base of the thumb.	20			
5. Count the beats for 1 full minute, using a watch with a second hand. Note* if measured for 30 seconds, multiply by two.	20			
6. Wash your hands.	10			
7. Record the count and any irregularities on the patient's medical record. Record as P = 72. Pulse is usually recorded immediately after temperature.	20			

Documentation in the Medical Record

____

____

____

____

Comments:

Total Points Earned ________ Divided by ________ Total Possible Points = ________ % Score

Instructor's Signature ____________________

Student Name ______________________ Date __________ Score __________

Procedure 28-7 Determining Respirations

Task: To determine and record a patient's respirations.

Equipment and Supplies:
- A watch with a second hand

Standards: Complete the procedure and all critical steps in __________ minutes with a minimum score of __________ % within three attempts.

Scoring: Divide points earned by total possible points. Failure to perform a critical step that is indicated with an asterisk (*), will result in an unsatisfactory overall score.

Time began __________ **Time ended** __________

Steps	**Possible Points**	**First Attempt**	**Second Attempt**	**Third Attempt**
1. Wash your hands.				
2. Identify your patient.				
3. The patient's arm will be in the same positions when counting the pulse. If having difficulty noticing breathing, place the arm across the chest to pick up movement.				
4. Count the respirations for 30 seconds, using a watch with a second hand, and multiply by 2.				
5. Release the patient's wrist.				
6. Record the respirations on the patient's medical record after the pulse recording. Record as R = 18.				

Documentation in the Medical Record

____

____

____

____

Comments:

Total Points Earned ________ Divided by ________ Total Possible Points = ________ % Score

Instructor's Signature ______________________

Student Name ______________________ Date __________ Score __________

Procedure 28-8 Determining a Patient's Blood Pressure

Task: To perform a blood pressure measurement that is correct in technique, accurate, and comfortable for the patient.

Equipment and Supplies:
- Sphygmomanometer
- Stethoscope
- Antiseptic wipes

Standards: Complete the procedure and all critical steps in __________ minutes with a minimum score of __________ % within three attempts.

Scoring: Divide points earned by total possible points. Failure to perform a critical step that is indicated with an asterisk (*), will result in an unsatisfactory overall score.

Time began __________ **Time ended** __________

Steps	Possible Points	First Attempt	Second Attempt	Third Attempt
1. Wash your hands.	5			
2. Assemble the equipment and supplies needed. Clean the earpieces of the stethoscope with alcohol swabs.	5			
3. Introduce yourself, identify the patient, and explain the procedure.	5			
4. Seat the patient in a comfortable position with legs uncrossed and arm resting at heart level on the lap or table.	5			
5. Determine the correct cuff size.	5			
6. Roll up the sleeve to about 5 inches above the elbow, or have the patient remove his or her arm from the sleeve.				
7. Palpate the brachial artery at the antecubital space in both arms. If one arm has a stronger pulse, use that arm. If the pulses are equal, select the right arm.	5			
8. Center the cuff bladder over the brachial artery, with the connecting tube away from the patient's body and the tube to the bulb close to the body.	5			
9. Place the lower edge of the cuff about 1 inch above the palpable brachial pulse, normally located in the natural crease of the inner elbow, and wrap it snugly and smoothly.	5			

Steps	Possible Points	First Attempt	Second Attempt	Third Attempt
10. Position the gauge of the sphygmomanometer so that it is at eye level.	5			
11. Take the patient's brachial pulse, and mentally add 40 mm to the reading.	5			
12. Insert the earpieces of the stethoscope turned down and forward into your ears.	5			
13. Place the stethoscope bell over the palpated brachial artery firmly enough to obtain a seal but not so tightly that you constrict the artery.	5			
14. Close the valve, and squeeze the bulb to inflate the cuff at a rapid but smooth rate to 20 mm above the palpated pulse level that was previously determined in step 12.	10			
15. Open the valve slightly and deflate the cuff at the constant rate of 2 mm Hg per second.	5			
16. Listen throughout the entire deflation until the sounds have stopped for at least 10 mm Hg.	10			
17. Remove the stethoscope from your ears, and record the systolic and diastolic readings as BP systolic/diastolic (e.g., BP 120/80).	10			
18. Note: If you are uncertain of your reading, release the air from the cuff, wait 1 to 2 minutes, then repeat the process. Wash your hands.*				

Documentation in the Medical Record

____

____

____

____

Comments:

Total Points Earned ________ Divided by ________ Total Possible Points = ________ % Score

Instructor's Signature ____________________

Student Name ______________________ Date ____________ Score ____________

Procedure 28-9 Measuring a Patient's Height and Weight

Task: To accurately weigh and measure a patient as part of the physical assessment.

Equipment and Supplies:
- A balance scale with a measuring bar

Standards: Complete the procedure and all critical steps in ____________ minutes with a minimum score of ____________ % within three attempts.

Scoring: Divide points earned by total possible points. Failure to perform a critical step that is indicated with an asterisk (*), will result in an unsatisfactory overall score.

Time began ____________ **Time ended** ____________

Steps	**Possible Points**	**First Attempt**	**Second Attempt**	**Third Attempt**
1. Wash your hands.	5			
2. Identify your patient and explain the procedure.	5			
3. If the patient is to remove his or her shoes for weighing, place a paper towel on the scale platform.	5			
4. Check to see that the balance bar pointer floats in the middle of the balance frame when all weights are at zero.	5			
5. Help the patient onto the scale. Be sure that the female patient is not holding a purse and that the male patient has removed any heavy objects from pockets.	5			
6. Move the large weight into the groove closest to the estimated weight of the patient.	5			
7. While the patient is standing still, slide the small upper weight to the right along the pound markers until the pointer balances in the middle of the balance frame.	10			
8. Leave the weights in place.	5			
9. Ask the patient to stand up straight and to look straight ahead. On some scales the patient may need to turn with the back to the scale.	5			

Steps	Possible Points	First Attempt	Second Attempt	Third Attempt
10. Adjust the height bar so that it just touches the top of the patient's head	**5**			
11. Leave the elevation bar set but fold down the horizontal bar.	**5**			
12. Assist the patient off the scale. Be sure all items removed for weighing are given back to the patient.	**5**			
13. Read the weight scale. Add the numbers at the markers of the large and the small weights and record the total to the nearest pound on the patient's medical record.	**15**			
14. Record the height. Read the marker at the movable point of the ruler, and record the measurement to the nearest quarter inch on the patient's medical record.	**15**			
15. Return the weights and the measuring bar to zero. Wash hands.	**5**			

Documentation in the Medical Record

____

____

____

____

Comments:

Total Points Earned ________ Divided by ________ Total Possible Points = ________ % Score

Instructor's Signature ________________

Student Name ______________________ Date ____________ Score ________

Procedure 29-1 Preparing for and Assisting with the Physical Examination

Task: To help the physician examine patients by preparing the necessary equipment and ensuring patient safety and comfort during the examination.

Equipment and Supplies:

- Stethoscope
- Scale
- Cotton balls
- Examination light
- Lubricating gel
- Sphygmomanometer
- Tape measure
- Pen light
- Tuning fork
- Laboratory request forms
- Patient gown
- Thermometer

Ophthalmoscope
Tongue depressor
Examination light
Percussion hammer
Latex gloves/finger cots
Otoscope
Gauze sponges
Nasal speculum
Biohazard container
Specimen bottles/glass slides
Drapes
Cotton-tipped applicators

Standards: Complete the procedure and all critical steps in ____________ minutes with a minimum score of ____________ % within three attempts.

Scoring: Divide points earned by total possible points. Failure to perform a critical step that is indicated with an asterisk (*), will result in an unsatisfactory overall score.

Time began ____________ **Time ended** ____________

Steps	Possible Points	First Attempt	Second Attempt	Third Attempt
1. Prepare the examining room according to acceptable medical aseptic rules.	5			
2. Wash hands.	6			
3. Locate the instruments for the procedure. Set them out in sequence.	5			
4. Identify the patient, and determine whether the patient understands the procedure.	6			
5. Review the medical history with the patient and investigate the purpose of the visit.	6			
6. Measure and record the patient's vital signs, height, and weight.	6			
7. Instruct the patient on how to collect the urine specimen, and hand the patient the properly labeled specimen container (see Chapter 49). Obtain any blood samples that are required (see Chapter 50). Obtain resting ECG if ordered (see Chapter 46).	6			

Steps	Possible Points	First Attempt	Second Attempt	Third Attempt
8. Hand the patient a gown and drape. Instruct the patient on how to put the gown on. Help patient with undressing as needed.	6			
9. Assist the patient in sitting on the narrow end of the examination table; place the drape over the patient's lap and legs. If the patient is elderly, confused, or feeling faint or dizzy, DO NOT leave him or her alone.	6			
10. Advise the physician that the patient is ready.	6			
11. Assist during the examination by handing the physician each instrument as it is needed and by positioning and draping the patient.	6			
12. When the physician has completed the examination, allow the patient to rest for a moment, then help the patient from the table. Assist with dressing, if necessary. Use proper body mechanics if assistance in transfer is needed.	6			
13. Record the necessary notes on the patient's chart and forward it to the physician for further notations.	6			
14. Return to the patient and ask him or her if there are any questions. Give the patient any final instructions, and schedule tests as ordered by the physician and/or the next appointment.	6			
15. Put on gloves and dispose of used supplies and linens in designated waste containers. Clean tabletop surfaces with disinfectant. Disinfect all equipment.	6			
16. Remove gloves and discard them in the biohazard waste container and wash hands.	6			
17. Replace used supplies and prepare room for next patient.	6			

Documentation in the Medical Record

____

____

____

____

Comments:

Total Points Earned ________ Divided by ________ Total Possible Points = ________ % Score

Instructor's Signature ____________________

Student Name ______________________ Date ____________ Score ________

Procedure 30-1 Preparing a Prescription for the Physician's Signature

Task: To accurately prepare a prescription for the physician's signature using appropriate abbreviations and prescription format.

Equipment and Supplies:
- Prescription pad
- Drug reference materials if needed
- Black pen
- Patient chart

Standards: Complete the procedure and all critical steps in ____________ minutes with a minimum score of ____________ % within three attempts.

Scoring: Divide points earned by total possible points. Failure to perform a critical step that is indicated with an asterisk (*), will result in an unsatisfactory overall score.

Time began ____________ **Time ended** ____________

Steps	**Possible Points**	**First Attempt**	**Second Attempt**	**Third Attempt**
1. Refer to the physician's written order for the prescription. If the physician gives a verbal order to write a prescription, write down the order and review it with the physician for accuracy.	**10**			
2. If unfamiliar with the medication, look up the drug in a drug reference book (such as the PDR). recommended dose, storage guidelines, drug-to-drug interactions, and possible side effects to make sure the transcription is correct and to be prepared to answer patient questions about the medication.	**10**			
3. Ask the patient about drug allergies.	**10**			
4. Using a prescription pad that has the physician's name, address, telephone number, and DEA registration number pre-printed on the slip, begin to transcribe the physician order.	**10**			
5. Record the patient's name, address, and date on which the prescription is being written.	**10**			
6. Next to the Rx write in legible handwriting the name of the drug (correctly spelled), the dosage form (such as tablet, capsule, etc., using correct abbreviations), and the strength ordered. For example, if the physician orders Lipitor, 40 mg tablets, by mouth, one tablet at bedtime then the first line of the prescription should read: Lipitor 40 mg tabs. This is the *inscription*.	**10**			

Steps	Possible Points	First Attempt	Second Attempt	Third Attempt
7. On the next line write *Disp*. This is the subscription which includes directions to the pharmacist on the amount to be dispensed and the form of the drug. For the Lipitor order, the subscription would read: Disp: #30	10			
8. Next comes the *signature*. This includes directions for the patient, such as how and when to take the medicine, and is usually preceded by the symbol *Sig*. For the Lipitor order the signature would read: Sig: i tab po hs	10			
9. The physician tells you the patient can get 3 refills of the prescription so this information should be added at the bottom of the prescription.	10			
10. The physician must sign the prescription before it is given to the patient.	10			
11. Document on the patient's chart the medication order and any pertinent details including patient education and refill information.	10			

Documentation in the Medical Record

____

____

____

____

Comments:

Total Points Earned ________ Divided by ________ Total Possible Points = ________ % Score

Instructor's Signature __________________

Student Name ______________________ Date ____________ Score ________

Procedure 31-1 Calculating the Correct Dosage for Administration

Task: To calculate the correct dosage amount and choose the correct equipment when the physician orders 2.4 million IU of penicillin G benzathine (Bicillin) administered to a patient.

Equipment and Supplies:
- Premixed syringes of Bicillin in the following two strengths are available:
    - 0.6 million IU/syringe
    - 1.2 million IU/syringe
- Paper and pencil

Standards: Complete the procedure and all critical steps in ____________ minutes with a minimum score of ____________ % within three attempts.

Scoring: Divide points earned by total possible points. Failure to perform a critical step that is indicated with an asterisk (*), will result in an unsatisfactory overall score.

Time began ____________ **Time ended** ____________

Steps	**Possible Points**	**First Attempt**	**Second Attempt**	**Third Attempt**
1. Read the order in quiet surroundings to make sure that you fully understand it.*	15	____	____	____
2. Write out the order.	15			
3. Examine the drug labels to see what strengths and amounts are available.	15	____	____	____
4. Write down the standard formula.	15	____	____	____
5. Rewrite the formula, replacing the unknown values with the known quantities. The unknown x will be the amount of the drug to give.	10	____	____	____
6. Work the proportion problem by cross-multiplying to solve for x.	10	____	____	____
7. State your answer by filling in the blanks, as follows: To administer 2.4 million IU of Bicillin, I would select ____________ of the premixed syringes labeled ____________.	20	____	____	____

Documentation in the Medical Record

____

____

____

____

Comments:

Total Points Earned ________ Divided by ________ Total Possible Points = ________ % Score

Instructor's Signature ____________________

Student Name ______________________ Date ____________ Score ____________

Procedure 31-2 Calculating the Correct Dosage for Administration Using Two Systems of Measurement

Task: To choose the correct system of measurement and calculate the correct dosage amount when the physician orders 120 mg of a drug to be administered to a patient.

Equipment and Supplies
- Tablets labeled 1 gr (grain) each
- Standard mathematical formula:

$$\frac{\text{Available strength}}{\text{Ordered strength}} = \frac{\text{Available amount}}{\text{Amount to give}}$$

- Conversion equivalent: 1 gr = 60 mg
- Paper and pencil

Standards: Complete the procedure and all critical steps in ____________ minutes with a minimum score of ____________ % within three attempts.

Scoring: Divide points earned by total possible points. Failure to perform a critical step that is indicated with an asterisk (*), will result in an unsatisfactory overall score.

Time began ____________ **Time ended** ____________

Steps	Possible Points	First Attempt	Second Attempt	Third Attempt
1. Read the order in quiet surroundings to make sure that you fully understand it.*	**15**			
2. Write out the order.	**10**			
3. Examine the drug labels to see what strengths and amounts are available.	**15**			
4. Convert the ordered system of measurement to the system of measurement on the label using the conversion formula. $\text{Have} \times \frac{\text{Wanted}}{\text{Have}}$ = Unit Wanted in New System (conversion)	**15**			
5. Write down the standard formula.	**10**			
6. Rewrite the formula, replacing the unknown values with the known quantities and using the system of measurement on the label. The unknown x will be the amount of the drug to give (amount to give).	**10**			

Steps	Possible Points	First Attempt	Second Attempt	Third Attempt
7. Work the proportion problem by cross-multiplying to solve for x.	10	______	______	______
8. By filling in the blank, as follows: State your answer To administer 120 mg of a drug from tablets labeled 1 gr (grain) each, give ________ tablet(s).	15	______	______	______

Documentation in the Medical Record

____

____

____

____

Comments:

Total Points Earned ________ Divided by ________ Total Possible Points = ________ % Score

Instructor's Signature ____________________

Student Name ______________________ Date ____________ Score ________

Procedure 31-3 Calculating the Correct Dosage for a Child when only Adult Medication is Available

Task: To calculate the correct dosage amount for a 90-pound child using Clark's rule when the adult dosage is 250 mg.

Equipment and Supplies:
- Adult dosage 250 mg/ml
- Clark's rule:

$$\text{Pediatric dose} = \frac{\text{Child's weight in pounds}}{150}$$

- Standard mathematical formula:

$$\frac{\text{Available strength}}{\text{Ordered strength}} = \frac{\text{Available amount}}{\text{Amount to give}}$$

- Paper and pencil

Standards: Complete the procedure and all critical steps in ____________ minutes with a minimum score of ____________ % within three attempts.

Scoring: Divide points earned by total possible points. Failure to perform a critical step that is indicated with an asterisk (*), will result in an unsatisfactory overall score.

Time began ____________ **Time ended** ____________

Steps	**Possible Points**	**First Attempt**	**Second Attempt**	**Third Attempt**
1. Read the order in quiet surroundings to make sure that you fully understand it.	**10**			
2. Write out the order.	**10**			
3. Examine the drug labels to see what strengths and amounts are available.	**10**			
4. Write down Clark's rule.	**10**			
5. Using Clark's rule, replace the unknown values with the known quantities. The unknown x will be the pediatric strength ordered (pediatric dose).	**20**			
6. Write down the standard formula.	**10**			
7. Rewrite the formula, replacing the unknown values with the available quantities and the pediatric strength just determined. The unknown x will be the amount of the drug to give (amount to give).	**10**			

Steps	Possible Points	First Attempt	Second Attempt	Third Attempt
8. Work the proportion problem by cross-multiplying to solve for x.	10	______	______	______
9. State your answer by filling in the blank, as follows: To administer an adult medication labeled 250 mg/mL to a 90-pound child, give ______ ml.	20	______	______	______

Documentation in the Medical Record

____

____

____

____

Comments:

Total Points Earned ________ Divided by ________ Total Possible Points = ________ % Score

Instructor's Signature ______________________

Student Name ________________ Date ________ Score ________

Procedure 31-4 Calculating the Correct Dosage for Administration Using Body Weight

Task: To calculate correct dosage by using body weight method. Ordered: Zovirax capsules 5 mg/kg every 8 hours for 7 days for a patient who has a diagnosis of herpes zoster. The patient weighs 176 pounds. The capsules are labeled 200 mg = 1 capsule.

Equipment and Supplies:
- Weight conversion: 2.5 lb = 1 kg
- Capsules labeled 200 mg/kg
- Balance scale
- Formula for conversion of pounds to kilograms
- Standard math formula:

$$\frac{\text{Available strength}}{\text{Ordered strength}} = \frac{\text{Available amount}}{\text{Amount to give}}$$

- Paper and pencil

Standards: Complete the procedure and all critical steps in ________ minutes with a minimum score of ________ % within three attempts.

Scoring: Divide points earned by total possible points. Failure to perform a critical step that is indicated with an asterisk (*), will result in an unsatisfactory overall score.

Time began ________ **Time ended** ________

Steps	**Possible Points**	**First Attempt**	**Second Attempt**	**Third Attempt**
1. Read the order in quiet surroundings to make sure that you fully understand it.	**10**			
2. Write out the order.	**10**			
3. Examine the drug label to check the strength and amount.	**10**			
4. Convert the patient's weight from pounds to kilograms.	**10**			
5. Write down the standard formula.	**10**			
6. Rewrite the formula, replacing the unknown values with the known quantities. The unknown x will be the amount of the drug to give.	**10**			
7. Work the problem by cross-multiplying to solve for x.	**10**			
8. State your answer by filling in the blank as follows: To administer 5 mg/kg of body weight of Zovirax from capsules labeled 200 mg each, I would give ________ capsule(s).	**30**			

Documentation in the Medical Record

____

____

____

____

Comments:

Total Points Earned ________ Divided by ________ Total Possible Points = ________ % Score

Instructor's Signature ____________________

Student Name ______________________ Date __________ Score __________

Procedure 32-1 Dispensing and Administering Oral Medications

Task: To safely dispense and administer an oral medication to a patient.

Equipment and Supplies:
- Container of ordered medication
- Medication cup
- A written physician order, including the drug name, strength, dose, and route

Standards: Complete the procedure and all critical steps in __________ minutes with a minimum score of __________ % within three attempts.

Scoring: Divide points earned by total possible points. Failure to perform a critical step that is indicated with an asterisk (*), will result in an unsatisfactory overall score.

Time began __________ **Time ended** __________

Steps	Possible Points	First Attempt	Second Attempt	Third Attempt
1. Read the order and clarify any questions with the physician.	5			
2. If unfamiliar with the drug, refer to the *PDR* or the package insert to determine the purpose of the drug, common side effects, typical dose, and any pertinent precautions or contraindications. Use the "seven rights" to prevent errors.	5			
3. Perform calculations needed to match the physician order. Confirm the answer with the physician if there are any questions.	5			
4. Dispense medication in a well-lit, quiet area.	5			
5. Wash your hands.*	5			
6. Compare the order with the label on the container of medicine when you remove it from storage. Check the expiration date on the container and dispose of the medication if it has expired.*	5			
7. Compare the order with the label on the container of medicine just before dispensing the ordered dose. Make sure that the strength on the label matches the order or that you dispense the correctly calculated dose.	5			
8. Gently tap the prescribed dose into the lid of the medication container. Avoid touching the inside of the lid, as well as the medication.	5			
9. Empty the medication in the container lid into a medicine cup.	5			

Steps	Possible Points	First Attempt	Second Attempt	Third Attempt
To Dispense Liquid Oral Preparations				
1. Shake medication well if required.	2			
2. When you pour liquid medications, hold the labeled side of the container toward the palm of your hand.	2			
3. Place the medicine cup on a flat surface and, at eye level, pour the medication to the prescribed dose mark on the medicine cup.	2			
For Both Solid and Liquid Oral Medications				
10. Recap the container and compare the label and the physician order before replacing the container in storage.	5			
11. Transport the medication to the patient.	3			
12. Greet and identify the patient by name.	3			
13. Mention the name of the drug, why it is being given, and ask the patient if she or he has any allergies to the medication.	5			
14. If necessary, help the patient into a sitting position.	3			
15. Administer tablets, capsules, or caplets with water. If the patient is receiving liquid medication, offer water after the medication has been taken, if appropriate. Make sure the patient swallows the entire dose.	5			
16. Conduct patient education on the purpose of the drug, typical side effects, and dosage and storage recommendations. Refer to the physician to clarify information if necessary.	5			
17. The patient must remain in the office for 20 to 30 minutes after drug administration as a precaution against untoward effects.	5			
18. If the patient experiences any discomfort after taking a medication, the physician should be notified immediately, and the incident should be documented completely and accurately.	5			
19. Wash hands.	5			
20. Document the administration of the drug including the date and time; the drug name, dose, strength, and route of administration; any side effects; and patient education conducted about the drug.*	5			

Documentation in the Medical Record

____

____

____

____

Comments:

Total Points Earned ________ Divided by ________ Total Possible Points = ________ % Score

Instructor's Signature ____________________

Student Name ______________________ Date ____________ Score ____________

Procedure 32-2 Filling a Syringe from a Vial

Task: To fill a syringe with 1.5 ml of sterile water from a multidose vial by using sterile technique.

Equipment and Supplies:

- A multidose vial containing the material to be injected
- Alcohol wipes
- A sterile needle and syringe unit
- A written order, including the drug name, strength, and route

Standards: Complete the procedure and all critical steps in ____________ minutes with a minimum score of ____________ % within three attempts.

Scoring: Divide points earned by total possible points. Failure to perform a critical step that is indicated with an asterisk (*), will result in an unsatisfactory overall score.

Time began ____________ **Time ended** ____________

Steps	Possible Points	First Attempt	Second Attempt	Third Attempt
1. Wash your hands.*	5			
2. Read the order and choose the correct vial of medication.	10			
3. Choose the correct syringe and needle size, depending on the site and the quantity of medication to be injected.	5			
4. Compare the order with both the name of the drug on the vial of medication and the amount to be withdrawn in the syringe.	10			
5. Gently agitate the medication by rolling the vial between your palms.	5			
6. Check the quality of the medication and the expiration date.*	5			
7. Cleanse the rubber stopper of the vial with the alcohol wipe, using a circular motion. Place the vial on a secure flat surface, leaving the alcohol wipe over the rubber stopper.*	5			
8. Grasp the syringe plunger and draw up an amount of air equal to the amount of medication ordered.	5			
9. Remove the needle cover and insert the needle into the center of the rubber stopper. Hold the vial firmly against a flat surface and make sure that the needle only touches the cleaned rubber area.	5			

Steps	Possible Points	First Attempt	Second Attempt	Third Attempt
10. Inject the aspirated air in the syringe into the vial.	5			
11. Pick the vial and syringe unit up and invert it. Slowly pull back on the plunger with the unit at eye level until the proper amount of medication is withdrawn.	10			
12. While the needle is still in the vial, check that there are no air bubbles in the syringe.	5			
13. If there are air bubbles, slip the fingers holding the vial down to grasp the vial and syringe as a single unit.	5			
14. With your free hand, tap the syringe until the air bubbles dislodge and float into the tip of the syringe.	5			
15. Gently expel these tiny air bubbles through the needle, then continue withdrawing the medication.	5			
16. Withdraw the needle from the vial, and replace the cover over the needle without the needle touching the sides.	5			
17. Return the medication to the shelf or the refrigerator, checking that you have the correct drug and dosage.	5			

Comments:

Total Points Earned ________ Divided by ________ Total Possible Points = ________ % Score

Instructor's Signature ____________________

Student Name ______________________ Date ____________ Score ____________

Procedure 32-3 Filling a Syringe from an Ampule

Task: To open an ampule.

Equipment and Supplies:
- Ampule
- Two alcohol pads (It is safer to use an unopened pad while breaking the neck of the ampule.)
- Filter needle
- Syringe

Standards: Complete the procedure and all critical steps in ____________ minutes with a minimum score of ____________ % within three attempts.

Scoring: Divide points earned by total possible points. Failure to perform a critical step that is indicated with an asterisk (*), will result in an unsatisfactory overall score.

Time began ____________ **Time ended** ____________

Steps	**Possible Points**	**First Attempt**	**Second Attempt**	**Third Attempt**
1. Wash your hands and gather appropriate syringe unit and filter needle.*	**20**	______	______	______
2. Gently tap the top of the ampule with your fingers to settle all the medication to the bottom portion of the flask.	**20**	______	______	______
3. Wipe the neck of the ampule clean with alcohol. It may be necessary to use a small file provided by the manufacturer to score an ampule at the breaking point to facilitate easier opening.	**10**	______	______	______
4. Wrap the top of the ampule with a gauze square or unopened alcohol pad to protect yourself from the glass. Hold the covered ampule between your thumb and finger, in front of you and above waist level.	**10**	______	______	______
5. Snap your wrist away from your body to break the neck of the ampule. You will hear a pop because the ampule is vacuum-sealed. The glass is designed not to shatter, and the medication will not spill out. Dispose of the glass pieces in the sharps container.	**10**	______	______	______
6. Without touching the sides, insert the syringe unit with the filter needle into the ampule and withdraw the ordered dose. The filter needle is designed to prevent aspiration of pieces of glass into the injection unit.	**20**	______	______	______

Steps	Possible Points	First Attempt	Second Attempt	Third Attempt
7. Change the needle for an appropriate length and gauge based on the physician order and patient characteristics.	10	____	____	____

Comments:

Total Points Earned ______ Divided by ______ Total Possible Points = ______ % Score

Instructor's Signature ____________

Student Name ______________________ Date __________ Score __________

Procedure 32-4 Giving an Intradermal Injection

Task: To inject 0.1 ml of purified protein derivative (PPD) to perform a Mantoux test as ordered by the physician.

Equipment and Supplies:
- A vial of tuberculin PPD
- Alcohol wipes
- A 3/8 inch, 27-gauge sterile needle and syringe unit
- Disposable gloves
- Gauze squares
- Sharps container
- Physician order, including the patient's name, when to give the drug, the route of administration, and the name and strength of the drug.

Standards: Complete the procedure and all critical steps in ____________ minutes with a minimum score of ____________ % within three attempts.

Scoring: Divide points earned by total possible points. Failure to perform a critical step that is indicated with an asterisk (*), will result in an unsatisfactory overall score.

Time began ____________ **Time ended** ____________

Steps	Possible Points	First Attempt	Second Attempt	Third Attempt
1. Wash your hands. Follow standard precautions. Glove yourself with nonsterile gloves.*	8			
2. Select the correct medication from the shelf or the refrigerator.	4			
3. Read the label to be sure that you have the right drug and the right strength. Perform the three label and order checks as the medication is dispensed.*	8			
4. Warm refrigerated medications by gently rolling the container between your palms.	4			
5. Prepare the syringe as described in Procedure 32-2, withdrawing the right dose.	4			
6. Transport the medication to the patient.	4			
7. Greet and identify the patient by name.	4			
8. Position the patient comfortably.	4			
9. Locate the antecubital space, then find a site several finger widths down the anterior aspect of the forearm. Avoid any scarred, discolored, or pigmented areas.	4			

Steps	Possible Points	First Attempt	Second Attempt	Third Attempt
10. Cleanse the patient's skin with an alcohol wipe, using a circular motion, moving from the center outward.	4			
11. Allow the antiseptic to dry.	4			
12. With the thumb and first two fingers of your nondominant hand, stretch the skin of the forearm apart and taut.	4			
13. Grasp the syringe between the thumb and first two fingers of your dominant hand, palm down, with the needle bevel upward. Hold the syringe close to the plunger end.	4			
14. At a 15-degree angle, carefully insert the needle through the skin just until the bevel point is under the skin surface.	4			
15. Slowly and steadily inject the medication by depressing the plunger with your little finger. A wheal should appear.	4			
16. After administering all of the medication, withdraw the needle.	4			
17. Immediately dispose of the contaminated syringe unit in a sharps container.	4			
18. Do not massage the area, but you may blot it with a cotton ball or gauze square.	4			
19. Make sure that your patient is comfortable and safe.	4			
20. Observe the patient for any adverse reaction. If you are performing allergy testing, the patient must be observed for 20 to 30 minutes.	4			
21. Dispose of the gloves in the biohazard container and wash your hands.	4			
22. Record the procedure and any reactions that occurred at the site of the injection on the patient's medical record. Include the exact site of the injection.	4			
23. Tell the patient when to return to the office for the reaction to be read or give the patient a postcard to be completed and returned.	4			

Documentation in the Medical Record

____

____

____

____

Comments:

Total Points Earned ________ Divided by ________ Total Possible Points = ________ % Score

Instructor's Signature ____________________

Student Name ______________ Date ______________ Score ______________

Procedure 32-5 Administering a Tuberculin Tine Test

Task: To Administer a Tuberculin Tine Test.

Equipment and Supplies:
- Tuberculin tine test stamp
- Alcohol wipe
- Disposable gloves
- Sharps container
- Physician order

Standards: Complete the procedure and all critical steps in ______________ minutes with a minimum score of ______________ % within three attempts.

Scoring: Divide points earned by total possible points. Failure to perform a critical step that is indicated with an asterisk (*), will result in an unsatisfactory overall score.

Time began ______________ **Time ended** ______________

Steps	**Possible Points**	**First Attempt**	**Second Attempt**	**Third Attempt**
1. Wash hands. Follow standard precautions. Glove with disposable nonsterile gloves.	10			
2. Greet the patient and verify patient name.	10			
3. Explain the procedure.	10			
4. Position the patient to reduce strain on the forearm.	5			
5. Cleanse the site with the alcohol wipe in a circular fashion from the inside outward. Allow alcohol to dry.	5			
6. Pull the site taut with the nondominant thumb and fingers.	5			
7. Press the prongs of the tine firmly against the cleansed area for 1 to 2 seconds.	10			
8. Immediately discard the stamp into the sharps container.	10			
9. Do not massage area.	5			
10. Dispose of the gloves in the biohazard container and wash hands.	10			

Steps	Possible Points	First Attempt	Second Attempt	Third Attempt
11. Observe patient for untoward reactions and document the procedure including the name of the test, time of administration, exact site of administration, and any patient complaints.	**10**	_____	_____	_____
12. Patient education to return to the office in 48 to 72 hours to have the results read or explain how to read results at home.	**10**	_____	_____	_____

Documentation in the Medical Record

____

____

____

____

Comments:

Total Points Earned ________ Divided by ________ Total Possible Points = ________ % Score

Instructor's Signature ____________________

Student Name ______________________ Date __________ Score __________

Procedure 32-6 Giving a Subcutaneous Injection

Task: To inject 0.5 ml of medication into the subcutaneous tissue using a 25 gauge, 5/8 inch needle and syringe of correct size and type, as directed by the physician.

Equipment and Supplies:
- A vial or ampule containing the medication to be injected
- Alcohol wipes
- Gauze squares or cotton balls
- A sterile needle and syringe unit
- Nonsterile disposable gloves
- Sharps container
- A written order, including the patient's name, when to give the drug, the route of administration, and the name and strength of the drug

Standards: Complete the procedure and all critical steps in __________ minutes with a minimum score of __________ % within three attempts.

Scoring: Divide points earned by total possible points. Failure to perform a critical step that is indicated with an asterisk (*), will result in an unsatisfactory overall score.

Time began __________ **Time ended** __________

Steps	Possible Points	First Attempt	Second Attempt	Third Attempt
1. Wash your hands. Follow Standard Precautions.*	5			
2. Select the correct medication from the shelf or the refrigerator.	5			
3. Read the label to be sure that you have the right drug and the right strength. Perform the 3 label and order checks while dispensing the medication and the 7 rights. Perform any necessary dose calculations.*	5			
4. Warm refrigerated medications by gently rolling the container between your palms.	5			
5. Prepare the syringe, withdrawing the right dose.	5			
6. Transport the medication to the patient.	2.5			
7. Greet and identify the patient by name.	2.5			
8. Position the patient comfortably.	5			
9. Expose the site and clean the area.	5			
10. Remove the cap from the needle.	5			

Steps	Possible Points	First Attempt	Second Attempt	Third Attempt
11. With the thumb and fingers of your nondominant hand, grasp the tissue of the posterior upper arm.	5			
12. Hold the syringe between the thumb and the first two fingers of your dominant hand, and with one swift movement, insert the entire needle up to the hub at a 45-degree angle.	5			
13. Aspirate (except when administering heparin or insulin) by withdrawing the plunger slightly to be sure that no blood enters the syringe.	5			
14. If blood appears, immediately withdraw the unit without injecting the medication, dispose of it in the sharps container. Compress the injection site with an alcohol swab or gauze bandage. Begin again with step 1.	2.5			
15. If no blood appears in the syringe, push in the plunger slowly and steadily until all medication has been administered.	2.5			
16. Place the gauze square next to the needle and withdraw it at the same angle of insertion.	5			
17. Gently massage the site with the gauze square (do not massage insulin or heparin injections).	5			
18. Discard the needle and syringe into the sharps container.	5			
19. Make sure that your patient is comfortable and safe.	5			
20. Dispose of the gloves in the biohazard waste and wash your hands.	5			
21. Observe the patient for any adverse reaction. You may need to keep the patient under observation for 20 to 30 minutes.	5			
22. Record the drug administration on the patient's medical record, and on the required DEA record if the medication is a controlled substance.	5			

Documentation in the Medical Record

____

____

____

____

Comments:

Total Points Earned ________ Divided by ________ Total Possible Points = ________ % Score

Instructor's Signature ____________________

Student Name ________________ Date ________ Score ________

Procedure 32-7 Giving an Intramuscular Injection

Task: To inject 2 ml of medication into the muscle, using a 22 gauge 1½ inch needle and 3 ml syringe, as directed by the physician.

Equipment and Supplies:
- A vial or ampule containing the medication to be injected
- Alcohol wipes
- Gauze squares or cotton balls
- A sterile needle and syringe unit
- Nonsterile disposable gloves
- Sharps container
- A written order, including the patient's name, when to give the drug, the route of administration, and the name and strength of the drug

Standards: Complete the procedure and all critical steps in ________ minutes with a minimum score of ________ % within three attempts.

Scoring: Divide points earned by total possible points. Failure to perform a critical step that is indicated with an asterisk (*), will result in an unsatisfactory overall score.

Time began ________ **Time ended** ________

Steps	**Possible Points**	**First Attempt**	**Second Attempt**	**Third Attempt**
1. Wash your hands. Follow Standard Precautions.*	5			
2. Select the correct medication from the shelf or the refrigerator.	5			
3. Read the label to be sure that you have the right drug and the right strength. Perform the 3 label and order checks while dispensing the medication and the 7 rights. Perform any necessary dose calculations.*	5			
4. Warm refrigerated medications by gently rolling the container between your palms.	5			
5. Prepare the syringe, withdrawing the right dose. Complete calculations.	5			
6. Transport the medication to the patient.	2.5			
7. Greet and identify the patient by name.	2.5			
8. Help the patient into an upright sitting position.	5			
9. Apply gloves. Expose the site.	5			
10. Clean skin. Remove the cap from the needle.	5			

Steps	Possible Points	First Attempt	Second Attempt	Third Attempt
11. With the thumb and fingers of your nondominant hand, grasp the tissue of the upper arm.	5			
12. Hold the syringe between the thumb and the first two fingers of your dominant hand, and with one swift movement, insert the entire needle up to the hub at a 90-degree* angle.	5			
13. Aspirate* by withdrawing the plunger slightly to be sure that no blood enters the syringe.	5			
14. If blood appears, immediately withdraw the unit without injecting the medication, dispose of it in the sharps container. Compress the injection site with an alcohol swab or gauze bandage. Begin again with step 1.	2.5			
15. If no blood appears in the syringe, push in the plunger slowly and steadily until all medication has been administered.	2.5			
16. Place the gauze square next to the needle and withdraw it at the same angle of insertion.	5			
17. Gently massage the site with a cotton ball.	5			
18. Discard the needle and syringe into the sharps container.	5			
19. Make sure that your patient is comfortable and safe.	5			
20. Dispose of the gloves in the biohazard waste and wash your hands.	5			
21. Observe the patient for any adverse reaction. You may need to keep the patient under observation for 20 to 30 minutes.	5			
22. Record the drug administration on the patient's medical record, and on the required DEA record if the medication is a controlled substance.	5			

Documentation in the Medical Record

____

____

____

____

Comments:

Total Points Earned ________ Divided by ________ Total Possible Points = ________ % Score

Instructor's Signature ____________________

Student Name ______________________ Date __________ Score __________

Procedure 32-8 Reconstituting a Powdered Drug for Administration

Task: To reconstitute a powdered drug for intramuscular injection as ordered by the physician.

Equipment and Supplies:
- A vial containing the ordered powdered medication
- Diluent: Sterile saline solution
- Alcohol wipes
- A cotton ball
- Two sterile needle and syringe units
- Nonsterile disposable gloves
- A sharps container
- A written order, including the patient's name, when to give the drug, the route of administration, and the name and strength of the drug.

Standards: Complete the procedure and all critical steps in __________ minutes with a minimum score of __________ % within three attempts.

Scoring: Divide points earned by total possible points. Failure to perform a critical step that is indicated with an asterisk (*), will result in an unsatisfactory overall score.

Time began __________ **Time ended** __________

Steps	**Possible Points**	**First Attempt**	**Second Attempt**	**Third Attempt**
1. Wash your hands. Follow standard precautions.*	10			
2. Select the correct vial of powdered medication from the shelf and the recommended diluent for reconstitution. Perform the three drug label and physician order checks during preparation and apply the seven rights throughout the procedure.*	15			
3. Read the label to determine the correct amount of diluent to add to create the dose ordered by the physician. Calculate the correct dose, if necessary, and continue with the three label checks.	15			
4. Remove the top from each vial and clean each with an alcohol wipe. Leave the wipes in place on top of each vial.	5			
5. Grasp the syringe plunger and draw up an amount of air equal to the amount of diluent needed to reconstitute the drug.	5			
6. Remove the needle cover and insert the needle into the center of the rubber stopper of the vial of diluent. Hold the vial firmly against a flat surface and watch carefully that the needle only touches the cleaned rubber area.	5			
7. Inject the aspirated air in the syringe into the diluent vial.	5			

Steps	Possible Points	First Attempt	Second Attempt	Third Attempt
8. Invert the diluent vial and aspirate the calculated or recommended amount of diluent.	5			
9. Remove the needle from the diluent vial and inject the diluent into the drug vial. Remove the needle and discard it in the sharps container.	5			
10. Roll the vial with the drug and diluent mixture between the palms of your hands to mix it thoroughly. Do not shake the vial unless directed to do so on the drug label. When the medication has been completely mixed, there will be no residue or crystals on the bottom of the vial.	5			
11. Aspirate air into the second syringe unit that is equal to the calculated amount of medication to be administered.	5			
12. Inject the air into the mixed drug vial, invert the vial, and withdraw the ordered amount of medication.	15			
13. Proceed as outlined in steps 6 to 22 in Procedure 32-6.	5			

Documentation in the Medical Record

____

____

____

____

Comments:

Total Points Earned ________ Divided by ________ Total Possible Points = ________ % Score

Instructor's Signature ____________________

Student Name ______________________ Date ____________ Score ________

Procedure 32-9 Giving a Z-Track Intramuscular Injection

Task: To inject 1 ml of medication into the muscle by using a 23-gauge, 2½-inch needle, and 3-ml syringe and the Z-track method, as directed by the physician.

Equipment and Supplies:
- A vial or ampule containing the medication to be injected
- Alcohol wipes
- Gauze squares or cotton balls
- A sterile needle and syringe unit
- Nonsterile disposable gloves
- Sharps container
- A written order, including the patient's name, when to give the drug, the route of administration, and the name and strength of the drug
- Package insert drug reference for safety precautions

Standards: Complete the procedure and all critical steps in ____________ minutes with a minimum score of ____________ % within three attempts.

Scoring: Divide points earned by total possible points. Failure to perform a critical step that is indicated with an asterisk (*), will result in an unsatisfactory overall score.

Time began ____________ **Time ended** ____________

Steps	Possible Points	First Attempt	Second Attempt	Third Attempt
1. Wash your hands. Follow standard precautions.*	5			
2. Select the correct medication from the shelf or the refrigerator.	5			
3. Read the label to be sure that you have the right drug and the right strength. Perform the three label and order checks while dispensing the medication and apply the seven rights. Perform any necessary dose calculations.*	5			
4. Warm refrigerated medications by gently rolling the container between your palms.	2			
5. Prepare the syringe, withdrawing the right dose. Complete calculations.	5			
6. Replace the needle cover and give a slight turn to loosen the needle. Secure a new needle, still in its sheath, to the tip of the syringe. Discard the drug-contaminated needle.	5			
7. Transport the medication to the patient.	2			
8. Greet and identify the patient by name.	2			
9. Help the patient into a semiprone position.	5			

Steps	Possible Points	First Attempt	Second Attempt	Third Attempt
10. Apply gloves. Expose the site.	2			
11. Clean skin. Remove the cap from the needle.	5			
12. Push the skin to one side and hold it firmly in place.* If the skin is slippery, use a dry gauze sponge to hold the skin in place.	5			
13. Grasp the syringe as you would a dart, and with one swift movement, insert the entire needle up to the hub, at a 90-degree angle* into the gluteal muscle.	5			
14. Aspirate* by withdrawing the plunger slightly to be sure that no blood enters the syringe.	5			
15. If blood appears, immediately withdraw the unit without injecting the medication, and dispose of it in the sharps container. Compress the injection site with an alcohol swab or gauze bandage. Begin again with step 1.	5			
16. If no blood appears in the syringe, push in the plunger slowly and steadily until all medication has been administered.	2			
17. Wait a few seconds, then withdraw the needle at the same angle of insertion. Wait 10 seconds, then release the skin.	5			
18. If recommended by the manufacturer, gently massage the site with a cotton ball.	5			
19. Discard the needle and syringe in the sharps container.	5			
20. Make sure that your patient is comfortable and safe.	5			
21. Dispose of the gloves in the biohazard waste container and wash your hands.	5			
22. Observe the patient for any adverse reaction. You may need to keep the patient under observation for 20 to 30 minutes.	5			
23. Record the drug administration on the patient's medical record and on the required Drug Enforcement Agency (DEA) record if the medication is a controlled substance.	5			

Documentation in the Medical Record

____

____

____

____

Comments:

Total Points Earned ________ Divided by ________ Total Possible Points = ________ % Score

Instructor's Signature ______________________

Student Name ______________________ Date ____________ Score ________

Procedure 33-1 Using an Automated External Defibrillator (AED)

Task: To defibrillate adult victims with cardiac arrest.

Equipment and Supplies:
- Practice AED
- Approved mannequin

Standards: Complete the procedure and all critical steps in ____________ minutes with a minimum score of ____________ % within three attempts.

Scoring: Divide points earned by total possible points. Failure to perform a critical step that is indicated with an asterisk (*), will result in an unsatisfactory overall score.

Time began ____________ **Time ended** ____________

Steps	**Possible Points**	**First Attempt**	**Second Attempt**	**Third Attempt**
1. Place the AED near the victim's left ear. Turn the AED on.	**20**			
2. Attach electrode pads as pictured on the AED electrodes at the sternum and apex of the heart. Make sure pads have complete contact with the victim's chest and they do not overlap.	**20**			
3. All rescuers must clear away from the victim. Press the ANALYZE button. The AED will analyze the victim's coronary status, will announce if the victim is going to be shocked, and automatically charges the electrodes.	**20**			
4. All rescuers must clear away from the victim.* Press the SHOCK button if the machine is not automated. May repeat 1 to 2 more analyze-shock cycles.	**20***			
5. If the machine gives the "no shock indicated" signal, assess the victim. Check the carotid pulse and breathing status and keep the AED attached until EMS arrives.	**20**			

Documentation in the Medical Record

____

____

____

____

Comments:

Total Points Earned ________ Divided by ________ Total Possible Points = ________ % Score

Instructor's Signature ____________________

Student Name ______________ Date ______________ Score ______________

Procedure 33-2 Responding to a Patient with an Obstructed Airway

Task: To remove an airway obstruction and restore ventilation.

Equipment and Supplies:
- Nonsterile gloves
- Ventilation mask (for unconscious victim)
- Approved mannequin to practice unconscious Foreign Body Airway Obstruction (FBAO).

Standards: Complete the procedure and all critical steps in ______________ minutes with a minimum score of ______________ % within three attempts.

Scoring: Divide points earned by total possible points. Failure to perform a critical step that is indicated with an asterisk (*), will result in an unsatisfactory overall score.

Time began ______________ **Time ended** ______________

Steps	Possible Points	First Attempt	Second Attempt	Third Attempt
1. Ask, "Are you choking?" If victim indicates yes, ask "Can you speak?". If unable to speak, tell the victim you are going to help.*	10			
2. Stand behind the victim with feet slightly apart.	5			
3. Reach around the victim's abdomen and place an index finger into the victim's navel or at the level of the belt buckle. Make a fist of the opposite hand (do not tuck the thumb into the fist) and place the thumb side of the fist against the victim's abdomen above the navel. If the victim is pregnant, place the fist above the enlarged uterus. If the victim is obese, it may be necessary to place the fist higher in the abdomen. It may be necessary to perform chest thrusts on a victim who is pregnant or obese.	5			
4. Place the opposite hand over the fist and give abdominal thrusts in a quick upward movement.	5			
5. Repeat the abdominal thrusts until the object is expelled or the victim becomes unresponsive.	5			
Unresponsive Victim				
6. Activate the emergency response system.*	10			
7. Put on gloves if available and get ventilation mask. Open the victim's mouth and perform a finger sweep to determine if the foreign object is in the mouth and to remove it.	5			

Steps	Possible Points	First Attempt	Second Attempt	Third Attempt
8. Open the airway with a head-tilt, jaw-thrust maneuver and attempt to ventilate with 2 slow breaths. If breaths do not go in (chest does not rise), retilt the head and try to ventilate again.	5			
9. If ventilation is unsuccessful, move to the victim's feet and kneel across the victim's thighs. Place the heel of one hand above the navel but below the xiphoid process of the sternum. Place the other hand on top of the first, with the fingers elevated off of the abdomen. Administer 5 abdominal thrusts.	5			
10. Move back beside the head of the victim and repeat the finger sweep. If the obstruction is not found, continue cycles of 2 rescue breaths, 5 abdominal thrusts, and finger sweep until either the obstruction is removed or EMS arrives.	5			
11. If the obstruction is removed, assess the victim for breathing and circulation. If a pulse is present, but no breathing, begin rescues breathing. If there is no pulse, begin CPR.	5			
12. Once patient is either stabilized or EMS has taken over care, remove gloves and the ventilator mask valve and dispose in the biohazard container. Disinfect the ventilator mask per manufacturer recommendations. Wash hands.	5			
13. Document the procedure and patient condition.	5			

Documentation in the Medical Record

____

____

____

____

Comments:

Total Points Earned ________ Divided by ________ Total Possible Points = ________ % Score

Instructor's Signature ____________________

Student Name ______________________ Date __________ Score __________

Procedure 33-3 Administering Oxygen

Task: To provide oxygen for a patient in respiratory distress.

Equipment and Supplies:
- Portable oxygen tank
- Pressure regulator
- Flow meter
- Nasal cannula with connecting tubing

Standards: Complete the procedure and all critical steps in __________ minutes with a minimum score of __________ % within three attempts.

Scoring: Divide points earned by total possible points. Failure to perform a critical step that is indicated with an asterisk (*), will result in an unsatisfactory overall score.

Time began __________ **Time ended** __________

Steps	**Possible Points**	**First Attempt**	**Second Attempt**	**Third Attempt**
1. Gather equipment and wash hands.	**10**			
2. Identify the patient and explain the procedure.	**10**			
3. Check the pressure gauge on the tank to determine the amount of oxygen in the tank.	**10**			
4. If necessary, open the cylinder on the tank one full counterclockwise turn and attach the cannula tubing to the flowmeter.	**20**			
5. Adjust the administration of the oxygen according to the physician's order. Check to make sure the oxygen is flowing through the cannula.	**10**			
6. Insert the cannula tips into the nostrils and adjust the tubing around the back of the patient's ears.	**10**			
7. Make sure the patient is comfortable and answer any questions.	**10**			
8. Wash hands.	**10**			
9. Document the procedure including the number of liters of oxygen being administered and the patient's condition. Continue to monitor the patient throughout the procedure and document any changes in condition.	**10**			

Documentation in the Medical Record

____

____

____

____

Comments:

Total Points Earned ________ Divided by ________ Total Possible Points = ________ % Score

Instructor's Signature ______________________

Student Name ______________ Date ______________ Score ______________

Procedure 33-4 Providing Rescue Breathing and Performing One Man CPR

Task: To restore a victim's breathing and blood circulation when respiration and pulse stop.

Equipment and Supplies:
- Nonsterile gloves
- CPR ventilator mask
- Approved mannequin

Standards: Complete the procedure and all critical steps in ______________ minutes with a minimum score of ______________ % within three attempts.

Scoring: Divide points earned by total possible points. Failure to perform a critical step that is indicated with an asterisk (*), will result in an unsatisfactory overall score.

Time began ______________ **Time ended** ______________

Steps	**Possible Points**	**First Attempt**	**Second Attempt**	**Third Attempt**
1. Establish unresponsiveness. Tap the victim and ask, Are you OK? Wait for victim to respond.	10			
2. Activate the emergency response system. Put on gloves and get ventilator mask.	5			
3. Tilt the victim's head and lift the chin. Look, listen, and feel for signs of breathing. Place your ear over the mouth and listen for breathing. Watch the rising and falling of the chest for evidence of breathing.	10			
4. If breathing is absent or inadequate, place the ventilator mask over the victim's mouth and give 2 slow breaths (2 seconds per breath), holding the ventilator mask tightly against the face while tilting the victim's chin back to open the airway. Allow time for exhalation between breaths.	10			
5. Check the carotid pulse. If a pulse is present, continue rescue breathing (1 breath every 5 seconds, about 10 to 12 breaths per minute). If no signs of circulation are present, begin cycles of 15 chest compressions (at a rate of about 100 compressions per minute) followed by 2 slow breaths.	10			
6. Kneel at the victim's side opposite the chest. Move your fingers up the ribs to the point where the sternum and the ribs join. Your middle fingers should fit into the area and your index finger should be next to it across the sternum.	10			

Steps	Possible Points	First Attempt	Second Attempt	Third Attempt
7. Place the heel of your hand on the chest midline over the sternum, just above your index finger.	5			
8. Place your other hand on top of your first hand and lift your fingers upward off of the chest.	5			
9. Bring your shoulders directly over the victim's sternum as you compress downward, and keep your arms straight.	5			
10. Depress the sternum $1\frac{1}{2}$ to 2 inches for an adult victim. Relax the pressure on the sternum after each compression but do not remove your hands from the victim's sternum.	10			
11. After performing 15 compressions (at a rate of about 100 compressions per minute), open the airway and give 2 slow breaths.	5			
12. After 4 cycles of compressions and breaths (15:2 ratio, about 1 minute) recheck breathing and carotid pulse. If there is a pulse but no breathing, continue rescue breathing (1 breath every 5 seconds, about 10 to 12 breaths per minute) and reevaluate the victim's breathing and pulse every few minutes. If there are no signs of circulation, continue 15:2 cycles of compressions and ventilations, starting with chest compressions. Continue giving CPR until the EMS relieves you.	5			
13. Remove gloves and the ventilator mask valve and dispose in the biohazard container. Disinfect the ventilator mask per manufacturer recommendations. Wash hands.	5			
14. Document the procedure and patient condition.	5			

Documentation in the Medical Record

____

____

____

____

Comments:

Total Points Earned ________ Divided by ________ Total Possible Points = ________ % Score

Instructor's Signature ______________________

Student Name ______________________ Date ____________ Score ________

Procedure 33-5 Caring for a Patient who Fainted

Task: To provide emergency care and assessment of a patient who has fainted.

Equipment and Supplies:
- Sphygmomanometer
- Stethoscope
- Watch with second hand
- Blanket
- Foot stool or box
- Physician may order oxygen:
  - Portable oxygen tank
  - Pressure regulator
  - Flow meter
  - Nasal cannula with connecting tubing

Standards: Complete the procedure and all critical steps in ____________ minutes with a minimum score of ____________ % within three attempts.

Scoring: Divide points earned by total possible points. Failure to perform a critical step that is indicated with an asterisk (*), will result in an unsatisfactory overall score.

Time began ____________ **Time ended** ____________

Steps	Possible Points	First Attempt	Second Attempt	Third Attempt
1. If warning is given that the patient feels faint, have the patient lower the head to the knees to increase blood supply to the brain. If this does not stop the episode, either have the patient lie down on the examination table or lower the patient to the floor. If the patient collapses to the floor when fainting, treat with caution due to possible head or neck injuries.	10			
2. Immediately notify the physician of the patient's condition and assess the patient for life-threatening emergencies such as respiratory or cardiac arrest. If the patient is breathing and has a pulse, monitor the patient's vital signs.	10			
3. Loosen any tight clothing and keep the patient warm, applying a blanket if needed.	20			
4. If there is no concern about a head or neck injury, elevate the patient's legs above the level of the heart.	10			
5. Continue to monitor vital signs and apply oxygen via nasal cannula if ordered by the physician.	10			

Steps	Possible Points	First Attempt	Second Attempt	Third Attempt
6. If vital signs are unstable or the patient does not respond quickly, activate emergency medical services.	10			
7. If the patient vomits, roll the patient on his or her side to avoid aspiration of vomitus into the lungs.	10			
8. Once the patient has completely recovered, assist the patient into a sitting position. *Do not* leave the patient unattended on the examination table.	10			
9. Document the incident including a description of the episode, patient symptoms, vital signs, length of time, and any complaints. If oxygen was administered, document the number of liters and length of administration.	10			

Documentation in the Medical Record

____

____

____

____

Comments:

Total Points Earned ________ Divided by ________ Total Possible Points = ________ % Score

Instructor's Signature ________________

Student Name ________________ Date ________ Score ________

Procedure 33-6 Controlling Bleeding

Task: To stop hemorrhaging from an open wound.

Equipment and Supplies:
- Gloves, sterile if available
- Appropriate Personal Protective Equipment according to OSHA guidelines including:
  - Impermeable gown
  - Goggles
  - Impermeable mask
- Sterile dressings
- Bandaging material
- Biohazard waste container

Standards: Complete the procedure and all critical steps in ________ minutes with a minimum score of ________ % within three attempts.

Scoring: Divide points earned by total possible points. Failure to perform a critical step that is indicated with an asterisk (*), will result in an unsatisfactory overall score.

Time began ________ **Time ended** ________

Steps	**Possible Points**	**First Attempt**	**Second Attempt**	**Third Attempt**
1. Wash hands and apply appropriate personal protective equipment.	**10**			
2. Assemble equipment and supplies.	**10**			
3. Apply several layers of sterile dressing material directly to the wound and exert pressure.	**10**			
4. Wrap the wound with bandage material. Add more dressing and bandaging material if bleeding continues.	**10**			
5. If bleeding persists and the wound is located on an extremity, elevate the extremity above the level of the heart. Notify the physician immediately if bleeding cannot be controlled.	**10**			
6. If bleeding still continues, apply pressure to the appropriate artery. If bleeding is in the arm, apply pressure to the brachial artery by squeezing the inner aspect of the upper mid-arm. If bleeding is in the leg apply pressure to the femoral artery on the affected side by pushing with the heel of the hand into the femoral crease at the groin. *If bleeding cannot be controlled, it may be necessary to activate the emergency medical system.*	**10**			

Steps	Possible Points	First Attempt	Second Attempt	Third Attempt
7. Once the bleeding is controlled and the patient is stabilized, dispose of contaminated materials into the biohazard waste container.	10			
8. Disinfect the area, remove gloves, and dispose into biohazard waste.				
9. Wash hands.	10			
10. Document the incident including the details of the wound, when and how it occurred, patient symptoms, vital signs, physician treatment, and the patient's current condition	10			

Documentation in the Medical Record

Comments:

Total Points Earned ________ Divided by ________ Total Possible Points = ________ % Score

Instructor's Signature ____________________

Student Name ____________ Date ________ Score ________

Procedure 34-1 Measuring Distance Visual Acuity with the Snellen Chart

Task: To determine the patient's degree of visual clarity at a measured distance by using the Snellen chart.

Equipment and Supplies:
- Snellen eye chart
- Eye occluder
- Pen or pencil and paper

Standards: Complete the procedure and all critical steps in ________ minutes with a minimum score of ________ % within three attempts.

Scoring: Divide points earned by total possible points. Failure to perform a critical step that is indicated with an asterisk (*), will result in an unsatisfactory overall score.

Time began ________ **Time ended** ________

Steps	**Possible Points**	**First Attempt**	**Second Attempt**	**Third Attempt**
1. Wash your hands.	10			
2. Prepare the examination room. Make sure that (a) the room is well lighted, (b) a distance marker is 20 feet from the chart, and (c) the chart is placed at the eye level of the patient.*	10			
3. Identify the patient and explain the procedure. Instruct the patient not to squint during the test, since this temporarily improves vision. The patient should not have an opportunity to study the chart before the test. If the patient wears corrective lenses, they should be worn during the test.	10			
4. Have the patient stand or sit at the 20-foot marker.*	10			
5. Position the Snellen chart at eye level to the patient.	5			
6. Instruct the patient to cover the left eye with the occluder and to keep both eyes open throughout the test to prevent squinting.	10			
7. Stand beside the chart and point to each row as the patient orally reads down the chart, starting with the 20/70 row.	10			
8. Proceed down the rows of the chart until the smallest row the patient can read with a maximum of two errors is reached. If one or two letters are missed, the outcome is recorded with a minus sign and the number of errors. If more than two errors are made, findings from reading the previous line should be documented.	10			

Steps	Possible Points	First Attempt	Second Attempt	Third Attempt
9. Record any patient reactions in reading the chart.	5			
10. Repeat the procedure with the left eye.	10			
11. Document the date and time, the procedure, visual acuity results, and any patient reactions on the patient's record. Also record whether corrective lenses were worn.	10			

Documentation in the Medical Record

Comments:

Total Points Earned ________ Divided by ________ Total Possible Points = ________ % Score

Instructor's Signature ____________________

Student Name ______________________ Date ____________ Score ____________

Procedure 34-2 Assessment of Color Acuity with the Ishihara Test

Task: To correctly assess a patient's color acuity and record the results.

Equipment and Supplies:
- Appropriate room area with natural light
- Ishihara color plate book
- Pen, pencil, and paper
- Watch with a second hand

Standards: Complete the procedure and all critical steps in ____________ minutes with a minimum score of ____________ % within three attempts.

Scoring: Divide points earned by total possible points. Failure to perform a critical step that is indicated with an asterisk (*), will result in an unsatisfactory overall score.

Time began ____________ **Time ended** ____________

Steps	**Possible Points**	**First Attempt**	**Second Attempt**	**Third Attempt**
1. Assemble the necessary equipment and prepare the room for testing. The room should be quiet and illuminated with natural light.	**10**			
2. Identify the patient and explain the procedure. Use a practice card during the explanation and be sure that the patient understands that he or she has 3 seconds to identify each plate.	**10**			
3. Hold up the first plate at a right angle to the patient's line of vision and 30 inches from the patient. Be sure both eyes are kept open during the test.	**20**			
4. Ask the patient to tell you what number is on the plate and record the plate number and the patient's answer.	**10**			
5. Continue this sequence until all 11 plates have been read. If the patient cannot identify the number on the plate, place an X in the record for that plate number. Your record should look like this: Plate 1 = pass, Plate 2 = pass, Plate 3 = x, Plate 4 = pass, and so on.	**10**			
6. Include any unusual symptoms such as eye rubbing, squinting, or excessive blinking in the record.	**10**			

Steps	Possible Points	First Attempt	Second Attempt	Third Attempt
7. Place the book back into its cardboard sleeve and return the book to its storage space. The Ishihara color plates need to be stored in a closed position away from external light to protect the colors.	10			
8. Record the procedure, including the date and time, the test results, and any patient symptoms exhibited during the test in the patient's record.	20			

Documentation in the medical record

Comments:

Total Points Earned ______ Divided by ______ Total Possible Points = ______ % Score

Instructor's Signature ______

Student Name ______________________ Date __________ Score __________

Procedure 34-3 Irrigating a Patient's Eyes

Task: To cleanse the eye(s), as ordered by the physician.

Equipment and Supplies:
- Prescribed sterile irrigation solution
- Sterile irrigating bulb syringe and sterile basin or prepackaged solution with dispenser
- Basin for drainage
- Sterile gauze squares
- Disposable drape
- Towel
- Nonsterile gloves
- Biohazard waste container

Standards: Complete the procedure and all critical steps in __________ minutes with a minimum score of __________ % within three attempts.

Scoring: Divide points earned by total possible points. Failure to perform a critical step that is indicated with an asterisk (*), will result in an unsatisfactory overall score.

Time began __________ **Time ended** __________

Steps	Possible Points	First Attempt	Second Attempt	Third Attempt
1. Wash your hands. Put on gloves.*	5			
2. Check the physician's orders to determine which eye (or both) requires irrigation and the type of solution to be used.*	5			
3. Assemble the materials needed.	5			
4. Check the expiration date of the solution and read the label three times.	5			
5. Identify the patient and explain the procedure.	5			
6. Assist the patient into a sitting or supine position, making certain that the head is turned toward the side of the affected eye. Place the disposable drape over the patient's neck and shoulder.	5			
7. Place or have the patient hold a drainage basin next to the affected eye to receive the solution from the eye. Place a polylined drape under the basin to avoid getting the solution on the patient.	5			
8. Moisten a gauze square with solution and cleanse the eyelid and lashes. Start at the inner canthus (near nose) and wipe toward the outer canthus (farthest from nose) and dispose of the gauze square after each wipe.	10			

Steps	Possible Points	First Attempt	Second Attempt	Third Attempt
9. If you are using a bulb syringe, pour the required volume of body-temperature irrigating solution into the basin and withdraw solution into the bulb syringe. If you are using an irrigating solution in a prepackaged dispenser, remove the lid.	10			
10. Separate and hold eyelids with the index finger and thumb of one hand. With the other hand, place the syringe or dispenser on the bridge of the nose parallel to the eye.	10			
11. Squeeze the bulb or dispenser, directing the solution toward the lower conjunctiva of the inner canthus, allowing the solution to flow steadily and slowly from the inner to outer canthus. Do not touch the eye or eyelids with the applicator.	10			
12. Refill the syringe or continue to gently squeeze the prepackaged bottle and continue the procedure until the amount of solution ordered by the physician has been administered or until the drainage is clear.	5			
13. Dry the eyelid from the inner canthus to the outer canthus with sterile gauze. Do not use cotton balls because fibers might remain in the eye.	5			
14. Clean the work area.	5			
15. Remove gloves and wash your hands.	5			
16. Document the procedure using appropriate abbreviations; include the date and time, the type and amount of solution used, which eye was irrigated, any significant patient reactions, and the results in the patient's record.	5			

Documentation in the Medical Record

___

___

___

___

Comments:

Total Points Earned ______ Divided by ______ Total Possible Points = ______ % Score

Instructor's Signature ______________

Student Name ______________________ Date ____________ Score ____________

Procedure 34-4 Instilling Eye Medication

Task: To apply medication to the eye(s), as ordered by the physician.

Equipment and Supplies:
- Sterile medication with sterile eye dropper or ophthalmic ointment
- Disposable drape
- Sterile gauze squares
- Nonsterile gloves

Standards: Complete the procedure and all critical steps in ____________ minutes with a minimum score of ____________ % within three attempts.

Scoring: Divide points earned by total possible points. Failure to perform a critical step that is indicated with an asterisk (*), will result in an unsatisfactory overall score.

Time began ____________ **Time ended** ____________

Steps	**Possible Points**	**First Attempt**	**Second Attempt**	**Third Attempt**
1. Wash your hands.*	10			
2. Check the physician's order to determine which eye(s) requires medication and the name and strength of the medication you will be using.	6			
3. Assemble equipment and supplies.	6			
4. Read the medication label three times.*	10			
5. Identify the patient and explain the procedure.	6			
6. Put on nonsterile gloves and rinse your gloved hands under warm water to remove all powder from gloves.	6			
7. Assist the patient into a sitting or supine position. Ask the patient to tilt the head backward and look up.	6			
8. Pull the lower conjunctival sac downward.*	10			
9. Insert the prescribed number of drops or amount of ointment into the eye. For eye drops, place drops in the center of the lower conjunctival sac with the tip of the dropper held parallel to the eye and ½ inch above the eye sac. For eye ointment (unguent), squeeze a thin ribbon along the lower conjunctival sac from inner to outer canthus, making sure not to touch the eye with the applicator.*	10			

Steps	Possible Points	First Attempt	Second Attempt	Third Attempt
10. Instruct the patient to *gently* close the eye and rotate the eyeball.	6			
11. Dry any excess drainage from inner to outer canthus and explain that the medication may temporarily blur vision.	6			
12. Discard the unused medication and clean the procedure area.	6			
13. Remove gloves and wash hands.	6			
14. Record the procedure on the patient's chart including the date and time, the name and strength of the medication, the amount of the dose administered, which eye was treated, teaching instructions given if the treatment is to continue at home, and any observations.	6			

Documentation in the medical record

____

____

____

____

Comments:

Total Points Earned ________ Divided by ________ Total Possible Points = ________ % Score

Instructor's Signature ____________________

Student Name ______________________ Date __________ Score __________

Procedure 34-5 Measuring Hearing Acuity Using an Audiometer

Task: To perform audiometric testing of hearing acuity.

Equipment and Supplies:
- Audiometer with adjustable headphones
- Quiet area

Standards: Complete the procedure and all critical steps in __________ minutes with a minimum score of __________ % within three attempts.

Scoring: Divide points earned by total possible points. Failure to perform a critical step that is indicated with an asterisk (*), will result in an unsatisfactory overall score.

Time began __________ **Time ended** __________

Steps	**Possible Points**	**First Attempt**	**Second Attempt**	**Third Attempt**
1. Wash hands, assemble equipment, and conduct patient into a quiet area.	**10**			
2. Explain the audiometer will measure if the patient can hear various sound wave frequencies through the headphones. Each ear will be tested separately. When the patient hears a frequency, he or she should raise a hand to signal the medical assistant.	**10**			
3. Place the headphones over the patient's ears, making sure they are adjusted for comfort.	**10**			
4. The audiometer tests each ear separately, starting at a low frequency. If the results are not automatically recorded by the machine, the medical assistant documents the patient response to the frequencies on a graph or audiogram. *The medical assistant requires specialized training to conduct this test.*	**20**			
5. Frequencies are gradually increased to test patient ability to hear. The medical assistant continues to document each response by the patient.	**10**			
6. The other ear is then tested and results documented.	**10**			
7. Patient results are given to the physician for interpretation.	**10**			
8. Disinfect the equipment according to manufacture guidelines.	**10**			
9. Wash hands.	**10**			

Documentation in the Medical Record

____

____

____

____

Comments:

Total Points Earned ________ Divided by ________ Total Possible Points = ________ % Score

Instructor's Signature ____________________

Student Name ______________ Date ______________ Score ______________

Procedure 34-6 Irrigating a Patient's Ear

Task: To irrigate a patient's ear.

Equipment and Supplies:
- Irrigating solution
- Basin for irrigating solution
- Bulb syringe or an approved otic irrigation device
- Gauze squares
- Otoscope
- Drainage basin
- Disposable drape with polylined barrier
- Cotton-tipped applicators
- Disposable gloves

Standards: Complete the procedure and all critical steps in ______________ minutes with a minimum score of ______________ % within three attempts.

Scoring: Divide points earned by total possible points. Failure to perform a critical step that is indicated with an asterisk (*), will result in an unsatisfactory overall score.

Time began ______________ **Time ended** ______________

Steps	Possible Points	First Attempt	Second Attempt	Third Attempt
1. Wash your hands.	5			
2. Check the physician's order and assemble the materials needed.	5			
3. Check the label of the solution three times: (a) when you remove it from the shelf, (b) when you pour it, and (c) when you return it to the shelf.	5			
4. Prepare the solution as ordered. The solution temperature should be at body temperature (98.6°F to 100°F) to help loosen the cerumen.	10			
5. Identify the patient and explain the procedure.	5			
6. View the affected ear with an otoscope to locate cerumen impaction.	5			
7. Place the patient in a sitting position with the head tilted toward the affected ear. Place a water-absorbent towel over a polylined barrier on the patient's shoulder, and place the collecting basin on the towel flush against the base of the ear.	5			
8. Apply gloves and wipe any particles from the outside of the ear with gauze squares.	5			
9. Test to be certain that the solution is warm,* fill the syringe, and expel air.	5			

Steps	Possible Points	First Attempt	Second Attempt	Third Attempt
10. Straighten the external ear canal.* For adults and children over the age of 3 years, gently pull the ear up and back; for children younger than 3 years, pull the ear down and back.	10			
11. Place the tip of the syringe into the meatus of the ear.	5			
12. Gently direct the flow of the solution toward the roof of the canal.	5			
13. Refill the syringe with warm solution and continue until the material has been removed. Note the particles in the collecting basin to be evaluated when the material has been successfully removed.	5			
14. Dry the patient's external ear with gauze squares and the visible ear canal gently with cotton-tipped applicators.	5			
15. Inspect the ear with an otoscope to determine the results.	5			
16. Place a clean, absorbent towel against the freshly irrigated ear and allow the patient to rest quietly while you wait for the physician to return to check the affected ear.	5			
17. Clean the work area, and return all equipment after it has been properly disinfected. Wash your hands.	5			
18. Record the procedure including the date and time, which ear was irrigated by using the appropriate abbreviations (AU – both ears, AD – right ear, AS – left ear), the type and amount of irrigating solution used, the characteristics of the material returned from the irrigation, the isibility of the tympanic membrane after irrigation, and any patient reactions.	5			

Documentation in the Medical Record

____

____

____

____

Comments:

Total Points Earned ________ Divided by ________ Total Possible Points = ________ % Score

Instructor's Signature ____________________

Student Name ______________________ Date __________ Score __________

Procedure 34-7 Instilling Medicated Ear Drops

Task: To instill the correct medication in the accurate dosage directly into the external auditory canal.

Equipment and Supplies:
- Prescribed otic drops in dispenser bottle
- Cotton balls
- Disposable gloves

Standards: Complete the procedure and all critical steps in __________ minutes with a minimum score of __________ % within three attempts.

Scoring: Divide points earned by total possible points. Failure to perform a critical step that is indicated with an asterisk (*) will result in an unsatisfactory overall score.

Time began __________ **Time ended** __________

Steps	**Possible Points**	**First Attempt**	**Second Attempt**	**Third Attempt**
1. Wash hands and gather the needed equipment and supplies.	**10**			
2. Check the medication label three times: (a) when you remove it from the shelf, (b) when you prepare it, and (c) when you return it to the shelf.	**10**			
3. Identify your patient and explain the procedure.	**10**			
4. Have the patient sit up and tilt the head away from the affected ear or lie down on the side with the affected ear upward.	**10**			
5. Check the temperature of the medication bottle. If it feels cold, gently roll the bottle back and forth between your hands to warm the drops.	**10**			
6. Hold the dropper firmly in your dominant hand. With the other hand, gently pull the pinna up and back if the patient is an adult or down and back if patient is younger than 3 years.*	**10**			
7. Place the tip of the dropper in the ear canal meatus and instill the medication drops along the side of the canal.	**10**			
8. Rest the patient on the opposite side of the affected ear and instruct him or her to remain in this position for about 3 minutes.	**10**			
9. If instructed to do so by the physician, place a moistened cotton ball into the ear canal.	**10**			
10. Clean the work area and wash your hands.	**10**			

Documentation in the Medical Record

____

____

____

____

Comments:

Total Points Earned ________ Divided by ________ Total Possible Points = ________ % Score

Instructor's Signature ____________________

Student Name ________________ Date ________ Score ________

Procedure 34-8 Collecting a Specimen for a Throat Culture

Task: To collect a specimen for throat culture with sterile technique for either immediate testing or transportation to the laboratory.

Equipment and Supplies:
- Nonsterile gloves
- Face protection barrier if the patient is coughing or if there is danger of splattering of body fluids
- Sterile swab
- Sterile tongue depressor
- Transport medium
- Biohazard waste container

Standards: Complete the procedure and all critical steps in ________ minutes with a minimum score of ________ % within three attempts.

Scoring: Divide points earned by total possible points. Failure to perform a critical step that is indicated with an asterisk (*), will result in an unsatisfactory overall score.

Time began ________ **Time ended** ________

Steps	**Possible Points**	**First Attempt**	**Second Attempt**	**Third Attempt**
1. Wash and dry your hands.	5			
2. Gather the materials needed.	5			
3. Don gloves and face protection if needed.	10			
4. Position the patient so that the light shines into the mouth.	10			
5. Remove the sterile swab from the sterile wrap with your dominant hand, and grasp the sterile tongue depressor with your nondominant hand.	10			
6. Instruct the patient to open the mouth and say "ah." Depress the tongue with the depressor.	10			
7. Swab the back of the throat between the tonsillar pillars and especially any reddened, patchy areas of the throat, white pus pockets, purulent areas, and the tonsils.	10			
8. Place the swab into the transport medium, label it, and send it to the outside laboratory. If direct slide testing is requested, return the labeled swab to the office laboratory.	10			
9. Dispose of contaminated supplies in a biohazard waste container.	5			

Steps	Possible Points	First Attempt	Second Attempt	Third Attempt
10. Disinfect the work area.	5			
11. Remove gloves; place in biohazard waste container.	5			
12. Wash your hands.	5			
13. Record procedure in the patient's record.	10			

Documentation in the Medical Record

____

____

____

____

Comments:

Total Points Earned ________ Divided by ________ Total Possible Points = ________ % Score

Instructor's Signature ____________________

Student Name ______________________ Date ____________ Score ____________

Procedure 35-1 Collecting a Wound Specimen for Testing and/or Culture

Task: To obtain an adequate, noncontaminated sample for culture.

Equipment and Supplies:
- Sterile culture kit containing tube, swabs, and transport media (for swabbing)
- Sterile culture kit containing syringe and transport media (for aspirating)
- Gauze flats
- Recommended wound cleansing solution
- Clean sterile dressing
- Gloves
- Biohazard container
- Face guard

Standards: Complete the procedure and all critical steps in ____________ minutes with a minimum score of ____________ % within three attempts.

Scoring: Divide points earned by total possible points. Failure to perform a critical step that is indicated with an asterisk (*), will result in an unsatisfactory overall score.

Time began ____________ **Time ended** ____________

Steps	**Possible Points**	**First Attempt**	**Second Attempt**	**Third Attempt**
1. Wash hands, gather supplies, and don gloves and face protection.	**10**	______	______	______
2. Remove dressing from the wound and dispose of dressing in biohazard waste container.	**10**	______	______	______
3. Observe the wound and make note of the color, odor, and amount of exudate present.	**10**	______	______	______
4. Swabbing. Remove the swab from the culture kit, insert the swab into the wound, and saturate it with the exudate. If necessary, use more than one swab, properly labeling each container, to obtain exudates from the entire wound. If doing an anaerobic culture, place the specimen in the culture tube as quickly as possible to avoid oxygen exposure and possible destruction of microbes.	**10**	______	______	______
5. Aspirating. Remove the syringe from the kit, insert the tip into the wound exudate, and pull back the plunger, drawing the exudate up into the syringe.	**10**	______	______	______
6. Place the swab into the culture tube and crush the transport media ampule, which is in the transport tube, by squeezing the walls of the transport tube slightly, or place the exudate-filled syringe directly into the transport tube.	**10**	______	______	______

Steps	Possible Points	First Attempt	Second Attempt	Third Attempt
7. Label the culture tube accurately. Include on the laboratory slip recent antibiotic therapy, the wound site, and the suspected organism.	10			
8. Clean the wound as ordered by the physician and apply a clean sterile dressing to the area.	10			
9. Clean area and dispose of all waste materials in biohazard waste container. Remove gloves and wash hands.	10			
10. Place culture tube in the laboratory collection area. Chart the procedure and all wound data on the patient's record.	10			

Documentation in the Medical Record

____

____

____

____

Comments:

Total Points Earned ________ Divided by ________ Total Possible Points = ________ % Score

Instructor's Signature ____________________

Student Name ______________________ Date __________ Score __________

Procedure 36-1 Inserting a Rectal Suppository

Task: To insert the prescribed medication accurately into the rectal mucosa.

Equipment and Supplies:
- Prescribed suppository medication
- Water-soluble lubricant
- Disposable tissues
- Biohazard waste container
- Disposable gloves

Standards: Complete the procedure and all critical steps in __________ minutes with a minimum score of __________ % within three attempts.

Scoring: Divide points earned by total possible points. Failure to perform a critical step that is indicated with an asterisk (*), will result in an unsatisfactory overall score.

Time began __________ **Time ended** __________

Steps	Possible Points	First Attempt	Second Attempt	Third Attempt
1. Wash your hands, read the order, and obtain the necessary supplies.	5			
2. Identify the patient and explain the procedure. Purpose: Proper identification saves time and avoids possible errors.	5			
3. Ask the patient to remove clothing covering the anal area.	5			
4. Assist the patient into a Sims' position and drape the exposed area.	5			
5. Don gloves. Purpose: Infection control.	10			
6. Remove the covering from the suppository and smooth any rough edges on the suppository. Purpose: Eliminates any possible trauma to the rectal mucosa.	5			
7. Generously lubricate the suppository with a water-soluble lubricant. Purpose: Promotes ease of insertion.	10			
8. With your free hand, gently lift the uppermost buttock.	20			
9. With your index finger, guide the suppository into the anus, directing it along the rectal wall and away from any fecal masses.	10			

Steps	Possible Points	First Attempt	Second Attempt	Third Attempt
10. To prevent immediate expulsion, be sure to insert the suppository beyond the internal sphincter.	5			
11. Use tissue to gently press on the anus for a few minutes to help the patient retain the rectal medication. Then, with the same tissue, wipe any excess lubricant from the rectal area. Dispose of used tissue in a biohazard container.	5			
12. Allow the patient to rest for 20 to 30 minutes before he or she gets up and leaves the office. Purpose: Medication retention.	5			
13. Clean up the area, remove gloves, and wash your hands. Purpose: Infection Control.	5			
14. Record the procedure and any pertinent information on the patient's record. Purpose: Procedures that are not recorded are considered not done.	5			

Documentation in the medical record

____

____

____

____

Comments:

Total Points Earned ________ Divided by ________ Total Possible Points = ________ % Score

Instructor's Signature ________________

Student Name ______________________ Date ____________ Score ____________

Procedure 36-2 Assisting with a Colon Endoscopic Examination

Task: To assist the physician with the examination, to prepare collected specimens as requested, and to promote patient comfort and safety.

Equipment and Supplies:
- Gloves (for medical assistant and physician)
- Appropriate instrument: sigmoidoscope, anoscope, or proctoscope
- Water-soluble lubricant
- Drape and patient gown
- Long cotton-tipped swabs
- Suction source
- Sterile biopsy forceps
- Rectal speculum
- Specimen containers with appropriate preservative added
- Laboratory requisition form
- Tissue wipes
- Biohazard container

Standards: Complete the procedure and all critical steps in ____________ minutes with a minimum score of ____________ % within three attempts.

Scoring: Divide points earned by total possible points. Failure to perform a critical step that is indicated with an asterisk (*), will result in an unsatisfactory overall score.

Time began ____________ **Time ended** ____________

Steps	Possible Points	First Attempt	Second Attempt	Third Attempt
1. Wash hands and assemble all needed equipment and supplies.	5			
2. Identify the patient and explain the procedure. Be sure patient has completed proper preparation procedures.	5			
3. Ask the patient to empty his or her bladder.	5			
4. Give the patient an examination gown and instruct him or her to remove all clothing below the waist and put on the gown with the opening to the back.	5			
5. Obtain and record the patient's vital signs.	10			
6. Assist the patient onto the table. When the physician is ready, place the patient in the appropriate position for the type of examination ordered.	5			
7. Drape the patient so that only the anus is exposed. A fenestrated drape (drape with a circular opening placed over the anus) may be used in place of the rectangular drape.	10			

Steps	Possible Points	First Attempt	Second Attempt	Third Attempt
8. Put on gloves and assist the physician as requested during the examination. This includes: • Lubricating the physician's gloved index finger for the digital examination • Lubricating the obturator tip of the instrument before insertion • Plugging in the scope's light source when the physician is ready • Handing the needed supplies to the physician • Collecting specimens by holding the container to accept the sample • Labeling specimens immediately because several specimens may be taken from different areas • Disposing of contaminated supplies as you are given them by the physician	**20**			
9. Throughout the examination, observe the patient for any adverse reactions. Encourage the patient to breathe slowly through pursed lips to facilitate relaxation.	**10**			
10. On completion of the examination, cleanse the patient's anal area with tissue wipes. Remove gloves and assist the patient into a resting position and allow the patient time to recover from the procedure.	**5**			
11. Assist patient off of table and instruct him or her to get dressed. Show the patient where the sink, towels, and tissues are and provide assistance if needed.	**5**			
12. Complete all laboratory request forms and specimen container labels, and place specimens in appropriate location for laboratory pickup.	**5**			
13. Clean work area and all equipment used. Endoscope is first sanitized and then sterilized according to manufacturer recommendations.	**5**			
14. Record procedure and any pertinent information on the patient's record.	**5**			

Documentation in the Medical Record

____

____

____

____

Comments:

Total Points Earned ________ Divided by ________ Total Possible Points = ________ % Score

Instructor's Signature ____________________

Student Name ______________________ Date ____________ Score ________

Procedure 37-1 Teaching Testicular Self-Examination

Task: To instruct the patient in the steps of testicular self-examination.

Equipment and Supplies:
- Self-examination pamphlet and shower card
- Demonstration model
- Nonsterile gloves

Standards: Complete the procedure and all critical steps in ____________ minutes with a minimum score of ____________ % within three attempts.

Scoring: Divide points earned by total possible points. Failure to perform a critical step that is indicated with an asterisk (*), will result in an unsatisfactory overall score.

Time began ____________ **Time ended** ____________

Steps	Possible Points	First Attempt	Second Attempt	Third Attempt
1. Wash your hands and collect needed supplies.	10			
2. Explain to the patient what you are going to do.	10			
3. Begin by explaining to the patient that testicular cancer may produce no symptoms in early stages so it is important to examine the testes once a month for abnormal changes and early detection of the disease. This should begin at puberty or about 15 years of age. It is best to do the examination in the shower or in a warm bath. The total examination takes about 3 minutes.	10			
4. Examination of the testes: Start by holding the scrotum in the palms of the hands. Then feel one testicle. Apply a small amount of pressure. Slowly roll it between the fingers and try to find hard, painless lumps.	10			
5. Examination of the epididymis: This comma-shaped cord is found behind the testis. Its job is to store and transport sperm. Tender when touched, it is the location of most noncancerous problems.	10			
6. Examination of the vas deferens: Continue by examining the sperm-carrying tube that runs up the epididymis. Normally, the vas feels like a firm, movable, smooth tube.	10			
7. Now repeat the entire examination on the other side, beginning with the opposite testis.	10			

Steps	Possible Points	First Attempt	Second Attempt	Third Attempt
8. After completing the examination on the model, ask the patient to do a return-examination using the model. A male assistant can have the patient do a self–testicular examination.	10			
9. Give the pamphlet to the patient along with the shower card with instructions regarding hanging it in the shower as a monthly reminder and guide.	10			
10. Record the instructional transaction in the patient's medical record.	10			

Documentation in the Medical Record

Comments:

Total Points Earned ________ Divided by ________ Total Possible Points = ________ % Score

Instructor's Signature ________________

Student Name ______________________ Date ____________ Score ____________

Procedure 37-2 Catheterization of the Female Patient

Task: To successfully empty the bladder by means of sterile catheterization.

Equipment and Supplies:
- Sterile urethral catheterization kit containing a straight catheter
- Sterile drapes
- Sterile lubricant
- Sterile tray
- Sterile gloves
- Sterile cotton balls or gauze squares
- Povidone-iodine (Betadine)
- Specimen container and laboratory slip
- Waterproof pad
- Gooseneck lamp
- Extra pair of sterile gloves

Standards: Complete the procedure and all critical steps in ____________ minutes with a minimum score of ____________ % within three attempts.

Scoring: Divide points earned by total possible points. Failure to perform a critical step that is indicated with an asterisk (*), will result in an unsatisfactory overall score.

Time began ____________ **Time ended** ____________

Steps	Possible Points	First Attempt	Second Attempt	Third Attempt
1. Wash your hands and collect necessary supplies.	4			
2. Explain the procedure to the patient and have the patient remove necessary clothing.	4			
3. Place your patient in the dorsal recumbent position.	4			
4. Drape the patient's upper body, leaving the genital area exposed.	4			
5. Position a gooseneck lamp over the genital area.	4			
6. Wash your hands and open the catheterization tray on a clean stable surface using sterile techniques. (A Mayo stand is often used.)	4			
7. Open the sterile underpad drape and hold the underpad so that the undersurface of the two corners encircles your hands. Slide it under the patient while she is lifting her hips off the table. Be careful not to touch the patient or the table with your hands. Ask patient to keep knees apart.	4			
8. Open the sterile drape and place it over the patient's exposed genital area so that the vulval area is exposed.	4			

Steps	Possible Points	First Attempt	Second Attempt	Third Attempt
9. Place the insertion kit and any other supplies on the sterile drape between the patient's legs.	4			
10. Put on sterile gloves following sterile procedure (see Chapter 54). Open the sterile povidone-iodine (Betadine) package and pour it over cotton balls or gauze squares in the tray.	8			
11. Open the sterile lubricant package and place it on the sterile field.	4			
12. Open all other items, including the catheter. Stand the specimen container on the tray.	4			
13. With the thumb and index finger of your nondominant hand, separate the patient's labia as widely as possible. Your nondominant hand must maintain this position throughout the balance of the procedure. Take care that your dominant hand does not touch the patient during the cleansing process. With your dominant hand, pick up one of the povidone-iodine–soaked gauze squares and wipe from top to bottom on one side of the labia. Discard the used gauze.	4			
14. Pick up another gauze square and wipe from top to bottom on the other side of the labia. Discard the used gauze.	4			
15. Pick up another gauze square, and using a circular motion, wipe over the urinary meatus from the inside outward. Discard the gauze.	4			
16. With your dominant hand, pick up the catheter about 3 inches from the insertion end and dip the tip into the sterile lubricant. Position the other end of the catheter in the collection compartment of the kit tray.	4			
17. Insert the lubricated tip into the urinary meatus and continue inserting the catheter 2 to 3 inches or until urine begins flowing out the catheter into the kit tray. Never force the catheter.	4			
18. Let some of the urine flow and then place the specimen container over the end of the catheter and collect the specimen.	4			
19. When the bladder is completely emptied and the urine stops flowing, gently remove the catheter. If more than 500 ml of urine drains into the collection tray, clamp the catheter and wait 10 to 15 minutes, then reopen the catheter and allow the bladder to empty.	4			
20. Secure the lid to the urine specimen container.	4			

Steps	Possible Points	First Attempt	Second Attempt	Third Attempt
21. Remove all supplies and dispose of them according to standard precautions.	4			
22. Assist patient off table and with dressing as needed.	4			
23. Complete the laboratory requisition and record the procedure; include the number of milliliters of urine removed from the bladder.	8			

Documentation in the Medical Record

___

___

___

___

Comments:

Total Points Earned ________ Divided by ________ Total Possible Points = ________ % Score

Instructor's Signature ________________

Student Name ______________________ Date ______________ Score ______________

Procedure 37-3 Catheterization of a Male Patient with a Straight Catheter

Task: To successfully empty the bladder by means of sterile catheterization.

Equipment and Supplies:
- Sterile urethral catheterization kit containing a straight catheter
- Sterile drapes
- Sterile lubricant
- Sterile tray
- Sterile gloves
- Sterile cotton balls or gauze squares
- Povidone-iodine (Betadine)
- Specimen container and laboratory slip
- Waterproof pad
- Gooseneck lamp
- Extra pair of sterile gloves

Standards: Complete the procedure and all critical steps in ______________ minutes with a minimum score of ______________ % within three attempts.

Scoring: Divide points earned by total possible points. Failure to perform a critical step that is indicated with an asterisk (*), will result in an unsatisfactory overall score.

Time began ______________ **Time ended** ______________

Steps	Possible Points	First Attempt	Second Attempt	Third Attempt
1. Wash your hands and collect necessary supplies.	5			
2. Explain the procedure to the patient and have the patient remove necessary clothing.	5			
3. Place your patient in the dorsal recumbent position.	5			
4. Drape the patient's upper body, leaving the genital area exposed.	5			
5. Position a gooseneck lamp over the genital area.	5			
6. Wash your hands and open the catheterization tray on a clean stable surface using sterile techniques. (A Mayo stand is often used.)	5			
7. Put on sterile gloves following sterile procedure (see Chapter 54). Open the sterile povidone-iodine (Betadine) package and pour it over cotton balls or gauze squares in the tray.	5			
8. Open the sterile lubricant package and place it on the sterile field.	5			

Steps	Possible Points	First Attempt	Second Attempt	Third Attempt
9. Open all other items, including the catheter. Stand the specimen container on the tray.	5			
10. Open the fenestrated drape and position it so the opening exposes the penis. Be careful not to touch the patient or the table.	5			
11. Place the sterile kit on the table on top of the sterile drape and open all the supplies as in Procedure 37-2, steps 10 through 12.	5			
12. Grasp the penis below the glans with your nondominant hand. In uncircumcised males, you must pull back the foreskin to see the meatus. You must do this and hold the penis upright with your nondominant hand only.	5			
13. Using your dominant hand and forceps, pick up a povidone-iodine (Betadine)–soaked cotton ball and clean around the meatus in circular motions from the center outward. Repeat this a total of three times using a fresh soaked cotton ball each time.	5			
14. With your dominant hand, lubricate the tip of the catheter at least 7 inches. Be sure to put the other end of the catheter into the collection compartment of the kit tray.	5			
15. Hold the shaft of the penis straight and upright with your dominant hand and apply gentle traction to straighten the urethra. Ask the patient to bear down as if to urinate. Gently insert the lubricated catheter tip into the urinary meatus 6 to 8 inches or until urine begins flowing out of the catheter. Never force the catheter; if you meet resistance, remove the catheter and notify the physician.	5			
16. Let some of the urine flow and then place the specimen container over the end of the catheter and collect the specimen.	5			
17. When the bladder is completely emptied and the urine stops flowing, gently remove the catheter. If more than 500 ml of urine drains into the collection tray, clamp the catheter and wait 10 to 15 minutes, then reopen the catheter and allow the bladder to empty.	5			
18. Secure the lid to the urine specimen container.	5			
19. Remove all supplies and dispose of them according to standard precautions.	2.5			

Steps	Possible Points	First Attempt	Second Attempt	Third Attempt
20. Assist patient off table and with dressing as needed.	2.5			
21. Complete the laboratory requisition and record the procedure; include the number of milliliters of urine removed from the bladder.	5			

Documentation in the Medical Record

Comments:

Total Points Earned ________ Divided by ________ Total Possible Points = ________ % Score

Instructor's Signature ____________________

Student Name ______________________ Date __________ Score __________

Procedure 38-1 Assisting with Examination of the Female Patient and Pap Smear

Task: To assist the physician in examination of a female patient and diagnostic Pap smear.

Equipment and Supplies:
- Patient gown
- Lubricant
- 44-inch gauze squares
- Laboratory requisition slips
- Drape sheet
- Examination light
- Cervical spatula and Cytobrush
- Microscopic slides
- Vaginal speculum
- Uterine sponge forceps
- Disposable gloves
- Fixative for Papanicolaou smear
- Urine specimen container if needed
- Stool for occult blood test if needed
- Biohazard waste container

Standards: Complete the procedure and all critical steps in ______________ minutes with a minimum score of ______________ % within three attempts.

Scoring: Divide points earned by total possible points. Failure to perform a critical step that is indicated with an asterisk (*), will result in an unsatisfactory overall score.

Time began ______________ **Time ended** ______________

Steps	**Possible Points**	**First Attempt**	**Second Attempt**	**Third Attempt**
1. Assemble the materials needed and prepare the room. Prepare the equipment and supplies needed for the Pap smear.	5			
2. Wash hands. Follow standard precautions. Don gloves.	5			
3. Identify the patient and briefly explain the procedure.	5			
4. Instruct the patient to empty the bladder and collect a urine specimen if needed.	5			
5. Instruct the patient to disrobe completely and to put on a gown. Explain that gown should open in the front.	5			
6. Assist the patient into a sitting position at the end of the examination table. Drape the patient and assist the physician with the examination. Provide reassurance to the patient as needed.	5			

Steps	Possible Points	First Attempt	Second Attempt	Third Attempt
7. When the physician is ready to examine the breasts and the abdomen in the supine position, assist the patient into the supine position and drape as needed.	5			
8. When the physician is ready to begin the vaginal examination, assist the patient into the lithotomy position. Patient's knees should be relaxed and rotated outward. Remember to always position the patient underneath the drape.	5			
9. Direct the light source toward the perineal area.	5			
10. Warm the stainless steel vaginal speculum in warm water (physician may prefer disposable plastic speculum). Pass the proper instruments to the physician in proper sequence. Physician will need the Cytobrush for cervical cells and the spatula for vaginal cells.	5			
11. Assist the physician with preparation of the slides and labeling (one marked *v* for vaginal, one marked *e* for endocervical). Spray fixative immediately about 6 inches from slide. Let dry for 10 minutes.	5			
12. Apply the water-soluble lubricant to the physician's fingers.	5			
13. Physician may obtain stool for occult blood test after rectal examination has been performed. Have materials ready.	5			
14. Instruct the patient to breathe deeply through the mouth with hands crossed over the chest.	5			
15. Place the soiled instruments in a basin.	5			
16. Assist the patient off the table and with dressing if needed.	5			
17. While patient is in the dressing room, clean the room, removing used equipment.	5			
18. Sanitize and sterilize stainless steel equipment. Remove gloves and wash your hands.	5			
19. Prepare the Pap smear for transportation to the laboratory. Include patient's last menstrual period (LMP) date and indicate whether patient is receiving hormone therapy.	5			
20. Record all procedures on the patient's medical record.	5			

Documentation in the Medical Record

____

____

____

____

Comments:

Total Points Earned ________ Divided by ________ Total Possible Points = ________ % Score

Instructor's Signature ____________________

Student Name ______________________ Date ____________ Score ________

Procedure 38-2 Teaching the Patient Breast Self-Examination

Task: To teach the patient how to palpate her breasts for possible abnormalities.

Equipment and Supplies:
- Instruction pamphlet
- Teaching model (to use to demonstrate the technique before a return demonstration by the patient)

Standards: Complete the procedure and all critical steps in ____________ minutes with a minimum score of ____________ % within three attempts.

Scoring: Divide points earned by total possible points. Failure to perform a critical step that is indicated with an asterisk (*), will result in an unsatisfactory overall score.

Time began ____________ **Time ended** ____________

Steps	**Possible Points**	**First Attempt**	**Second Attempt**	**Third Attempt**
1. Assemble equipment.	10			
2. Tell patient to always examine breasts while bathing or showering in warm water. The best time to perform this examination is immediately after the menstrual period is completed because at this time there is minimal breast engorgement. Nonmenstruating women should examine breasts on the first day of the month.	20			
3. Have patient raise one arm. With her fingers flat, she should press gently in small circles, starting at the outermost top edge of the breast and spiraling in toward the nipple. Instruct her to touch every part of each breast, including the axillary region, gently feeling for a lump or thickening. The right hand should be used to examine the left breast, and the left hand, to examine the right breast.	20			
4. After the bath/shower is completed, the patient should continue the examination in front of a mirror with arms at the sides. Then with arms raised above the head, she should look carefully for changes in the size, shape, and contour of each breast. She should look for puckering, dimpling, or changes in skin texture.	20			
5. The patient should gently squeeze both nipples and look for discharge.	10			

Steps	Possible Points	First Attempt	Second Attempt	Third Attempt
6. Before dressing, the patient should lie on a bed, place a towel or pillow under the right shoulder, and place the right hand behind the head. The right breast should be examined by using the left hand. Instruct the patient to press gently in small circles, starting at the outermost top edge, including the axillary region, and spiraling in toward the nipple. The procedure should be repeated with left breast.	**10**			
7. The patient should return the demonstration of how to do the breast examination to confirm understanding.	**10**			
8. Give the patient the instruction pamphlet to use at home.	**10**			

Documentation in the Medical Record

Comments:

Total Points Earned ________ Divided by ________ Total Possible Points = ________ % Score

Instructor's Signature ____________________

Student Name ______________________ Date __________ Score __________

Procedure 38-3 Preparing the Patient for Cryosurgery

Task: To prepare the patient for cryosurgery and assist the physician in cryosurgery.

Equipment and Supplies:
- Cryosurgery machine equipped with liquid nitrogen canister
- Cryoprobe
- Cervical tenaculum
- Cervical ring forceps or disposable cervical swabs
- Vaginal speculum
- 44-inch gauze squares
- Gloves
- Gowns and face protection
- Specimen containers
- Biohazard waste container
- Cytology request forms

Standards: Complete the procedure and all critical steps in __________ minutes with a minimum score of __________ % within three attempts.

Scoring: Divide points earned by total possible points. Failure to perform a critical step that is indicated with an asterisk (*), will result in an unsatisfactory overall score.

Time began __________ **Time ended** __________

Steps	Possible Points	First Attempt	Second Attempt	Third Attempt
1. Assemble equipment.	5			
2. Wash hands and don gloves.	10			
3. Obtain the patient's temperature and blood pressure and record them on the patient's record.	10			
4. Drape and assist the patient into the lithotomy position. Don gloves.	10			
5. Assist the physician with the procedure by handing the equipment needed.	10			
6. Encourage the patient to take deep breaths to promote relaxation of the pelvic muscles during the procedure. Observe patient for any sign of distress.	10			
7. When the procedure has been completed, place the patient in a supine position and allow her to rest while you tidy the room and remove the used supplies. Retake temperature and blood pressure.	10			
8. Help patient sit up and assist her in dressing if necessary.	5			

Steps	Possible Points	First Attempt	Second Attempt	Third Attempt
9. Remove gloves and wash hands.	**10**			
10. Return equipment to the proper storage area.	**10**			
11. Record procedure and final vital sign measurements on the patient's record.	**10**			

Documentation in the Medical Record

____

____

____

____

Comments:

Total Points Earned ________ Divided by ________ Total Possible Points = ________ % Score

Instructor's Signature ________________

Student Name ______________________ Date ____________ Score ________

Procedure 38-4 Assisting with the Prenatal Examination

Task: To promote a healthy pregnancy for the mother and fetus and screen for potential problems.

Equipment and Supplies:
- Scale with height measurement
- Sphygmomanometer
- Stethoscope
- Tape measure
- Doppler fetoscope
- Urine specimen container
- Latex gloves, vaginal speculum, and lubricant if vaginal examination conducted
- Biohazard waste container

Standards: Complete the procedure and all critical steps in ____________ minutes with a minimum score of ____________ % within three attempts.

Scoring: Divide points earned by total possible points. Failure to perform a critical step that is indicated with an asterisk (*), will result in an unsatisfactory overall score.

Time began ____________ **Time ended** ____________

Steps	Possible Points	First Attempt	Second Attempt	Third Attempt
1. Wash hands, assemble equipment, and identify the patient.	5			
2. Measure and record the patient's weight.	10			
3. Collect a urine specimen, perform, and record urinalysis results to determine the presence of protein, glucose, or ketones in the urine.	10			
4. Measure and record the mother's blood pressure.	10			
5. Instruct the patient to disrobe form the waist down and put on a gown open to the front so the uterine fundal height can be measured.	10			
6. Assist the patient onto the examination table if needed and provide a drape for privacy.	10			
7. Assist the physician as needed throughout the examination.	10			
8. After the examination is completed, assist the patient off the examination table, making sure to observe for signs of dizziness or problems with balance.	10			
9. Answer patient questions and provide patient education materials needed.	10			

Steps	Possible Points	First Attempt	Second Attempt	Third Attempt
10. Discard supplies and disinfect the equipment according to manufacture guidelines. Wear latex gloves and follow OSHA guidelines if handling any contaminated items.	5			
11. Wash hands.	5			
12. Document pertinent information in the patient chart.	5			

Documentation in the Medical Record

Comments:

Total Points Earned ________ Divided by ________ Total Possible Points = ________ % Score

Instructor's Signature ________________________

Student Name ______________________ Date ____________ Score ____________

Procedure 38-5 Establishing the Estimated Day of Delivery with Nagele's Rule and the Lunar Method

Task: To establish the patient's due date.

Equipment and Supplies:
- Calendar for present and following year
- Paper and pencil
- Commercial estimated day of delivery (EDD) wheel (optional)

Standards: Complete the procedure and all critical steps in ____________ minutes with a minimum score of ____________ % within three attempts.

Scoring: Divide points earned by total possible points. Failure to perform a critical step that is indicated with an asterisk (*), will result in an unsatisfactory overall score.

Time began ____________ **Time ended** ____________

Steps	Possible Points	First Attempt	Second Attempt	Third Attempt
1. Ask patient for the date of the onset of the last menstrual period (LMP). Be sure that this is the date of the onset and not the date of the termination of the menses.	20			
2. Patient informs you that her LMP was April 12, 20XX.	20			
3. Calculate her EDD by using Nagele's method. Begin with the date of the first day of her LMP. Count back 3 months and add 1 year plus 7 days.	20			
4. Using the same LMP, calculate her EDD with the lunar rule. Example: LMP = June 7, 2002 + 9 months = March 7, 2002 + 7 days = March 14, 2003.	20			
5. Compare the results for accuracy. Did you obtain the same EDD with both methods?	20			

Documentation in the Medical Record

____

____

____

____

Comments:

Total Points Earned ________ Divided by ________ Total Possible Points = ________ % Score

Instructor's Signature ____________________

Student Name ______________________ Date ______________ Score ______________

Procedure 39-1 Measuring the Circumference of an Infant's Head

Task: To obtain an accurate measurement of the circumference of an infant's head.

Equipment and Supplies:
- Flexible disposable tape measure
- Age-specific and gender-specific growth chart
- Patient's chart
- Pen or pencil

Standards: Complete the procedure and all critical steps in ______________ minutes with a minimum score of ______________ % within three attempts.

Scoring: Divide points earned by total possible points. Failure to perform a critical step that is indicated with an asterisk (*), will result in an unsatisfactory overall score.

Time began ______________ **Time ended** ______________

Steps	Possible Points	First Attempt	Second Attempt	Third Attempt
1. Wash hands.	**10**			
2. Identify the patient and gain infant cooperation through conversation.	**10**			
3. Place the infant in the supine position; an older child may sit on the examination table; alternatively, the infant may be held by the parent.	**10**			
4. Hold the tape measure with the zero mark against the infant's forehead, slightly above the eyebrows and the top of the ears. Ask the parent for assistance if necessary.	**10**			
5. Bring the tape measure around the head, just above the ears, to meet at the mid forehead.	**10**			
6. Read to the nearest 0.01 cm or ¼ inch.	**20**			
7. Record the measurement on the growth chart and the patient's chart.	**10**			
8. Dispose of the tape measure.	**10**			
9. Wash hands.	**10**			

Documentation in the Medical Record

____

____

____

____

Comments:

Total Points Earned ________ Divided by ________ Total Possible Points = ________ % Score

Instructor's Signature ____________________

Student Name ______________________ Date ____________ Score ____________

Procedure 39-2 Measuring Infant Length and Weight

Task: To accurately measure infant length and weight so growth patterns can be monitored and recorded.

Equipment and Supplies:
- Infant scale with paper cover
- Flexible measuring tape
- Examination table paper
- Pen
- Infant growth chart
- Biohazard waste container

Standards: Complete the procedure and all critical steps in ____________ minutes with a minimum score of ____________ % within three attempts.

Scoring: Divide points earned by total possible points. Failure to perform a critical step that is indicated with an asterisk (*), will result in an unsatisfactory overall score.

Time began ____________ **Time ended** ____________

Steps	Possible Points	First Attempt	Second Attempt	Third Attempt
Measuring Infant Length				
1. Wash hands, assemble equipment, and explain the procedure to the infant's caregiver.	5			
2. Undress infant in preparation for measurement of length and height. May leave diaper on until length measurement is taken but it must be removed before weighing the infant.	10			
3. Ask the caregiver to place the infant on his or her back on the examination table that is covered with paper. If it is a pediatric table with a headboard, ask the caregiver to gently hold the infant's head against the board while you straighten the infant's leg and mark on the paper the location of the heel. If there is no headboard ask the caregiver to gently hold the infant's head still while you extend the leg for measurement.	10			
4. Measure and record the infant's length with the tape measure.	10			
5. Document the results in either inches or centimeters depending on office policy on the infant's growth chart, in the progress notes, and in the caregiver's record if requested. Complete the growth chart graph by connecting the dot from the last visit.	5			

Steps	Possible Points	First Attempt	Second Attempt	Third Attempt
Measuring Infant Weight				
1. Wash hands, assemble equipment, and explain the procedure to the infant's caregiver.	5			
2. Completely undress the infant including the diaper.	10			
3. Place the infant gently onto the center of the scale, keeping your hand directly above the infant's trunk for safety.	10			
4. Slide the weights across the scale until balance is achieved. Attempt to read the infant's weight while he or she is still.	10			
5. Return the weights to the far left of the scale and remove the baby. Caregiver can apply a diaper while you discard the paper covering the scale. If it has become contaminated during the procedure, follow OSHA guidelines for gloves and disposal of contaminated waste. Disinfect the equipment according to manufacturer's guidelines.	10			
6. Wash hands.	5			
7. Document the results in either pounds or kilograms dependent on office policy on the infant's growth chart, in the progress notes, and in the caregiver's record if requested. Complete the growth chart graph by connecting the dot from the last visit.	5			

Documentation in the Medical Record

____

____

____

____

Comments:

Total Points Earned ________ Divided by ________ Total Possible Points = ________ % Score

Instructor's Signature ____________________

Student Name ______________________ Date __________ Score __________

Procedure 39-3 Obtaining Pediatric Vital Signs and Vision Screening

Task: To accurately obtain vital signs and screen vision in a pediatric patient.

Equipment and Supplies:
- Digital or tympanic thermometer
- Pediatric blood pressure cuff
- Wristwatch with sweep second-hand
- Weight scale
- Stethoscope
- Pediatric E eye chart and oculator
- Pencil and paper

Standards: Complete the procedure and all critical steps in __________ minutes with a minimum score of __________ % within three attempts.

Scoring: Divide points earned by total possible points. Failure to perform a critical step that is indicated with an asterisk (*), will result in an unsatisfactory overall score.

Time began __________ **Time ended** __________

Steps	**Possible Points**	**First Attempt**	**Second Attempt**	**Third Attempt**
1. Gather equipment.	5			
2. Wash hands.	5			
3. Explain the procedure to the parent, and if you want the parent to help by holding the child, explain the technique you want him or her to use.	5			
4. Help child stand in the center of the scale and weigh the child. Ask child to turn around and obtain the child's height. Record your findings.	5			
5. Obtain tympanic or axillary temperature by using the procedure explained in Chapter 28.	5			
6. Record temperature. Indicate the method used: A = axillary.	5			
7. Place stethoscope on child's chest at the midpoint between the sternum and the left nipple and listen for the apical beat.	5			
8. Count the apical beat for 1 full minute.	10			
9. Record the apical pulse. Be sure to write "(A)" after the rate to indicate that this is an apical pulse reading.	5			

Steps	Possible Points	First Attempt	Second Attempt	Third Attempt
10. Place the palm of your hand flat on the child's chest and count the respirations for 1 full minute.	5			
11. Record the respiration rate.	5			
12. Check to be sure that you have the correct-size blood pressure cuff and then proceed with taking the blood pressure. Follow procedure in Chapter 28.	10			
13. Record the blood pressure.	5			
14. If vision screening is to be done, familiarize the child with the E by asking him to make an E point the same way as your E is pointing. Then position the child in front of the pediatric E Snellen chart and have him or her match the E, by using his or her hands, with the one to which you are pointing.	5			
15. Record the vision results: OD = right eye, OS = left eye, OU = both eyes.	5			
16. Compliment the child on his or her performance, and if the parent is present, share the praise with the parent.	5			
17. Wash hands.	5			
18. Return all equipment used to proper storage area.	5			

Documentation in the Medical Record

____

____

____

____

Comments:

Total Points Earned ________ Divided by ________ Total Possible Points = ________ % Score

Instructor's Signature ________________

Student Name ______________________ Date __________ Score __________

Procedure 39-4 Applying a Urinary Collection Device

Task: To properly apply a pediatric urinary collection device.

Equipment and Supplies:
Pediatric urine collection bag
Labeled laboratory urine specimen container
Laboratory test request form
Antiseptic wipes
Biohazard waste container
Disposable examination gloves

Standards: Complete the procedure and all critical steps in __________ minutes with a minimum score of __________ % within three attempts.

Scoring: Divide points earned by total possible points. Failure to perform a critical step that is indicated with an asterisk (*), will result in an unsatisfactory overall score.

Time began __________ **Time ended** __________

Steps	**Possible Points**	**First Attempt**	**Second Attempt**	**Third Attempt**
1. Assemble all needed supplies.	**5**			
2. Wash hands and don gloves.	**5**			
3. Ask parent to remove the diaper from the child or lay the child in a supine position on the examination table and remove the diaper.	**10**			
4. Cleanse the genitalia with antiseptic wipes. Male: Cleanse the urinary meatus in a circular motion, starting directly on the meatus, and work in an outward pattern. Repeat with a clean wipe. If the child is not circumcised, retract the foreskin to expose the meatus, and when you have completed cleansing, return the foreskin to its natural position. Female: Hold the labia open with your left hand and with your right hand, cleanse the inner labia, from the clitoris to the vaginal meatus, in a superior to inferior pattern. Discard the first wipe and repeat with a clean wipe.	**10**			
5. Make sure the area is dry. Unfold the collection device, remove the paper from the upper portion, place this portion over the mons pubis, and press it securely into place. Continue by removing the lower portion of the paper and securing this portion against the perineum. Be sure that the device is attached smoothly and that you have not taped it to part of the infant's thigh.	**10**			

Steps	Possible Points	First Attempt	Second Attempt	Third Attempt
6. Re-diaper the infant, or if the parent is helping, the parent may re-diaper the infant at this time. The diaper will help hold the bag in place.	**5**			
7. Suggest that the parent give the child liquids if allowed and check the bag for urine at frequent intervals.	**5**			
8. When there is a noticeable amount of urine in the bag, remove the device, cleanse the skin area that was attached to the device, and rediaper the child.	**10**			
9. Pour the urine carefully into the laboratory urine container and handle the sample in a routine manner.	**10**			
10. Dispose of all used equipment in a biohazard waste container.	**10**			
11. Remove gloves, dispose of them in a biohazard container, and wash hands.	**10**			
12. Record the procedure in the patient's record.	**10**			

Documentation in the Medical Record

____

____

____

____

Comments:

Total Points Earned ________ Divided by ________ Total Possible Points = ________ % Score

Instructor's Signature ________________

Student Name ______________________ Date ____________ Score ________

Procedure 40-1 Assisting with Cold Application

Task: To instruct a patient in the correct application of cold to a body area to decrease pain, prevent further swelling, and/or decrease inflammation.

Equipment and Supplies:
- Ice bag or closeable disposable plastic kitchen food bag
- Small ice cubes or ice chips
- Towel

Standards: Complete the procedure and all critical steps in ____________ minutes with a minimum score of ____________ % within three attempts.

Scoring: Divide points earned by total possible points. Failure to perform a critical step that is indicated with an asterisk (*), will result in an unsatisfactory overall score.

Time began ____________ **Time ended** ____________

Steps	**Possible Points**	**First Attempt**	**Second Attempt**	**Third Attempt**
1. Wash your hands.	**10**			
2. Explain the procedure to the patient and answer any questions.	**10**			
3. Check the bag for possible leaks.	**10**			
4. Fill the bag with small cubes or chips of ice until it is about two thirds full.	**10**			
5. Push down on the top of the bag to expel excess air and apply the cap.	**10**			
6. Dry the outside and cover it with one or two layers of the towel.	**10**			
7. Help the patient position the ice bag on the injured area.	**10**			
8. Advise the patient to leave the ice bag in place for about 20 to 30 minutes or until the area feels numb, whichever is first.	**10**			
9. Check the skin for color, sensation, and pain.	**10**			
10. Record the procedure in the patient's chart.	**10**			

Documentation in the Medical Record

____

____

____

____

Comments:

Total Points Earned ________ Divided by ________ Total Possible Points = ________ % Score

Instructor's Signature ____________________

Student Name ______________________ Date ____________ Score ____________

Procedure 40-2 Assisting with Hot Moist Heat Application in the Office

Task: To instruct a patient in the correct application of moist heat to a body area to increase circulation, increase metabolism, and relax muscles.

Equipment and Supplies:
- Commercial hot moist heat packs
- Towel

Standards: Complete the procedure and all critical steps in ____________ minutes with a minimum score of ____________ % within three attempts.

Scoring: Divide points earned by total possible points. Failure to perform a critical step that is indicated with an asterisk (*), will result in an unsatisfactory overall score.

Time began ____________ **Time ended** ____________

Steps	**Possible Points**	**First Attempt**	**Second Attempt**	**Third Attempt**
1. Wash your hands.	**10**			
2. Explain the procedure to the patient and answer any questions.	**10**			
3. Ask the patient to remove all jewelry in the area to be treated.	**20**			
4. Place one or two layers of towel over the area to be treated.	**20**			
5. Apply the commercial heated moist heat packs.	**20**			
6. Cover with the remaining portion of the towel.	**20**			

Documentation in the Medical Record

____

____

____

____

Comments:

Total Points Earned ________ Divided by ________ Total Possible Points = ________ % Score

Instructor's Signature ____________________

Student Name ______________ Date ______________ Score ______________

Procedure 40-3 Assisting with Therapeutic Ultrasound Application

Task: To apply ultra–high-frequency sound waves to the patient's deep tissues for therapy.

Equipment and Supplies:
- Ultrasound machine
- Ultrasound gel or lotion (the coupling agent)

Standards: Complete the procedure and all critical steps in ______________ minutes with a minimum score of ______________ % within three attempts.

Scoring: Divide points earned by total possible points. Failure to perform a critical step that is indicated with an asterisk (*), will result in an unsatisfactory overall score.

Time began ______________ **Time ended** ______________

Steps	Possible Points	First Attempt	Second Attempt	Third Attempt
1. Prepare the equipment and wash your hands.	5			
2. Confirm the patient's identity.	5			
3. Explain the procedure and tell the patient to notify you of any discomfort immediately during the procedure.	5			
4. Question the patient about the presence of any internal or external metal objects.	5			
5. Position the patient comfortably, with the area to be treated exposed.	5			
6. Apply a warmed ultrasound gel (the coupling agent) liberally over the area to be treated and to the applicator head.	5			
7. Begin the treatment with the intensity control at the lowest setting.	5			
8. Set the timer on the machine to the ordered time.	5			
9. Slowly increase the intensity control to the ordered amount.	5			
10. Hold the applicator with the head firmly and completely against the patient's skin over the area to be treated.	5			
11. Work the applicator over the area to be treated by moving it continuously in a circular fashion at a speed of 2 inches per second or as directed by the physician.	5			

Steps	Possible Points	First Attempt	Second Attempt	Third Attempt
12. Keep the applicator head in contact with the patient's skin at all times while the machine is on and keep it moving continuously during the treatment time.	5			
13. When the timer sounds, it shuts off the machine automatically. Then you can safely lift the applicator head away from the patient.	5			
14. Return the intensity control to zero.	5			
15. Remove the ultrasound gel from the patient's skin and from the applicator head with a tissue or paper wipe.	5			
16. Assist the patient in getting dressed if necessary.	5			
17. Record the procedure in the patient's chart including the date, area treated, intensity setting, duration of treatment, and any unusual occurrences or reactions during treatment. If none occurred, indicate that also.	20			

Documentation in the Medical Record

___

___

___

___

Comments:

Total Points Earned ________ Divided by ________ Total Possible Points = ________ % Score

Instructor's Signature ____________________

Student Name ______________________ Date ____________ Score ____________

Procedure 40-4 Assisting with Cast Application

Task: To assist the physician in applying a plaster cast.

Equipment and Supplies:
- Tubular stockinette to fit the limb to be casted
- Sheet wadding or roller padding
- Roller plaster or other appropriate casting material
- Bucket of cool or room temperature water
- Cast knife or heavy bandage scissors (used only for casting)
- Gloves

Standards: Complete the procedure and all critical steps in ____________ minutes with a minimum score of ____________ % within three attempts.

Scoring: Divide points earned by total possible points. Failure to perform a critical step that is indicated with an asterisk (*), will result in an unsatisfactory overall score.

Time began ____________ **Time ended** ____________

Steps	Possible Points	First Attempt	Second Attempt	Third Attempt
1. Assemble equipment and supplies. Be sure that the stockinette is correct size to fit comfortably over the fractured area.	5			
2. Explain the procedure to the patient.	5			
3. Assist the physician in covering the injured limb with the stockinette leaving extra fabric above and below the proposed casting area.	5			
4. Hand the physician the sheet wadding and support the patient's limb as directed.	5			
5. Wet the roller plaster by holding it in the bucket of water until bubbles no longer appear around the ends of the roller, then gently squeeze the roller.	5			
6. Press out the extra water and hand the saturated rollers on at a time as requested.	5			
7. When the plaster cast application has been completed, hand the physician the plaster knife or heavy bandage scissors and assist as needed in trimming the rough plaster edges.	5			
8. After the edges are smooth, assist in folding the extra stockinette over the cast ends toward the center of the cast to for a cuff of stockinette at each end of the cast.	5			

Steps	Possible Points	First Attempt	Second Attempt	Third Attempt
9. Place the casted limb carefully on a pillow to begin drying. Avoid squeezing the soft cast.	10			
10. Clean the skin of all casting material.	5			
11. Instruct the patient to report odors, staining, undue warmth, changes in limb color, swelling, and numbness and to keep the limb elevated for at least the first 24 hours.	5			
12. Review case care instructions with the patient and a family member if the cast was placed on a child. Give the patient a copy of the cast care instructions and if the physician has ordered a form of isometric exercises, be certain to demonstrate the exercise technique. Be sure to reinforce any precautions the physician has informed the patient.	5			
13. Discard water down the sink drain but keep all plaster residues from the bottom of the bucket out of the drain. Discard the used plaster bandage and plaster residue in the regular trash or in a designated disposal container.	5			
14. Check the limb in 20 to 30 minutes for color, swelling, numbness, and temperature. Advise the physician and chart your finding.*	10			
15. If arm has been casted, and the physician has ordered a sling, apply the sling as ordered.	10			
16. If a foot has been casted and crutches are ordered, continue instructions with the patient in the use of crutches after fitting them appropriately.	10			

Documentation in the Medical Record

____

Comments:

Total Points Earned ________ Divided by ________ Total Possible Points = ________ % Score

Instructor's Signature ________________

Student Name ______________________ Date __________ Score __________

Procedure 40-5 Triangular Arm Sling Application

Task: To properly place a casted arm in a triangular sling.

Equipment and Supplies:
- Triangular-shaped arm sling

Standards: Complete the procedure and all critical steps in __________ minutes with a minimum score of __________ % within three attempts.

Scoring: Divide points earned by total possible points. Failure to perform a critical step that is indicated with an asterisk (*), will result in an unsatisfactory overall score.

Time began __________ **Time ended** __________

Steps	Possible Points	First Attempt	Second Attempt	Third Attempt
1. Be sure that you have a physician's order for a triangular arm sling.	**10**			
2 Wash your hands and obtain the desired sling.	**10**			
3. Explain the procedure to the patient.	**10**			
4. Position the patient's injured arm across the chest so that it is parallel to the floor and the patient's waist with the hand slightly elevated.	**10**			
5. Carefully slide the triangular sling between the patient's chest and the affected arm.	**10**			
6. Bring the lower front corner up over the shoulder of the affected side to the neck.	**10**			
7. Grab the opposite corner and tie or pin the ends together at the side of the neck.	**20**			
8. Fold the sling edge to form a smooth edge along the wrist.	**10**			
9. Record the procedure in the patient's record.	**10**			

Documentation in the Medical Record

____

____

____

____

Comments:

Total Points Earned ________ Divided by ________ Total Possible Points = ________ % Score

Instructor's Signature ______________________

Student Name ______________________ Date ____________ Score ____________

Procedure 40-6 Assisting with Cast Removal

Task: To remove a cast.

Equipment and Supplies:
- Cast cutter
- Cast spreader
- Large bandage scissors

Standards: Complete the procedure and all critical steps in ____________ minutes with a minimum score of ____________ % within three attempts.

Scoring: Divide points earned by total possible points. Failure to perform a critical step that is indicated with an asterisk (*), will result in an unsatisfactory overall score.

Time began ____________ **Time ended** ____________

Steps	**Possible Points**	**First Attempt**	**Second Attempt**	**Third Attempt**
1. Explain the procedure to the patient.	10			
2. Provide adequate support for the limb throughout the entire procedure.	10			
3. Make a cut on both the medial side and the lateral side of the long axis of the cast.	10			
4. Pry the two halves apart using the cast spreader.	10			
5. Carefully remove the two parts of the cast.	10			
6. Use the large bandage scissors to cut away the stockinette and padding remaining.	10			
7. Gently wash the area that was covered by the cast with mild soap and warm water.	10			
8. Dry and apply a gentle skin lotion.	10			
9. Give the patient appropriate instructions as to exercising and using the limb.	10			
10. Record the procedure in the patient's medical record.	10			

Documentation in the Medical Record

____

____

____

____

Comments:

Total Points Earned ________ Divided by ________ Total Possible Points = ________ % Score

Instructor's Signature ______________________

Student Name ______________________ Date ______________ Score ______________

Procedure 40-7 Assisting the Patient with Crutch Walking

Task: To properly fit crutches for your patient and teach them how to use them properly in three point walking.

Equipment and Supplies:
- Crutches

Standards: Complete the procedure and all critical steps in ______________ minutes with a minimum score of ______________ % within three attempts.

Scoring: Divide points earned by total possible points. Failure to perform a critical step that is indicated with an asterisk (*), will result in an unsatisfactory overall score.

Time began ______________ **Time ended** ______________

Steps	**Possible Points**	**First Attempt**	**Second Attempt**	**Third Attempt**
1. Fit the crutches to the patient so the armrest is 2 inches below the armpit.	**20**			
2. Be sure that all wing nuts are tight.	**10**			
3. Make sure the foam pads at the armpits and around the handgrips are comfortable.	**10**			
4. Instruct the patient to keep the injured leg as relaxed as possible and slightly bent at the knee.	**10**			
5. The patient's elbow should be bent from 23 to 30 degrees when holding the handgrip.	**10**			
6. Place the crutch tips about 6 inches away from and parallel to the toes.	**10**			
7. Ask the patient to push down on the crutches and lift the body slightly, nearly straightening the arms.	**10**			
8. Swing the body forward about 12 inches.	**10**			
9. Standing on the good leg, move the crutches just ahead of the good foot and repeat	**10**			

Documentation in the Medical Record

Comments:

Total Points Earned ________ Divided by ________ Total Possible Points = ________ % Score

Instructor's Signature ____________________

Student Name ______________________ Date ____________ Score ________

Procedure 41-1 Assisting with the Neurological Examination

Task: To assist the physician in obtaining an accurate neurological examination of the patient.

Equipment and Supplies:
- Otoscope
- Ophthalmoscope
- Percussion hammer
- Disposable pinwheel
- Penlight
- Tuning fork
- Cotton ball
- Tongue depressor
- Small vials of warm and cold liquids prepared according to the physician's instructions
- Small vials of sweet and salty tasting liquids prepared according to the physician's instructions
- Small vials containing substances with distinct odors such as instant coffee, cinnamon, vanilla, etc. prepared according to the physician's instructions

Standards: Complete the procedure and all critical steps in ____________ minutes with a minimum score of ____________ % within three attempts.

Scoring: Divide points earned by total possible points. Failure to perform a critical step that is indicated with an asterisk (*), will result in an unsatisfactory overall score.

Time began ____________ **Time ended** ____________

Steps	Possible Points	First Attempt	Second Attempt	Third Attempt
1. Greet the patient and help them onto the examination table. Explain the procedure to the patient.	25			
2. During the examination, be prepared to assist the patient in changing positions as necessary, have the necessary examination instruments ready for the physician at the appropriate time during the examination, and record all results from the examination as indicated by the physician.	25			
3. The neurological examination will generally follow the following order but can be modified according to physician preference. a. Mental status examination b. Proprioception and cerebellar function c. Cranial nerve assessment d. Sensory nerve function e. Reflexes	25			
4. Complete the documentation of the examination in the patient's medical record.	25			

Documentation in the Medical Record

____

____

____

____

Comments:

Total Points Earned ________ Divided by ________ Total Possible Points = ________ % Score

Instructor's Signature ____________________

Student Name ______________________ Date __________ Score __________

Procedure 41-2 Preparing the Patient for an EEG

Task: To properly prepare a patient physically and psychologically to obtain an accurate and useful EEG recording.

Equipment and Supplies:
- Collodion

Standards: Complete the procedure and all critical steps in __________ minutes with a minimum score of __________ % within three attempts.

Scoring: Divide points earned by total possible points. Failure to perform a critical step that is indicated with an asterisk (*), will result in an unsatisfactory overall score.

Time began __________ **Time ended** __________

Steps	Possible Points	First Attempt	Second Attempt	Third Attempt
1. Greet patient and introduce yourself. Explain to the patient you will go over what is going to happen step by step to ensure the best results.	**5**			
2. Explain to the patient the purpose of the EEG, how the procedure will be carried out, and what will be expected of the patient during the test.	**5**			
3. Tell the patient that the electrodes pick up tiny electrical signals from the body and that there is no danger of electrical shock.	**10**			
4. Explain that the test is painless because the electrodes are attached to the scalp with collodion.	**10**			
5. If this is a sleep EEG, suggest the patient stay up later than usual the night before the test so that it will be easier to fall asleep.	**10**			
6. Go over the physical preparation including the diet to be followed for the 48 hours before the test. This usually includes no stimulants like coffee, chocolate or sodas and no meal skipping.	**10**			
7. Tell the patient that at the beginning of the test a baseline EEG will be taken and during this time the patient will be asked to avoid all movement, even eye and tongue movement.	**10**			
8. Explain that the brain will be stimulated by the patient viewing flickering lights. The EEG will be measuring the brain's response to this stimulation.	**10**			
9. Ask the patient if they have any questions. If so, answer them so the patient understands the procedure clearly.	**10**			

Documentation in the Medical Record

____

____

____

____

Comments:

Total Points Earned ________ Divided by ________ Total Possible Points = ________ % Score

Instructor's Signature ______________________

Student Name ______________________ Date ____________ Score ____________

Procedure 41-3 Preparing the Patient for and Assisting with a Lumbar Puncture

Task: To properly prepare a patient physically and mentally for a lumar puncture in order to obtain a specimen of CSF for testing.

Equipment and Supplies:
- Local anesthetic
- Sterile, disposable lumbar puncture kit
- Mayo stand
- Sterile gloves
- Permanent marker to label tubes

Standards: Complete the procedure and all critical steps in ____________ minutes with a minimum score of ____________ % within three attempts.

Scoring: Divide points earned by total possible points. Failure to perform a critical step that is indicated with an asterisk (*), will result in an unsatisfactory overall score.

Time began ____________ **Time ended** ____________

Steps	Possible Points	First Attempt	Second Attempt	Third Attempt
1. Greet patient and introduce yourself. Explain to the patient you will go over what is going to happen step by step to ensure the best results.	5			
2. Explain to the patient the purpose of the lumbar puncture, how the procedure will be carried out, and what will be expected of the patient during the test.	5			
3. Have the patient void just prior to the procedure.	5			
4. Give the patient a hospital gown and have them put it on with the opening down the back.	5			
5. Place the patient in a left, side-lying fetal position for the lumbar puncture.	5			
6. Support the patient's head with a pillow as needed and provide a pillow for between the knees if needed also.	5			
7. Do a sterile skin prep of the patient's lumbar region in the usual manner.	10			
8. Place the sterile disposable lumbar puncture kit on the mayo stand and open it establishing a sterile field. Put on sterile gloves and take the fenestrated drape from the kit and drape the lumbar region of the patient so that only the L3-L4 region of the lower spine is exposed.	10			

Steps	Possible Points	First Attempt	Second Attempt	Third Attempt
9. When the physician is ready to do the lumbar puncture, provide the local anesthetic by holding the vial for the physician or pouring it into the sterile medicine cup on the sterile field on the mayo stand.	5			
10. Reassure the patient and help them to hold still during the injection of the local anesthetic and the insertion of the spinal needle.	5			
11. Be prepared to hold the top of the manometer steady if requested by the physician.	5			
12. Using the permanent marker, label the specimens #1, #2, and #3 in the order that they were collected. This is a critically important step in this procedure.	10			
13. Complete the laboratory requisition form and prepare the CSF specimens for transport to the laboratory.	5			
14. Break down the mayo stand by disposing of the sharps, biohazard and regular waste in the normal manner.	5			
15. Monitor the patient and give liquids as directed by the physician.	5			
16. Document the procedure in the patient's chart.	10			

Documentation in the Medical Record

Comments:

Total Points Earned ________ Divided by ________ Total Possible Points = ________ % Score

Instructor's Signature ____________________

Student Name ______________________ Date ____________ Score ____________

Procedure 43-1 Performing Spirometry Testing

Task: To perform volume capacity testing.

Equipment and Supplies:
- Balance scale with measuring device
- Volume capacity spirometer with recording paper in place
- External spirometric tubing
- Disposable mouthpiece
- Noseclip
- Biohazard waste container

Standards: Complete the procedure and all critical steps in ____________ minutes with a minimum score of ____________ % within three attempts.

Scoring: Divide points earned by total possible points. Failure to perform a critical step that is indicated with an asterisk (*), will result in an unsatisfactory overall score.

Time began ____________ **Time ended** ____________

Steps	Possible Points	First Attempt	Second Attempt	Third Attempt
1. Introduce yourself and confirm the identity of the patient. Ascertain if any special preparation was needed by this patient and if it was followed.	5			
2. Explain the purpose of the test.	5			
3. Obtain the patient's vital signs.	5			
4. Explain the actual maneuver.	5			
5. Be certain the patient is comfortable and in proper sitting or standing position.	5			
6. Loosen any tight clothing, such as a necktie, bra, or belt. Show the patient the proper chin and neck position.	10			
7. Practice the maneuver with the patient and tell the patient, "Inhale."	10			
8. Use active, forceful coaching during testing. Begin by saying, "Blow." Then say, "Blow out hard." Then say, "Keep blowing, keep blowing." Then say, "Don't stop-blow harder."	10			
9. Give the patient feedback after the maneuver is completed.	5			

Steps	Possible Points	First Attempt	Second Attempt	Third Attempt
10. Continue testing until three acceptable maneuvers have been obtained.	**10**			
11. Dismiss the patient only if results are satisfactory.	**5**			
12. Clean and disinfect the equipment. Discard waste in a biohazard waste container.	**5**			
13. Wash hands.	**5**			
14. Record testing information on the patient's chart and place the chart with the test results on the physician's desk for interpretation.	**5**			

Documentation in the Medical Record

___

___

___

___

Comments:

Total Points Earned ________ Divided by ________ Total Possible Points = ________ % Score

Instructor's Signature ____________________

Student Name ____________________ Date __________ Score __________

Procedure 43-2 Obtaining Sputum for Culture

Task: To collect a sputum sample while observing standard precautions.

Equipment and Supplies:
- Sterile laboratory specimen cup, accurately labeled
- Plastic laboratory specimen bag
- Biohazard waste container

Standards: Complete the procedure and all critical steps in __________ minutes with a minimum score of __________ % within three attempts.

Scoring: Divide points earned by total possible points. Failure to perform a critical step that is indicated with an asterisk (*), will result in an unsatisfactory overall score.

Time began __________ **Time ended** __________

Steps	Possible Points	First Attempt	Second Attempt	Third Attempt
1. Assemble the equipment.	5			
2. Greet the patient and explain the procedure.	5			
3. Wash hands and put on gloves, face shield, and lab coat.	5			
4. Have the patient rinse his or her mouth with water.	10			
5. Instruct the patient to take three deep breaths and then cough deeply to bring up secretions from the lower respiratory tract.	10			
6. Tell the patient to spit directly into the specimen container and to avoid getting any sputum on the sides of the container.	10			
7. Place the lid on the container securely and then place the container into the plastic specimen bag.	10			
8. Offer the patient a glass of water or ginger ale.	10			
9. If another test is ordered for tomorrow morning, instruct the patient when to come and remind him or her to follow the same instructions for preparation.	10			
10. Clean the work area and properly dispose of all supplies.	5			

Steps	Possible Points	First Attempt	Second Attempt	Third Attempt
11. Wash your hands.	10			
12. Process the specimen immediately to ensure optimal test results.	5			
13. Record the procedure in the patient's record.	5			

Documentation in the Medical Record

____

____

____

____

Comments:

Total Points Earned ________ Divided by ________ Total Possible Points = ________ % Score

Instructor's Signature ________________

Student Name ______________________ Date ____________ Score ____________

Procedure 45-1 Sensorimotor Changes of Aging

Task: Role play to better understand the needs of aging persons.

Equipment and Supplies:
- Yellow glasses, ski goggles, or lab goggles
- Pink, white, yellow "pills" (various colors of tic tacs work)
- Vaseline
- Cotton balls
- Eye patches
- Tape
- Thick gloves
- Utility glove
- Tongue depressors
- Ace bandages
- Medical forms in small print
- Pennies
- Button shirts
- Walker

Standards: Complete the procedure and all critical steps in ____________ minutes with a minimum score of ____________ % within three attempts.

Scoring: Divide points earned by total possible points. Failure to perform a critical step that is indicated with an asterisk (*), will result in an unsatisfactory overall score.

Time began ____________ **Time ended** ____________

Steps	**Possible Points**	**First Attempt**	**Second Attempt**	**Third Attempt**
1. **Role play vision and hearing loss:** • Put 2 cotton balls in each ear and eye patch over 1 eye. Follow your partner's instructions. • Partner: stand out of line of vision (to prevent lip reading) and without gestures, without change in voice volume, tell your partner to cross the room and pick up a book.	**10**			
2. **Role play yellowing of lens:** • Line up "pills" of different pastel colors. • Partner: pick out the different colors while wearing the yellow glasses.	**10**			
3. **Role-play difficulty with focusing:** • Put on goggles smeared with Vaseline and follow your partner's directions. • Partner: stand at least 3 feet in front of your partner and motion for them to come to you (your partner is deaf so talking will not help).	**10**			

Steps	Possible Points	First Attempt	Second Attempt	Third Attempt
4. **Loss of peripheral vision:** • Put on goggles with black paper taped to sides. • Partner: stand to the side out of the field of vision and motion for your patient to follow you.	**10**			
5. **Simulating aphasia and partial paralysis:** • You are unable to use your right arm or leg. Place tape over your mouth. Let your partner know you need to go to the bathroom. • Stand at least 3 feet away with your back to your partner and wait for instructions.	**10**			
6. **Problems with dexterity:** • Put thick gloves on your hands and try to sign your name, button a shirt, tie your shoes, and pick up pennies.	**10**			
7. **Problems with mobility:** • Use the walker to cross the room. • Partner: after your partner starts to use the walker, hand them a book to carry.	**10**			
8. **Changes in sensation:** • Put a rubber utility glove on; turn on hot water; test the difference in temperature between the gloved hand and non-gloved hand.	**10**			
9. **Summarize and share with the group your impressions of the affect of sensorimotor changes and aging.**	**20**			

Documentation in the Medical Record

____

____

____

____

Comments:

Total Points Earned ________ Divided by ________ Total Possible Points = ________ % Score

Instructor's Signature ____________________

Student Name ______________________ Date ____________ Score ____________

Procedure 46-1 Obtaining a 12-lead ECG

Task: To obtain an accurate, artifact-free recording of the electrical activity of the heart.

Equipment and Supplies:
- ECG machine with patient lead cable
- 10 disposable, self-adhesive electrodes
- Patient gown and drape
- ECG mounting card if necessary

Standards: Complete the procedure and all critical steps in ____________ minutes with a minimum score of ____________ % within three attempts.

Scoring: Divide points earned by total possible points. Failure to perform a critical step that is indicated with an asterisk (*), will result in an unsatisfactory overall score.

Time began ____________ **Time ended** ____________

Steps	**Possible Points**	**First Attempt**	**Second Attempt**	**Third Attempt**
1. Wash hands.	5			
2. Explain the procedure to the patient.	5			
3. Ask the patient to disrobe to the waist and remove socks, stockings, or pantyhose as necessary.	5			
4. Position the patient on the exam table and drape appropriately.	5			
5. Turn on the machine to allow the stylus to warm up.	5			
6. Label the beginning of the tracing paper with the patient's name, date, and time.	5			
7. At each site where you will place an electrode, clean the skin with an alcohol wipe.	5			
8. Apply the self-adhesive electrodes to clean, dry fleshy areas of the extremities.	10			
9. Apply the self-adhesive electrodes to clean areas on the chest	10			
10. Carefully connect the lead wires to the correct electrode with the alligator clips on the end of each lead.	10			
11. Press the AUTO button on the machine and run the ECG tracing.	5			

Steps	Possible Points	First Attempt	Second Attempt	Third Attempt
12. Watch for artifacts during the recording.	5			
13. Remove the lead wires from the electrodes, and then remove the electrodes from the patient.	5			
14. Assist the patient with getting dressed as needed. Clean and return the ECG machine to its storage area.	5			
15. Mount the ECG tape or give the unmounted ECG tape to the physician as directed.	5			
16. Wash hands.	5			
17. Record the procedure in patient's chart.	5			

Documentation in the Medical Record

____

____

____

____

Comments:

Total Points Earned ________ Divided by ________ Total Possible Points = ________ % Score

Instructor's Signature ____________________

Student Name ______________ Date ______________ Score ______________

Procedure 46-2 Applying a Holter Monitor

Task: To establish possible correlation between coronary disorders and daily activity.

Equipment and Supplies:
- Holter monitor and blank magnetic recording tape
- Disposable electrodes
- Razor
- Tape
- Activity diary
- Carrying case with belt or shoulder strap
- Alcohol wipes
- Cloth tape (nonallergenic)

Standards: Complete the procedure and all critical steps in ______________ minutes with a minimum score of ______________ % within three attempts.

Scoring: Divide points earned by total possible points. Failure to perform a critical step that is indicated with an asterisk (*), will result in an unsatisfactory overall score.

Time began ______________ **Time ended** ______________

Steps	Possible Points	First Attempt	Second Attempt	Third Attempt
1. Wash your hands.	5			
2. Assemble equipment needed.	5			
3. Install new battery or fully charged rechargeable battery in the monitor.	5			
4. Greet the patient and explain the procedure.	5			
5. Ask the patient to disrobe to the waist and sit at the end of the examination table or to lie down.	5			
6. If the patient has a hairy chest, dry shave the area at each of the electrode sites.	5			
7. Clean each electrode application site with an alcohol wipe and allow the sites to air dry.	5			
8. Fold a gauze pad over your index finger and briskly rub the sites.	5			
9. Apply the electrodes to the appropriate sites, making sure to use enough pressure so that each adheres completely to the skin.	5			
10. Attach the lead wires to the electrodes and connect the end terminal to the patient cable.	5			

Steps	Possible Points	First Attempt	Second Attempt	Third Attempt
11. Place a strip of cloth tape over each electrode.	5			
12. Attach the test cable to the monitor and plug it into the electrocardiograph. Run a baseline test tracing.	5			
13. Help the patient get dressed without disturbing the connected electrodes. Be certain that the cable extends through the buttoned front or out the bottom of the shirt or blouse.	5			
14. Place the monitor in the carrying case, and attach it to the patient's belt or place it over the shoulder. Be sure the wires are not being pulled or bent in half.	5			
15. Plug the electrode cable into the monitor.	5			
16. Record the patient's name, date of birth, and starting date and time of the patient's activity diary.	5			
17. Give the patient the activity diary and advise him or her to begin by writing in the present activity.	5			
18. Give patient appointment for return in 24 hours.	5			
19. Wash hands.	5			
20. Record the procedure in patient's chart.	5			

Documentation in the Medical Record

____

____

____

____

Comments:

Total Points Earned ________ Divided by ________ Total Possible Points = ________ % Score

Instructor's Signature ____________________

Student Name ______________________ Date ______________ Score ______________

Procedure 47-1 General Procedure for X-Ray Examination

Task: To assist with an x-ray examination under the supervision of a physician.

Equipment and Supplies:
- Physician's order for an x-ray examination
- Patient identification card to imprint radiographs
- X-ray machine
- X-ray cassettes, loaded with film
- X-ray darkroom with automatic processor

Standards: Complete the procedure and all critical steps in ______________ minutes with a minimum score of ______________ % within three attempts.

Scoring: Divide points earned by total possible points. Failure to perform a critical step that is indicated with an asterisk (*), will result in an unsatisfactory overall score.

Time began ______________ **Time ended** ______________

Steps	Possible Points	First Attempt	Second Attempt	Third Attempt
1. Check order and equipment needed. Ascertain if any special preparations were needed.	5			
2. Introduce yourself, and confirm the identity of the patient. Ascertain if any necessary preparations were implemented.	5			
3. Explain the procedure and place the x-ray cassette correctly.	5			
4. Check to make certain that the patient has removed all metal objects from the area to be examined.	5			
5. Drape the patient as necessary, and shield the pelvic area.	5			
6. Position the patient properly, and immobilize the part, if necessary.	5			
7. Align the x-ray tube to the cassette at the proper distance.	10			
8. Measure the patient's thickness through the path of the central ray and set the control panel for he correct exposure.	10			
9. Stand behind a lead shield during the exposure.	10			

Steps	Possible Points	First Attempt	Second Attempt	Third Attempt
10. Ask the patient to assume a comfortable position after the examination is completed, and wait until the films are processed.	10			
11. In the darkroom, remove the film from the cassette, identify the film, and process the film in the automatic processor.	10			
12. Dismiss the patient if all films are satisfactory.	10			
13. Place the dry, finished x-ray film in a properly labeled envelope and present it to the physician for interpretation. When it has been read, file it according to the policies of the office.	10			
14. Record the x-ray examination on the patient's chart, along with the final written x-ray findings.	10			

Documentation in the Medical Record

____

____

____

____

Comments:

Total Points Earned ________ Divided by ________ Total Possible Points = ________ % Score

Instructor's Signature ________________

Student Name ______________________ Date ____________ Score ____________

Procedure 48-1 Using the Microscope

Task: To focus the microscope properly, using a prepared slide, under low power, high power, and oil immersion

Equipment and Supplies:
- Microscope
- Lens tissue
- Lens cleaner
- Slide with stained specimen

Standards: Complete the procedure and all critical steps in ____________ minutes with a minimum score of ____________ % within three attempts.

Scoring: Divide points earned by total possible points. Failure to perform a critical step that is indicated with an asterisk (*), will result in an unsatisfactory overall score.

Time began ____________ **Time ended** ____________

Steps	Possible Points	First Attempt	Second Attempt	Third Attempt
1. Wash your hands.	4			
2. Gather the materials needed.	4			
3. Clean the lenses with lens tissue and lens cleaner. Clean the 100x lens (oil immersion) last.	4			
4. Adjust seating to a comfortable height.	4			
5. Plug the microscope into an electric outlet, and turn on the light switch.	4			
6. Place the slide specimen on the stage and secure it.	4			
7. Turn the revolving nosepiece to low power.	4			
8. Carefully raise the stage while observing with the naked eye from the side.	4			
9. Focus the specimen, using the coarse-adjustment knob.	4			
10. Switch to fine adjustment, and focus the specimen in detail.	4			
11. Adjust the amount of light by closing the iris diaphragm and lowering the condenser.	4			
12. Turn the revolving nosepiece between the high-power objective and oil immersion.	4			

Steps	Possible Points	First Attempt	Second Attempt	Third Attempt
13. Place a small drop of oil on the slide.	4			
14. Carefully swing the oil immersion objective into place.	4			
15. Adjust the focus with the fine-adjustment knob.	4			
16. Increase the light by opening the iris diaphragm and raising the condenser.	4			
17. Identify the specimen.	4			
18. Return to low power.	4			
19. Lower the stage.	4			
20. Center the stage. Remove the slide.	4			
21. Switch off the light and unplug the microscope.	4			
22. Clean the lenses with lens tissue, and remove oil with lens cleaner.	4			
23. Wipe the microscope with a cloth.	4			
24. Cover the microscope. Clean the work area.	4			
25. Wash your hands.	4			

Documentation in the Medical Record

____

____

____

____

Comments:

Total Points Earned ________ Divided by ________ Total Possible Points = ________ % Score

Instructor's Signature ____________________

Student Name ______________________ Date ____________ Score ____________

Procedure 49-1 Collecting a Clean-catch Urine Specimen

Task: To collect a contaminant-free urine sample for culture or analysis using midstream clean-catch technique.

Equipment and Supplies:
- Sterile container with lid and label
- Antiseptic towelettes
- Set of written patient instructions

Standards: Complete the procedure and all critical steps in ____________ minutes with a minimum score of ____________ % within three attempts.

Scoring: Divide points earned by total possible points. Failure to perform a critical step that is indicated with an asterisk (*), will result in an unsatisfactory overall score.

Time began ____________ **Time ended** ____________

Steps	Possible Points	First Attempt	Second Attempt	Third Attempt
1. Label the container and give the patient the supplies.	10			
2. Explain the instructions to adult patients or to the guardians of child patients.	10			
OBTAINING A CLEAN-CATCH MIDSTREAM SPECIMEN FROM A FEMALE PATIENT	40			
1. Wash hands and remove underclothing.				
2. Expose the urinary meatus by spreading apart the labia with one hand.				
3. Cleanse each side of the urinary meatus with a front-to-back motion, from the pubis to the anus. Use a fresh cotton ball on each side. (If the midstream specimen kit is used, an antiseptic wipe is provided to cleanse each side of the meatus.)				
4. Cleanse directly across the meatus, front-to-back, using a third cotton ball or antiseptic wipe				
5. Rinse with water to remove traces of the soap used to prevent its entrance into the specimen.				
6. Dry the area with a clean cotton ball using front-to-back motion. If a midstream kit has been used, the rinsing and drying procedure can be omitted.				
7. Hold the labia apart throughout this procedure.				
8. Void a small amount of urine into the toilet.				

Steps	Possible Points	First Attempt	Second Attempt	Third Attempt
9. Move the specimen container into position and void the next portion of urine into it. Remember this is a sterile container. Do not put your fingers on the inside of the container				
10. Remove the cup and void the last amount of urine into the toilet. (This means that the first part and the last part of the urinary flow have been excluded from the specimen. Only the middle portion of the flow is included.)				

Comments:

OBTAINING A CLEAN-CATCH MIDSTREAM SPECIMEN FROM A MALE PATIENT	**40**			
1. Wash your hands and expose the penis.				
2. Retract the foreskin of the penis (if not circumcised).				
3. Cleanse the area around the glans penis (meatus) and the urethral opening by washing each side of the glans with a separate cotton ball. If a midstream kit is used, antiseptic wipes are provided.				
4. Cleanse directly across the urethral opening using a third cotton ball or antiseptic wipe.				
5. If soap and cotton balls are used, rinse with water to remove all traces of soap.				
6. Dry the area using a front-to-back motion.				
7. Void a small amount of urine into the toilet or urinal.				
8. Collect the next portion of the urine in the sterile container without touching the inside of the container with hands or penis.				
9. Void the last amount of urine into the toilet or urinal.				
10. Wipe and redress.				
11. Return the specimen to the designated area provided.				

Comments:

Documentation in the Medical Record

____

____

____

____

Comments:

Total Points Earned ________ Divided by ________ Total Possible Points = ________ % Score

Instructor's Signature ____________________

Student Name ______________________ Date ____________ Score ____________

Procedure 49-2 Assessing Urine for Color and Turbidity

Task: To assess and record the color and clarity of a urine specimen.

Equipment and Supplies:
- Urine specimen
- Centrifuge tube

Standards: Complete the procedure and all critical steps in ____________ minutes with a minimum score of ____________ % within three attempts.

Scoring: Divide points earned by total possible points. Failure to perform a critical step that is indicated with an asterisk (*), will result in an unsatisfactory overall score.

Time began ____________ **Time ended** ____________

Steps	Possible Points	First Attempt	Second Attempt	Third Attempt
1. Wash and dry your hands and apply gloves.	10			
2. Mix the urine by swirling.	10			
3. Label a centrifuge tube if a complete urinalysis is being done.	10			
4. Pour the specimen into a standard-size centrifuge tube.	10			
5. Assess and record the color. • Pale straw • Yellow • Dark yellow • Amber	20			
6. Assess clarity. • Clear—no cloudiness • Slightly cloudy—can see light print through tube • Moderately cloudy—can see only dark print through tube • Very cloudy—cannot see through tube	20			
7. Clean the work area, remove gloves, and wash your hands.	10			
8. Record the results in the patient's record.	10			

Documentation in the Medical Record

____

____

____

____

Comments:

Total Points Earned ________ Divided by ________ Total Possible Points = ________ % Score

Instructor's Signature ____________________

Student Name ____________ Date ____________ Score ____________

Procedure 49-3 Measuring Specific Gravity Using a Urinometer

Task: To calibrate the urinometer to perform a quality control check and to obtain duplicate specific gravity readings.

Equipment and Supplies:
- Urine specimen
- Distilled water
- Urinometer and cylinder

Standards: Complete the procedure and all critical steps in ____________ minutes with a minimum score of ____________ % within three attempts.

Scoring: Divide points earned by total possible points. Failure to perform a critical step that is indicated with an asterisk (*), will result in an unsatisfactory overall score.

Time began ____________ **Time ended** ____________

Steps	**Possible Points**	**First Attempt**	**Second Attempt**	**Third Attempt**
1. Wash and dry your hands and put on nonsterile gloves and eye protection.	5			
2. Fill the glass cylinder two-thirds full with distilled water at 20° C (room temperature).	5			
3. Read the specific gravity of the distilled water.	10			
4. Allow the specimen to come to room temperature if it was refrigerated.	10			
5. Mix the specimen well by swirling.	10			
6. Pour the specimen into the clean glass cylinder to two-thirds to three-fourths full.	10			
7. Remove any foam using filter paper.	5			
8. With the cylinder on a level surface, gently insert the urinometer in the specimen with a spinning motion.	10			
9. While the urinometer stops rotating in the specimen, read the lower curve of the meniscus, at eye level.	10			

Steps	Possible Points	First Attempt	Second Attempt	Third Attempt
10. Clean and dry the equipment, and return it to proper storage.	5			
11. Clean the work area. Wash your hands.	5			
12. Record the results on the laboratory form or in the patient's record.	15			

Documentation in the Medical Record

____

____

____

____

Comments:

Total Points Earned ________ Divided by ________ Total Possible Points = ________ % Score

Instructor's Signature ________________________

Student Name ______________________ Date ______________ Score ______________

Procedure 49-4 Measuring Specific Gravity Using a Refractometer

Task: To measure the refractive index of urine using a refractometer. A refractometer is also known as a total solids (TS) meter.

Equipment and Supplies:
- Urinary refractometer
- Disposable pipet
- Distilled water
- Biohazard waste container

Standards: Complete the procedure and all critical steps in ______________ minutes with a minimum score of ______________ % within three attempts.

Scoring: Divide points earned by total possible points. Failure to perform a critical step that is indicated with an asterisk (*), will result in an unsatisfactory overall score.

Time began ______________ **Time ended** ______________

Steps	Possible Points	First Attempt	Second Attempt	Third Attempt
1. Wash hands and assemble equipment while the urine specimen reaches room temperature.	10			
2. Apply gloves and mix the urine specimen in the collection container.	10			
3. Using a disposable pipet, apply a drop of water to the prism of the refractometer by lifting the plastic cover. Close the cover and point the device toward a light source such as a window or lamp. Look into the refractometer and rotate the eyepiece so the scale can be clearly read. The scale reads from 1.000 to 1.035 in increments of 0.001; distilled water should read 1.000.	30			
4. Adjust the refractometer using the small screw-driver provided by the manufacturer if the scale does not read 1.000.	10			
5. Wipe the prism with a soft, lint-free tissue and apply a drop of mixed urine. Close the cover, point the device at a light source and read the specific gravity on the scale. Discard the pipet in a biohazard waste container.	10			
6. Wipe the urine from the prism with a disposable soft, lint-free tissue between samples. When finished, clean with tissue moistened with distilled water. Discard these tissues in a biohazard waste container.	10			

Steps	Possible Points	First Attempt	Second Attempt	Third Attempt
7. Record the results and discard the urine sample.	10			
8. Remove and discard gloves and wash the hands.	10			

Documentation in the Medical Record

Comments:

Total Points Earned ________ Divided by ________ Total Possible Points = ________ % Score

Instructor's Signature ________________

Student Name ______________________ Date ____________ Score ____________

Procedure 49-5 Testing Urine with Chemical Reagent Strips

Task: To test urine with chemical reagent strips

Equipment and Supplies:
- Urine specimen
- Reagent strips
- Timer

Standards: Complete the procedure and all critical steps in ____________ minutes with a minimum score of ____________ % within three attempts.

Scoring: Divide points earned by total possible points. Failure to perform a critical step that is indicated with an asterisk (*), will result in an unsatisfactory overall score.

Time began ____________ **Time ended** ____________

Steps	Possible Points	First Attempt	Second Attempt	Third Attempt
1. Wash and dry your hands. Put on nonsterile gloves and eye protection.	5			
2. Check the time of collection, the container, and the mode of preservation.	5			
3. If the specimen has been refrigerated, allow it to warm to room temperature.	5			
4. Check the reagent strip container for the expiration date.	5			
5. Remove the reagent strip from the container. Hold it in your hand, or place it on a clean paper towel. Recap the container tightly.	5			
6. Compare nonreactive test pads with the negative color blocks on the color chart on the container.	10			
7. Thoroughly mix the specimen by swirling or inverting.	5			
8. Following manufacturer's directions, note the time, and simultaneously dip the strip into the urine and remove it.	10			
9. Quickly remove the excess urine from the strip.	10			
10. Hold the strip horizontally. After the exact amount of time specified by the manufacturer has elapsed, compare the strip with the appropriate color chart on the reagent container.	10			

Steps	Possible Points	First Attempt	Second Attempt	Third Attempt
11. Read the concentration.	10			
12. Clean the work area, remove your gloves, and wash your hands.	10			
13. Record the results in the patient's chart.	10			

Documentation in the Medical Record

Comments:

Total Points Earned ________ Divided by ________ Total Possible Points = ________ % Score

Instructor's Signature ________________

Student Name ______________________ Date ____________ Score ________

Procedure 49-6 Testing Urine for Glucose with the Clinitest Method

Task: To perform confirmatory testing for glucose in the urine with the Clinitest procedure for reducing substances.

Equipment and Supplies:
- Urine specimen
- Clinitest tablet, tube, and dropper
- Distilled water
- Test tube rack
- Color chart

Standards: Complete the procedure and all critical steps in ____________ minutes with a minimum score of ____________ % within three attempts.

Scoring: Divide points earned by total possible points. Failure to perform a critical step that is indicated with an asterisk (*), will result in an unsatisfactory overall score.

Time began ____________ **Time ended** ____________

Steps	**Possible Points**	**First Attempt**	**Second Attempt**	**Third Attempt**
1. Wash and dry your hands and put on nonsterile gloves and eye protection.	**5**			
2. Holding a Clinitest dropper vertically, add 10 drops of distilled water and then 5 drops of urine to a Clinitest tube.	**10**			
3. Place the prepared tube in the rack.	**5**			
4. With dry hands, remove a Clinitest tablet from the bottle by pouring the tablet into the bottle cap.	**10**			
5. Tap the tablet into the test tube and recap the container.	**10**			
6. Observe the entire reaction to detect the rapid pass-through phenomenon, which means that the glucose level in the urine is very high.	**10**			
7. When reaction ceases, time exactly 15 seconds; then gently shake the tube to mix the entire contents.	**10**			
8. Immediately compare the color of the specimen with the five-drop color chart and record your findings.	**10**			
9. If an orange color briefly develops during the reaction, rapid pass-through has occurred, and the test must be repeated with the use of the two-drop color chart.	**10**			

Steps	Possible Points	First Attempt	Second Attempt	Third Attempt
10. Clean the work area, remove gloves, and wash hands.	10			
11. Record the results in the patient's chart. Negative—Clear Trace—Slightly cloudy 1+—Can see light print through tube 2+—Can see dark print through tube 3+—Cannot see through tube 4+—Large, fluffy precipitate forms and settles on standing	10			

Documentation in the Medical Record

Comments:

Total Points Earned ________ Divided by ________ Total Possible Points = ________ % Score

Instructor's Signature ________________

Student Name ______________________ Date ____________ Score ________

Procedure 49-7 Testing Urine for Protein Using the Sulfosalicylic Acid (SSA)

Task: To test urine for protein by using the sulfosalicylic acid (SSA) precipitation test.

Equipment and Supplies:
- Urine specimen
- 3% sulfosalicylic acid
- Centrifuge tube and centrifuge
- Test tube and rack
- Dropper

Standards: Complete the procedure and all critical steps in ____________ minutes with a minimum score of ____________ % within three attempts.

Scoring: Divide points earned by total possible points. Failure to perform a critical step that is indicated with an asterisk (*), will result in an unsatisfactory overall score.

Time began ____________ **Time ended** ____________

Steps	**Possible Points**	**First Attempt**	**Second Attempt**	**Third Attempt**
1. Wash and dry your hands. Put on nonsterile gloves and eye protection.	**10**			
2. If the urine is cloudy, filter the specimen or use a centrifuged specimen.	**20**			
3. In a clear test tube, mix equal volumes of urine and 3% SSA.	**20**			
4. Observe for cloudiness and record: Negative—Clear Trace—Slightly cloudy 1+—Can see light print through tube 2+—Can see dark print through tube 3+—Cannot see through tube 4+—Large, fluffy precipitate forms and settles on standing	**20**			
5. Clean the work area, remove gloves and face protection, and wash hands.	**10**			
6. Record the results in the patient's chart.	**20**			

Documentation in the Medical Record

____

____

____

____

Comments:

Total Points Earned ________ Divided by ________ Total Possible Points = ________ % Score

Instructor's Signature ____________________

Student Name ______________________ Date ____________ Score ________

Procedure 49-8 Analyzing Urine Specimen for Microscopic Examination

Task: To perform a microscopic examination of urine to determine the presence of normal and abnormal elements.

Equipment and Supplies:
- Urine specimen
- Centrifuge tube
- Centrifuge
- Disposable pipette
- Microscope slide and coverslip
- Microscope
- Permanent marker

Standards: Complete the procedure and all critical steps in ____________ minutes with a minimum score of ____________ % within three attempts.

Scoring: Divide points earned by total possible points. Failure to perform a critical step that is indicated with an asterisk (*), will result in an unsatisfactory overall score.

Time began ____________ **Time ended** ____________

Steps	**Possible Points**	**First Attempt**	**Second Attempt**	**Third Attempt**
1. Wash and dry your hands. Put on face protection and nonsterile gloves.	5			
2. Gently mix the urine specimen.	5			
3. Pour 10 mL of urine into a labeled centrifuge tube and cap the tube.	5			
4. Place the tube in the centrifuge.	5			
5. Place another tube containing 10 mL of water in the opposite cup.	5			
6. Secure the lid, and centrifuge for 5 minutes or for the time specified for your instrument.	5			
7. Remove the tube from the centrifuge after the instrument has come to a full stop.	5			
8. Pour off the clear supernatant from the top of the specimen by inverting the centrifuge tube over the sink drain.	5			
9. Prevent the loss of sediment down the drain.	5			

Steps	Possible Points	First Attempt	Second Attempt	Third Attempt
10. Thoroughly mix the sediment by grasping the tube near the top and rapidly flicking it with the fingers of the other hand until all sediment is thoroughly resuspended.	5			
11. Transfer one drop of sediment to a clean, labeled slide.	5			
12. Place a clean coverslip over the drop, and place the slide on the microscope stage. Remove face protection.	5			
13. Focus under low power, and reduce the light.	5			
14. First, scan the entire coverslip for abnormal findings.	5			
15. Examine five low-power fields. Count and classify each type of cast seen, if any, and note mucus if present.	5			
16. Switch to high-power magnification, and adjust the light.	5			
17. In five high-power fields, count the following elements: red blood cells, white blood cells, and round, transitional, and squamous epithelial cells.	5			
18. In the same five fields, report the following as few, moderate, or many: crystals (identify and report each type seen separately), bacteria (identify as rods or cocci), sperm, yeast, and parasites.	5			
19. Average the five fields, and report the results. Do not remove the slide from the microscope until the physician has verified the results.	5			
20. Clean up the work area, remove face protection and gloves, and wash hands.	2.5			
21. Record the verified results in the patient's chart.	2.5			

Documentation in the Medical Record

____

____

____

____

Comments:

Total Points Earned ________ Divided by ________ Total Possible Points = ________ % Score

Instructor's Signature ______________________

Student Name ____________________ Date __________ Score __________

Procedure 49-9 Performing a Pregnancy Test

Task: To perform a pregnancy testing of urine with the QuickVue by Quidel pregnancy test method.

Equipment and Supplies:
- Urine specimen
- QuickVue test kit

Standards: Complete the procedure and all critical steps in __________ minutes with a minimum score of __________ % within three attempts.

Scoring: Divide points earned by total possible points. Failure to perform a critical step that is indicated with an asterisk (*), will result in an unsatisfactory overall score.

Time began __________ **Time ended** __________

Steps	**Possible Points**	**First Attempt**	**Second Attempt**	**Third Attempt**
1. Wash and dry hands. Put on face protection and nonsterile gloves.	**10**			
2. Prepare the testing equipment.	**10**			
3. Collect the needed specimen.	**10**			
4. Remove the test cassette from the foil pouch.	**10**			
5. Add 3 drops of urine using the dropper that accompanies the kit. Dispose of the dropper in a biohazard bag.	**10**			
6. Wait 3 minutes and read the test results.	**10**			
7. Interpret the results. NEGATIVE: A blue control line will be present next to the letter C. No line will be present next to the letter T. POSITIVE: A blue control line will appear next to the letter C along with a pink line next to the letter T. If a blue line does not appear in the "C" area, the test is invalid and the specimen must be retested with another kit. Check the expiration date of the kit before proceeding.	**20**			
8. Discard the cassette in a biohazard waste container, remove gloves, and wash hands.	**10**			
9. Record the results in the patient's chart as either positive or negative.	**10**			

Documentation in the Medical Record

____

____

____

____

Comments:

Total Points Earned ________ Divided by ________ Total Possible Points = ________ % Score

Instructor's Signature ____________________

Student Name ______________________ Date ____________ Score ________

Procedure 49-10 Performing a Rapid Urine Culture Test

Task: To assess the level of bacteriuria to aid in diagnosis of urinary tract infections.

Equipment and Supplies:
- Clean-catch midstream urine specimen
- Uricult test kit
- Incubator
- Biohazard waste container

Standards: Complete the procedure and all critical steps in ____________ minutes with a minimum score of ____________ % within three attempts.

Scoring: Divide points earned by total possible points. Failure to perform a critical step that is indicated with an asterisk (*), will result in an unsatisfactory overall score.

Time began ____________ **Time ended** ____________

Steps	**Possible Points**	**First Attempt**	**Second Attempt**	**Third Attempt**
1. Wash hands and assemble equipment and specimen. Check the expiration date on the test kit. Label the vial with the patient information.	**10**			
2. Put on gloves. Remove the slide from the test kit. Do not touch the slide or lay it down.	**10**			
3. Dip the slide into the urine specimen, tipping the cup carefully if necessary. Alternatively, the urine may be poured over the slide and caught in another container.	**10**			
4. Allow excess urine to drain, then replace the slide in the protective vial. Screw the cap on loosely.	**10**			
5. Incubate the vial upright in a 35°-37° C incubator for 18 to 24 hours.	**10**			
6. After incubation, read the test results by removing the slide from its protective vial and assessing bacterial colony density by comparing the slide with the density chart provided. No actual colony counting is necessary.	**10**			
7. Interpret the results as follows NORMAL: Less than 10,000 colony-forming units (cfu)/ml of urine; no UTI is present. BORDERLINE: 10,000 to 100,000 cfu/ml of urine; a chronic or relapsing infection may be present and the test should be repeated. POSITIVE: More than 100,000 cfu/ml of urine; a UTI is likely.	**10**			

Steps	Possible Points	First Attempt	Second Attempt	Third Attempt
8. Return the vial to the protective case and replace the cap.	**5**			
9. Dispose of the test kit in a biohazard waste container.	**5**			
10. Remove gloves and wash hands.	**5**			
11. Record the results.	**5**			

Documentation in the Medical Record

Comments:

Total Points Earned ________ Divided by ________ Total Possible Points = ________ % Score

Instructor's Signature ____________________

Student Name ____________________ Date __________ Score __________

Procedure 50-1 Collecting a Venous Blood Sample Using the Syringe Method

Task: To collect a venous blood specimen.

Equipment and Supplies:
- Needle, syringe with 21- or 22-gauge needle
- Evacuated tubes appropriate to tests ordered
- 70% isopropyl alcohol
- Sterile gauze pads
- Tourniquet
- Nonallergenic tape

Standards: Complete the procedure and all critical steps in __________ minutes with a minimum score of __________ % within three attempts.

Scoring: Divide points earned by total possible points. Failure to perform a critical step that is indicated with an asterisk (*), will result in an unsatisfactory overall score.

Time began __________ **Time ended** __________

Steps	Possible Points	First Attempt	Second Attempt	Third Attempt
1. Check the requisition form to determine the tests ordered. Gather the correct tubes and supplies that you will need.	5			
2. Wash and dry your hands, and put on face protection and nonsterile gloves.	5			
3. Identify the patient and explain the procedure.	5			
4. Assist the patient to a seated position with the arm well supported in a slightly downward position.	2.5			
5. Assemble equipment. Choice of syringe and needle size depends on your inspection of the patient's veins. Attach the needle to the syringe. Keep the cover on the needle.	5			
6. Apply the tourniquet around the patient's arm 3 to 4 inches above the elbow. The tourniquet should never be tied so tightly that it restricts blood flow in the artery.	5			
7. Ask the patient to open and close his or her hand several times.	5			
8. Cleanse the site, starting in the center of the area and working outward in a circular pattern.	5			
9. Dry the site with a sterile gauze pad.	5			

Steps	Possible Points	First Attempt	Second Attempt	Third Attempt
10. Remove the needle sheath.	5			
11. Grasp the patient's arm with the nondominant hand while using your thumb and forefinger to draw the skin taut over the site to anchor the vein.	5			
12. Insert the needle through the skin and into the vein with the bevel of the needle up, aligned parallel to the vein, at a 15-degree angle, rapidly, and smoothly.	5			
13. Slowly pull back the plunger of the syringe with the nondominant hand. Make sure that you do not move the needle after entering the vein. Allow the syringe or tube to fill to optimum capacity.	5			
14. Release the tourniquet when venipuncture is complete. It must be released before the needle is removed from the arm.*	5			
15. Place sterile gauze over the puncture site at the time of needle withdrawal.	5			
16. Instruct the patient to apply direct pressure on the puncture site with sterile gauze. The patient may elevate the arm.	5			
17. Transfer the blood to a tube. Gently invert tubes to mix anticoagulants and blood.	5			
18. Check the puncture site for bleeding.	5			
19. Apply a hypoallergenic bandage.	2.5			
20. Dispose of the needle safely. Allow it to drop directly into the disposal unit without touching it with your fingers. Do not recap used needles.	2.5			
21. Clean the work area, remove gloves and face protection, and wash your hands.	2.5			
22. Complete the laboratory requisition form, and route the specimen to the proper place. Record the procedure in the patient's chart.	5			

Documentation in the Medical Record

____

____

____

____

Comments:

Total Points Earned ________ Divided by ________ Total Possible Points = ________ % Score

Instructor's Signature ____________________

Student Name ______________ Date ________ Score ________

Procedure 50-2 Collecting a Venous Blood Sample Using the Evacuated Tube Method

Task: To collect a venous blood specimen.

Equipment and Supplies:
- Vacutainer needle, adapter, and proper tubes for requested tests
- 70% isopropyl alcohol
- Sterile gauze pads
- Tourniquet
- Nonallergenic tape
- Permanent marking pen

Standards: Complete the procedure and all critical steps in ____________ minutes with a minimum score of ____________ % within three attempts.

Scoring: Divide points earned by total possible points. Failure to perform a critical step that is indicated with an asterisk (*), will result in an unsatisfactory overall score.

Time began ____________ **Time ended** ____________

Steps	Possible Points	First Attempt	Second Attempt	Third Attempt
1. Check the requisition form to determine the tests ordered. Gather the correct tubes and supplies that you will need.	4			
2. Wash and dry your hands, and put on face protection and nonsterile gloves.*	5			
3. Identify the patient and explain the procedure.	4			
4. Assist the patient to sit with the arm well supported in a slightly downward position.	4			
5 Assemble equipment.	4			
6. Apply the tourniquet around the patient's arm 3 to 4 inches above the elbow.	4			
7. Select the venipuncture site by palpating the antecubital space, and use your index finger to trace the path of the vein and to judge its depth.	4			
8. Ask the patient to open and close his or her hand several times.	4			
9. Cleanse the site, starting in the center of the area and working outward in a circular pattern.	4			

Steps	Possible Points	First Attempt	Second Attempt	Third Attempt
10. Dry the site with a sterile gauze pad.	4			
11. Remove the needle sheath.	4			
12. Anchor the vein.	4			
13. Insert the needle through the skin and into the vein with the bevel of the needle up, aligned parallel to the vein, at a 15-degree angle, rapidly, and smoothly.	5			
14. Push the tube onto the needle inside the holder.	4			
15. Allow the tube to fill to optimum capacity.	4			
16. Remove the Vacutainer tube from the adapter before removing the needle from the vein.	4			
17. Release the tourniquet when venipuncture is complete. It must be released before the needle is removed from the arm.*	5			
18. Place sterile gauze over the puncture site at the time of needle withdrawal.	4			
19. Instruct the patient to apply direct pressure on the puncture site with a sterile gauze pad.	4			
20. Gently invert tubes to mix anticoagulants and blood.	4			
21. Check the puncture site for bleeding.	4			
22. Apply a hypoallergenic bandage.	4			
23. Dispose of the needle safely.*	5			
24. Clean the work area, remove gloves and face protection, and wash your hands.	4			
25. Complete the laboratory requisition and route to the proper place. Record the procedure in the patient's record.	4			

Documentation in the Medical Record

____

____

____

____

Comments:

Total Points Earned ________ Divided by ________ Total Possible Points = ________ % Score

Instructor's Signature ____________________

Student Name ______________________ Date ____________ Score ____________

Procedure 50-3 Collecting a Venous Blood Sample Using the Butterfly Method

Task: To accurately obtain the venous sample from a hand vein using the butterfly method.

Equipment and Supplies:
- Tourniquet
- Alcohol pads or other antiseptic preps
- Gauze pads
- Butterfly needle set
- Appropriate pediatric tubes arranged in the order of the draw or
- Luer-Lok syringe
- Sharps disposal container
- Nonallergenic bandage
- Permanent marking pen

Standards: Complete the procedure and all critical steps in ____________ minutes with a minimum score of ____________ % within three attempts.

Scoring: Divide points earned by total possible points. Failure to perform a critical step that is indicated with an asterisk (*), will result in an unsatisfactory overall score.

Time began ____________ **Time ended** ____________

Steps	**Possible Points**	**First Attempt**	**Second Attempt**	**Third Attempt**
1. Check the requisition and gather the appropriate tubes for the needed tests. Assemble the balance of your supplies.	**4**			
2. Wash your hands, and put on face protection and gloves.*	**4**			
3. Prepare your patient as for an antecubital draw.	**4**			
4. Remove the butterfly device from the package and stretch it slightly.	**4**			
5. Attach the butterfly device to the syringe or evacuated tube holder.	**4**			
6. Seat the first tube into the evacuated tube holder.	**4**			
7. Apply a tourniquet to the patient's wrist, just proximal to the wrist bone.	**4**			
8. Hold the hand in your nondominant hand with the fingers lower than the wrist.	**4**			
9. Select a vein and cleanse the site at the bifurcation.	**4**			

Steps	Possible Points	First Attempt	Second Attempt	Third Attempt
10. Using your thumb, pull the patient's skin taut over the knuckles.	4			
11. With the needle at a 10- to 15-degree angle, bevel up, align it with the vein.	4			
12. Insert the needle gently by threading it up the lumen of the vein.	12			
13. Push the blood collecting tube onto the end of the holder or draw blood into the syringe. Note the position of the hands while drawing the blood.	4			
14. Release the tourniquet when the blood appears in the tube.*	12			
15. Always keep the tube and the holder in a downward position so that the tube will fill from the bottom up.	4			
16. Place a gauze pad over the puncture site and gently remove the needle.	4			
17. Instruct the patient to apply direct pressure on the puncture site with a sterile gauze pad.	4			
18. Gently invert tubes to mix anticoagulants and blood.	4			
19. Check the puncture site for bleeding.	4			
20. Apply a hypoallergenic bandage.	4			
21. Dispose of the needle safely.*	12			
22. Clean the work area, remove gloves and face protection, and wash your hands.	4			

Documentation in the Medical Record

____

____

____

____

Comments:

Total Points Earned ________ Divided by ________ Total Possible Points = ________ % Score

Instructor's Signature ____________________

Student Name ______________________ Date ______________ Score ________

Procedure 50-4 Collecting a Capillary Blood Sample

Task: To collect a capillary blood specimen suitable for testing, using fingertip puncture technique.

Equipment and Supplies:
- Sterile disposable manual lancet or Autolet with Autolet platforms
- 70% alcohol
- Sterile gauze pads
- Nonallergenic tape
- Supplies for requested test (e.g., Unopettes or capillary tubes)
- Sealing clay or caps for capillary tubes
- Permanent marking pen

Standards: Complete the procedure and all critical steps in ______________ minutes with a minimum score of ______________ % within three attempts.

Scoring: Divide points earned by total possible points. Failure to perform a critical step that is indicated with an asterisk (*), will result in an unsatisfactory overall score.

Time began ______________ **Time ended** ______________

Steps	**Possible Points**	**First Attempt**	**Second Attempt**	**Third Attempt**
1. Wash and dry your hands. Put on face protection and nonsterile gloves.	5			
2. Explain the procedure to your patient.	5			
3. Assemble the needed materials, based on the physician's requisition.	5			
4. Select a puncture site.	5			
5. Milk, or very gently rub, the finger along the sides.	5			
6. Milk, or very gently rub, the finger along the sides.	5			
7. Grasp the patient''s finger on the sides near the puncture site, with your nondominant forefinger and thumb.	5			
8. Hold the lancet at a right angle to the patient's finger, and make a rapid, deep puncture on the patient's fingertip.	5			
9. Wipe away the first drop of blood.	5			
10. Apply gentle pressure to cause the blood to flow freely.	5			

Steps	Possible Points	First Attempt	Second Attempt	Third Attempt
11. Collect blood samples. a. Express a large drop of blood, fill capillary tubes, and seal the end of the tube in clay. b. Wipe the finger with a clean sterile gauze pad, and fill a Unopette.	**10**			
12. Apply pressure to the site with clean sterile gauze.	**5**			
13. Label all samples and requisitions correctly, and forward them to the laboratory for testing.	**10**			
14. Check the patient for bleeding, and apply a nonallergenic bandage if indicated.	**5**			
15. Dispose of used materials in proper containers.	**10**			
16. Clean the work area. Remove face protection and gloves. Wash your hands.	**5**			
17. Record the procedure in the patient's record.	**5**			

Documentation in the Medical Record

____

____

____

____

Comments:

Total Points Earned ________ Divided by ________ Total Possible Points = ________ % Score

Instructor's Signature ____________________

Student Name ______________________ Date ____________ Score ____________

Procedure 51-1 Performing a Microhematocrit

Task: To accurately perform a microhematocrit.

Equipment and Supplies:
- EDTA anticoagulant blood
- Capillary tubes
- Sealing clay
- Centrifuge

Standards: Complete the procedure and all critical steps in ____________ minutes with a minimum score of ____________ % within three attempts.

Scoring: Divide points earned by total possible points. Failure to perform a critical step that is indicated with an asterisk (*), will result in an unsatisfactory overall score.

Time began ____________ **Time ended** ____________

Steps	**Possible Points**	**First Attempt**	**Second Attempt**	**Third Attempt**
1. Wash and dry your hands. Put on face protection and nonsterile gloves.	**5**			
2. Assemble the materials needed.	**5**			
3. Fill two plain (blue-tipped) capillary tubes three fourths full with well-mixed EDTA anticoagulant blood.	**10**			
4. Plug the dry end of each tube with a sealing clay.	**10**			
5. Place the tubes opposite each other in the centrifuge, with sealed ends securely against the gasket.	**10**			
6. Note the numbers on the centrifuge slots and record them.	**10**			
7. Secure the locking top, fasten the lid down, and lock.	**10**			
8. Set the timer, and adjust the speed as needed.	**10**			
9. Allow the centrifuge to come to a complete stop. Unlock the lids.	**5**			
10. Remove the tubes immediately.	**5**			

Steps	Possible Points	First Attempt	Second Attempt	Third Attempt
11. Determine the microhematocrit values, using one of the following methods: a. Centrifuge with built-in reader using calibrated capillary tubes. 1) Position the tubes as directed by manufacturer's instructions. 2) Read both tubes. 3) The average of the two results is reported. 4) The two values should not vary by more than 2%. b Centrifuge without built-in reader. 1) Carefully remove the tubes from the centrifuge. 2) Place a tube on the microhematocrit reader. 3) Align the clay–red blood cell junction with the zero line on the reader. Align the plasma meniscus with the 100% line. The value is read at the junction of the red cell layer and the buffy coat.* 4) Read both tubes. 5) The average of the two results is reported. 6) The two values should not vary by more than 2%.	5			
12. Dispose of the capillary tubes in a biohazard container.	5			
13. Clean the work area and properly dispose of all biohazard materials. Remove gloves and face protection and wash your hands.	5			
14. Record the results in the patient's medical record.	5			

Documentation in the Medical Record

____

____

____

____

Comments:

Total Points Earned ________ Divided by ________ Total Possible Points = ________ % Score

Instructor's Signature ____________________

Student Name ____________ Date ____________ Score ____________

Procedure 51-2 Performing a Hemoglobin Test

Task: To accurately determine the level of hemoglobin present in a blood sample with the hemoglobinometer method.

Equipment and Supplies:
- Hemoglobinometer
- Reagent applicators
- Autolet or blood lancet
- Alcohol preps
- Gauze squares

Standards: Complete the procedure and all critical steps in ____________ minutes with a minimum score of ____________ % within three attempts.

Scoring: Divide points earned by total possible points. Failure to perform a critical step that is indicated with an asterisk (*), will result in an unsatisfactory overall score.

Time began ____________ **Time ended** ____________

Steps	Possible Points	First Attempt	Second Attempt	Third Attempt
1. Wash and dry hands.	5			
2. Collect and assemble all equipment and supplies needed.	5			
3. Explain the procedure to the patient.	5			
4. Put on gloves.*	5			
5. Prepare the clipped chamber by slightly offsetting the cover slide to expose the chamber slide surface.	5			
6. Examine the fingers and choose the site to be used to obtain the blood sample.	5			
7. Clean the site with alcohol or other recommended antiseptic preparation.	5			
8. Perform a capillary puncture and obtain the blood sample.	5			
9. Wipe away the first drop of blood.	5			
10. Place one large drop of blood on the chamber slide. Do not touch the slide with the finger.	5			
11. Agitate the blood with a reagent stick until the blood appears shiny or transparent.	5			

Steps	Possible Points	First Attempt	Second Attempt	Third Attempt
12. Close the chamber and insert the chamber into the hemoglobinometer.	5			
13. Hold the device horizontally at eye level and turn on the light at the base of the unit with the left hand.	5			
14. Visualize the split green field through the viewer and with the right hand move the slide adjustment until there is no visible difference between the two hemispheres in the viewer.	10			
15. Read the scale on the right side of the instrument. Your reading will be in grams of hemoglobin per 100 ml of blood.	10			
16. Dispose of the biohazard waste in correct containers, and properly clean the hemoglobinometer chamber and work area. Return equipment to proper storage location.	5			
17. Remove gloves and wash hands.	5			
18. Record the test results in the patient's medical record.	5			

Documentation in the Medical Record

Comments:

Total Points Earned ________ Divided by ________ Total Possible Points = ________ % Score

Instructor's Signature ________________

Student Name ______ Date ______ Score ______

Procedure 51-3 Filling a Unopette©

Task: To properly fill a Unopette pipette with blood and to transfer the sample to a Unopette reservoir.

Equipment and Supplies:
- Unopette unit: capillary pipette, pipette shield, reservoir
- EDTA anticoagulant blood
- Gauze squares
- Test tube rack

Standards: Complete the procedure and all critical steps in ______ minutes with a minimum score of ______ % within three attempts.

Scoring: Divide points earned by total possible points. Failure to perform a critical step that is indicated with an asterisk (*), will result in an unsatisfactory overall score.

Time began ______ **Time ended** ______

Steps	**Possible Points**	**First Attempt**	**Second Attempt**	**Third Attempt**
1. Wash and dry your hands, and put on face protection and nonsterile gloves.	5			
2. Remove a Unopette reservoir from the storage container, and recap the container tightly.	5			
3. Use the pipette shield to puncture the diaphragm of the Unopette reservoir. The hole must be large enough to allow the pipette to enter freely.	5			
4. Remove the pipette shield.	5			
5. Hold the pipette nearly horizontal.	5			
6. Place the tip of the pipette into a well-mixed tube of blood, and allow the pipette to fill by capillary action until blood reaches the end of the pipette. It will stop by itself.	5			
7. Place a finger over the hole in the end of the pipette to prevent loss of any sample, and carefully wipe the outside of the pipette with gauze to remove all traces of blood.	5			
8. Squeeze the reservoir with one hand.	5			
9. While holding your index finger over the hole in the top of the pipette, insert the pipette into the reservoir and seat it firmly in place with a twisting motion.	5			

Steps	Possible Points	First Attempt	Second Attempt	Third Attempt
10. Release the pressure on the reservoir, and remove your finger from the top of the pipette. The sample will be drawn into the reservoir.	**10**			
11. Gently squeeze and release the reservoir several times to rinse all blood from the pipette into the reservoir. Liquid should rise to the overflow chamber but should not be forced out of the top of the pipette.	**10**			
12. Mix the contents of the Unopette gently by inversion or by rolling between the palms of your hands.	**5**			
13. Identify the Unopette.	**10**			
14. Allow the Unopette to sit for the specified amount of time, as stated in the directions.	**5**			
15. Place the shield on the top of the prepared Unopette to prevent evaporation.	**5**			
16. Clean the work area by properly disposing of all biohazard materials. Remove the face protection and gloves and wash your hands.	**5**			
17. Record the test results in the patient's medical record.	**5**			

Documentation in the Medical Record

______

______

______

______

Comments:

Total Points Earned ______ Divided by ______ Total Possible Points = ______ % Score

Instructor's Signature ______

Student Name ______________________ Date ____________ Score ________

Procedure 51-4 Charging (Filling) a Hemacytometer

Task: To fill the hemacytometer for a manual cell count.

Equipment and Supplies:
- Neubauer ruled hemacytometer
- Hemacytometer coverslip
- Lint-free tissue
- 70% alcohol
- Blood-diluting pipette or Unopette

Standards: Complete the procedure and all critical steps in __________ minutes with a minimum score of __________ % within three attempts.

Scoring: Divide points earned by total possible points. Failure to perform a critical step that is indicated with an asterisk (*), will result in an unsatisfactory overall score.

Time began __________ **Time ended** __________

Steps	**Possible Points**	**First Attempt**	**Second Attempt**	**Third Attempt**
1. Wash and dry your hands. Put on face protection and nonsterile gloves.	**5**			
2. Clean the hemacytometer and coverslip with 70% alcohol and lint-free tissue and thoroughly dry.	**10**			
3. Align the coverslip on the chamber.	**10**			
4. Convert to dropper assembly by withdrawing the pipette from the reservoir and reseating it securely in reverse position.	**10**			
5. To clean the capillary bore, invert the reservoir and gently squeeze the sides, expelling two drops from the well-mixed pipette or Unopette.	**10**			
6. Touch the tip of the pipette to the edge of the coverslip in the loading area of the chamber.	**10**			
7. Controlling the flow with the finger on the pipette or by gentle squeezing of the Unopette, fill the chamber in one smooth motion.	**10**			
8. Stop filling when the ruled area is full, and do not overfill.	**10**			
9. Fill both sides of the hemacytometer.	**10**			

Steps	Possible Points	First Attempt	Second Attempt	Third Attempt
10. Allow the chamber to sit undisturbed for 1 or 2 minutes so that the cells settle, but do not allow the sample to dry.	5			
11. Clean the work area by properly disposing of all biohazard materials.	5			
12. Record the test results in the patient's record.	5			

Documentation in the Medical Record

____

____

____

____

Comments:

Total Points Earned ________ Divided by ________ Total Possible Points = ________ % Score

Instructor's Signature ________________

Student Name ______________________ Date ____________ Score ________

Procedure 51-5 Counting Cells in the Neubauer Ruled Hemacytometer

Task: To properly focus a hemacytometer, to locate the appropriate areas to count, and to direct your field of vision through the chamber in the proper manner while counting cells.

Equipment and Supplies:
- Properly filled hemacytometer
- Microscope
- Hand tally counter

Standards: Complete the procedure and all critical steps in ____________ minutes with a minimum score of ____________ % within three attempts.

Scoring: Divide points earned by total possible points. Failure to perform a critical step that is indicated with an asterisk (*), will result in an unsatisfactory overall score.

Time began ____________ **Time ended** ____________

Steps	**Possible Points**	**First Attempt**	**Second Attempt**	**Third Attempt**
1. Wash and dry your hands.	5			
2. Place the hemacytometer on the lowered microscope stage under low-power magnification.	5			
3. Center the ruled area over the opening in the stage.	5			
4. Reduce the light intensity by closing the diaphragm and lowering the condenser.	5			
5. Raise the stage carefully while watching from the side to be certain that the objective lens does not hit the coverslip.	5			
6. Focus and center the correct area (top left large W square for counting white blood cells), using the coarse adjustment and mechanical stage simultaneously.	5			
7. Adjust the light until the cells are easily visible.	5			

Steps	Possible Points	First Attempt	Second Attempt	Third Attempt
8. Count white blood cells under low power, by depressing the hand tally once for each cell seen. a) Begin in the top row, on the far left. b) Count the top row, moving visually from left to right. c) Count all cells within the boundaries of the square and also cells touching the top and the left-hand lines of the square. d) Do not count cells touching the right-hand lines or the bottom lines of the square. e) When you come to the end of the top row, drop to the second row. f) Count the second row, moving visually from right to left. g) Continue counting in this zigzag pattern, ending at the bottom left small square.	25			
9. When you have finished counting a large square, record the number.	5			
10. Return the tally to zero, move to the next large square, and begin to count.	5			
11. Switch to high power and focus with the fine adjustment for counting red blood cells (top left R square).	5			
12. Locate the remaining squares to be counted and determine the number of cells in each. For white blood cells, the counts from each square should vary by no more than 10 cells. For red blood cells, the numbers should vary by no more than 20 cells. Greater variation indicates an unevenly filled hemacytometer. In such cases, the chamber should be cleaned and refilled.	5			
13. Total the cells counted in all four squares for white blood cells and in five squares for red blood cells.	5			
14. Count the second side of the chamber in the same manner.	5			
15. Average the counts from both sides.	5			
16. Calculate the results. For red blood cells: average times 10,000 For white blood cells: average times 50	5			
17. Record the results in the patient's medical record.	5			

Documentation in the Medical Record

____

____

____

____

Comments:

Total Points Earned ________ Divided by ________ Total Possible Points = ________ % Score

Instructor's Signature ____________________

Student Name ______________________ Date ____________ Score ____________

Procedure 51-6 Staining a Blood Smear with Wright's Stain

Task: To prepare and stain a slide that meets the criteria for the performance of a differential examination.

Equipment and Supplies:
- Clean glass slides
- Transfer pipette or capillary tube
- Wright's stain materials
- EDTA anticoagulant blood specimen

Standards: Complete the procedure and all critical steps in ____________ minutes with a minimum score of ____________ % within three attempts.

Scoring: Divide points earned by total possible points. Failure to perform a critical step that is indicated with an asterisk (*), will result in an unsatisfactory overall score.

Time began ____________ **Time ended** ____________

Steps	Possible Points	First Attempt	Second Attempt	Third Attempt
1. Wash and dry your hands. Put on face protection and nonsterile gloves.	5			
2. Assemble the materials needed.	5			
3. Mix the blood specimen.	5			
4. Use a transfer pipette or capillary tube to dispense a small drop of blood onto a slide, about ½ to ¾ inch from the right end.	5			
5. Hold one side of this slide with your nondominant hand.	5			
6. Use your dominant hand to place the spreader slide in front of the drop of blood at an angle of 30° to 35°.	5			
7. Pull back the spreader slide into the drop of blood and allow the blood to spread to the edges of the slide.	5			
8. Push the spreader slide forward with a quick smooth motion, maintaining the same angle throughout.	5			
9. Rapidly but gently wave the slide to accelerate the drying process.	5			
10. Stand the slide with the thick end down, and allow the slide to complete drying.	5			

Steps	Possible Points	First Attempt	Second Attempt	Third Attempt
11. Label the slide when it is dry. Use a pencil and write the name in the thick end of the smear.	5			
12. Stain according to method used. Two-step method: a) Place the smear on a staining rack, with the blood side up. b) Flood the smear with Wright's stain. c) Wait for 1 to 3 minutes. d) Add an equal amount of buffer, drop by drop, on top of the Wright's stain. e) Blow gently, and mix the two solutions until a green metallic sheen appears. This should appear within 2 to 4 minutes. f) Rinse thoroughly with distilled water. g) Drain water from the slide. h) Wipe the back of the smear with gauze. i) Stand the smear to dry. Quick stain: a) Place the smear into solutions according to the manufacturer's instructions b) Proceed with steps f through i just listed.	35			
13. Clean the work area. Properly dispose of all biohazard materials. Remove face protection and gloves. Wash your hands.	5			
14. Record the test results in the patient's medical record.	5			

Documentation in the Medical Record

____

____

____

____

Comments:

Total Points Earned ________ Divided by ________ Total Possible Points = ________ % Score

Instructor's Signature ____________________

Student Name ______________________ Date ____________ Score ____________

Procedure 51-7 Performing Differential Examination of a Smear Stained with Wright's Stain

Task: To perform a differential cell count, evaluate the red blood cell morphology, and estimate the number of platelets.

Equipment and Supplies:
- Microscope
- Immersion oil
- Lens tissue
- Lens cleaner

Standards: Complete the procedure and all critical steps in ____________ minutes with a minimum score of ____________ % within three attempts.

Scoring: Divide points earned by total possible points. Failure to perform a critical step that is indicated with an asterisk (*), will result in an unsatisfactory overall score.

Time began ____________ **Time ended** ____________

Steps	**Possible Points**	**First Attempt**	**Second Attempt**	**Third Attempt**
1. Wash and dry your hands.	5			
2. Assemble the materials needed.	5			
3. Clean the microscope with lens tissue and lens cleaner.	5			
4. Place the slide on the stage, with the smear facing up.	5			
5. Locate an area of the smear where the red blood cells barely touch each other or slightly overlap, using the low-power objective.	5			
6. Focus under oil immersion with the fine-adjustment knob and increased light.	5			
7. Count 100 consecutive white blood cells in a winding pattern, identifying each cell encountered.	10			
8. Record each white cell on the differential cell counter by depressing the appropriate key for each cell.	15			

Steps	Possible Points	First Attempt	Second Attempt	Third Attempt
9. Evaluate the red blood cells observed in 10 fields. Record any variations in: Size—microcytosis, macrocytosis, anisocytosis Shape—poikilocytosis, ovalocytosis, target cells, sickle cells, etc. Content—normochromic or hypochromic	**20**			
10. Count the platelets in 10 fields, obtain an average, and multiply that average by 15,000 to give an estimate of the platelet count. The normal platelet count is 150,000 to 400,000/mm^3. Report the count as normal, decreased, or increased.	**10**			
11. Clean the microscope with lens tissue and lens cleaner.	**5**			
12. Clean the work area and properly dispose of all materials. Wash your hands.	**5**			
13. Record the testing results in the patient's record.	**5**			

Documentation in the Medical Record

Comments:

Total Points Earned ________ Divided by ________ Total Possible Points = ________ % Score

Instructor's Signature ____________________

Student Name ______________________ Date ______________ Score __________

Procedure 51-8 Determining a Sedimentation Rate by the Wintrobe Method

Task: To properly fill a Wintrobe tube and observe and record the findings of an erythrocyte sedimentation rate, using the Wintrobe method.

Equipment and Supplies:
- EDTA anticoagulant blood specimen
- Wintrobe tube
- Wintrobe rack
- Timer
- Pasteur pipette
- Bulb

Standards: Complete the procedure and all critical steps in ______________ minutes with a minimum score of ______________ % within three attempts.

Scoring: Divide points earned by total possible points. Failure to perform a critical step that is indicated with an asterisk (*), will result in an unsatisfactory overall score.

Time began ______________ **Time ended** ______________

Steps	**Possible Points**	**First Attempt**	**Second Attempt**	**Third Attempt**
1. Wash and dry your hands. Put on face protection and nonsterile gloves.	5			
2. Assemble the materials needed.	5			
3. Check the leveling bubble of the Wintrobe rack.	10			
4. Mix the blood well.	10			
5. Fill the Pasteur pipette with blood, and insert the tip of the pipette to the bottom of the Wintrobe tube.	10			
6. Fill the Wintrobe tube to the 0 mark by squeezing the bulb of the pipe.	10			
7. Slowly remove the pipette from the tube while keeping the tip of the pipette below the level of the blood.	10			
8. Place the tube in a numbered slot in the Wintrobe rack, and set the timer for 1 hour. The tube must be in a vertical position and free from all vibration.	10			
9. Measure the distance the erythrocytes have fallen after 1 hour. The ESR scale measures from 0 at the top to 100 at the bottom. Each line is 1 mm.	10			

Steps	Possible Points	First Attempt	Second Attempt	Third Attempt
10. Clean the work area and properly dispose of all biohazard materials. Remove face protection and gloves and wash your hands.	**10**	______	______	______
11. Record the findings in the patient's medical record. Remember: The ESR is reported in millimeters per hour.	**10**	______	______	______

Documentation in the Medical Record

____

____

____

____

Comments:

Total Points Earned ________ Divided by ________ Total Possible Points = ________ % Score

Instructor's Signature ____________________

Student Name ______________________ Date ____________ Score ____________

Procedure 51-9 Performing Mono-Test for Infectious Mononucleosis

Task: To perform and interpret a slide test for infectious mononucleosis.

Equipment and Supplies:
- Mono-test kit
- Blood specimen (serum or plasma)

Standards: Complete the procedure and all critical steps in ____________ minutes with a minimum score of ____________ % within three attempts.

Scoring: Divide points earned by total possible points. Failure to perform a critical step that is indicated with an asterisk (*), will result in an unsatisfactory overall score.

Time began ____________ **Time ended** ____________

Steps	**Possible Points**	**First Attempt**	**Second Attempt**	**Third Attempt**
1. Wash and dry your hands. Glove and put on face protection.	5			
2. Remove the test kit from the refrigerator, and allow the reagents to warm to room temperature. Check the expiration date of the kit.	10			
3. Fill a disposable capillary tube to the calibration mark with serum or plasma. Using the rubber bulb included in the kit, deposit the specimen in the first circle of the clean glass slide also provided in the kit.	10			
4. Place one drop of negative control in the second circle and one drop of positive control in the third circle.	10			
5. Thoroughly mix the Mono-Test reagent by rolling the bottle gently between the palms of the hands. Squeeze the enclosed dropper to mix all the contents of the bottle.	10			
6. Hold the dropper in a vertical position, and add one drop of Mono-Test reagent to each area of the slide. Do not touch the dropper to the slide.	10			
7. Using separate stirrers, quickly and thoroughly mix each area, spreading each area out to 1 inch in diameter.	10			
8. Rock the slide gently for exactly 2 minutes; observe immediately for agglutination. A dark background is best for viewing.	10			

Steps	Possible Points	First Attempt	Second Attempt	Third Attempt
9. Interpret the test results, and record them. Agglutination is positive, and no agglutination is negative.	10			
10. Clean the work area. Remove gloves, and wash your hands.	10			
11. Record the test results in the patient's medical record.	5			

Documentation in the Medical Record

Comments:

Total Points Earned ________ Divided by ________ Total Possible Points = ________ % Score

Instructor's Signature ____________________

Student Name ______________________ Date ____________ Score ____________

Procedure 51-10 Determining ABO Group Using a Slide Test

Task: To accurately determine a patient's ABO group using the slide test technique.

Equipment and Supplies:
- Glass slide with frosted ends
- Anti-A and anti-B serum
- Applicator sticks
- Lancet and automatic finger puncture device
- Alcohol preps
- Sterile gauze squares

Standards: Complete the procedure and all critical steps in ____________ minutes with a minimum score of ____________ % within three attempts.

Scoring: Divide points earned by total possible points. Failure to perform a critical step that is indicated with an asterisk (*), will result in an unsatisfactory overall score.

Time began ____________ **Time ended** ____________

Steps	**Possible Points**	**First Attempt**	**Second Attempt**	**Third Attempt**
1. Reread the physician's orders and assemble all of the supplies and equipment needed to complete the testing procedure.	5			
2. Wash your hands and put on face protection and gloves.	5			
3. Explain the procedure to the patient.	5			
4. Label the slides in the frosted area with the patient's name.	5			
5. Place 1 drop of anti-A serum on slide #1, 1 drop of anti-B serum on slide #2, and 1 drop of anti-A and anti-B on slide #3.	10			
6. Select the puncture site and perform a finger puncture procedure.	10			
7. Wipe away the first drop of blood.	5			
8. Place one large drop of blood on each of the three prepared slides.	10			
9. Cover the puncture site with a sterile gauze square and instruct the patient to apply gentle pressure to the site.	10			
10. Mix the antiserum and blood thoroughly, using a clean applicator stick for each slide.	10			

Steps	Possible Points	First Attempt	Second Attempt	Third Attempt
11. Read and interpret the results of the reaction for all slides.	**10**			
12. Discard all biohazard testing waste in the appropriate container.	**5**			
13. Clean the testing area.	**5**			
14. Record the testing results in the patient's medical record.	**5**			

Documentation in the Medical Record

____

____

____

____

Comments:

Total Points Earned ________ Divided by ________ Total Possible Points = ________ % Score

Instructor's Signature ____________________

Student Name ________________ Date ________ Score ________

Procedure 51-11 Determining Rh Factor Using the Slide Method

Task: To accurately determine the presence or absence of anti-D agglutinations.

Equipment and Supplies:
- Two glass slides with frosted ends
- Anti-D serum
- Applicator sticks
- Lancet and automatic finger puncture device
- Alcohol preps
- Sterile gauze squares
- Laboratory marker or pencil

Standards: Complete the procedure and all critical steps in ________ minutes with a minimum score of ________ % within three attempts.

Scoring: Divide points earned by total possible points. Failure to perform a critical step that is indicated with an asterisk (*), will result in an unsatisfactory overall score.

Time began ________ **Time ended** ________

Steps	Possible Points	First Attempt	Second Attempt	Third Attempt
1. Check the physician's order and assemble all of the equipment and supplies needed to complete the testing procedure.	5			
2. Wash your hands and put on face protection and gloves.	5			
3. Label one slide "D" and one slide "C."	5			
4. Place 1 drop of anti-D serum on the "D" slide.	5			
5. Place 1 drop of the appropriate control reagent on the "C" slide.	10			
6. Perform a capillary puncture to secure a blood specimen.	10			
7. To each slide, add 2 drops of the patient's blood.	10			
8. Thoroughly mix the blood with the anti-D serum, using a clean applicator stick for each slide, and spread the reaction mixture over an area measuring approximately 20 × 40 mm on each slide.	10			
9. Read the results immediately.	10			

Steps	Possible Points	First Attempt	Second Attempt	Third Attempt
10. Discard all disposable equipment in the proper biohazardous waste containers.	**10**			
11. Clean area. Remove gloves and wash your hands.	**10**			
12. Record the testing results in the patient's medical record.	**10**			

Documentation in the Medical Record

____

____

____

____

Comments:

Total Points Earned _______ Divided by _______ Total Possible Points = _______ % Score

Instructor's Signature _______________

Student Name ______________________ Date __________ Score __________

Procedure 51-12 Performing a Blood Glucose Accu-Check Test

Task: To accurately perform a blood test for possible diabetes mellitus.

Equipment and Supplies:
- Accu-Check glucose monitor or similar glucose monitoring device
- Accu-Check glucose testing strip
- Lancet and autoloading finger-puncturing device
- Alcohol preps
- Gauze squares

Standards: Complete the procedure and all critical steps in ______________ minutes with a minimum score of ______________ % within three attempts.

Scoring: Divide points earned by total possible points. Failure to perform a critical step that is indicated with an asterisk (*), will result in an unsatisfactory overall score.

Time began ______________ **Time ended** ______________

Steps	Possible Points	First Attempt	Second Attempt	Third Attempt
1. Reread the physician's order and collect the necessary equipment and supplies needed to complete the testing procedure.	5			
2. Wash your hands and put on gloves.	5			
3. Ask the patient to wash his or her hands in warm soapy water, then to rinse them in warm water, and dry them completely.	5			
4. Check the patient's index and ring fingers and select the site for puncture.	5			
5. Turn on the Accu-Check monitor by pressing the ON button.	5			
6. Make sure the code number on the LED display matches the code number on the container of testing strips.	5			
7. Remove a testing strip from the vial and immediately replace the vial cover.	5			
8. Check the strip for discoloration by comparing the color of the round window on the back of the testing strip with the designated "unused" color chart provided on the test strip vial label.	5			

Steps	Possible Points	First Attempt	Second Attempt	Third Attempt
9. When the test strip symbol begins flashing in the lower right-hand corner of the display screen, insert the test strip into the designated testing slot until it locks into place. When the test strip is inserted correctly, the arrows on the test strip will be facing up and pointing toward the monitor.	5			
10. Cleanse the selected site on the patient's fingertip with the alcohol wipe and allow the finger to air dry.	5			
11. Perform the finger puncture and wipe away the first drop of blood.	5			
12. Apply a large hanging drop of blood to the center of the yellow testing pad. a. Do not touch the pad with the patient's finger. b. Do not apply a second drop of blood. c. Do not smear the blood with your finger. d. Be certain the yellow test pad is saturated with blood.	30			
13. Give the patient a gauze square to hold securely over the puncture site.	5			
14. The monitor will automatically begin the measurement process as soon as it senses the drop of blood.	5			
15. Read the test result when it is displayed in the display window in milligrams per deciliter. Turn off the monitor by pressing the "O" button.	5			

Documentation in the Medical Record

____

____

____

____

Comments:

Total Points Earned ________ Divided by ________ Total Possible Points = ________ % Score

Instructor's Signature ____________________

Student Name ______________________ Date __________ Score __________

Procedure 51-13 Determining Cholesterol Level Using a ProAct Testing Device

Task: To accurately perform and report a ProAct test for cholesterol level.

Equipment and Supplies:
- ProAct testing device
- Lithium heparin capillary tube and capillary pipettor
- Lancets and lancet device
- Sterile gauze
- Alcohol preps
- Biohazard waste container
- Biohazard sharps container

Standards: Complete the procedure and all critical steps in __________ minutes with a minimum score of __________ % within three attempts.

Scoring: Divide points earned by total possible points. Failure to perform a critical step that is indicated with an asterisk (*), will result in an unsatisfactory overall score.

Time began __________ **Time ended** __________

Steps	Possible Points	First Attempt	Second Attempt	Third Attempt
1. Reread the physician's order and assemble all the supplies and equipment needed to complete the test.	5			
2. Wash your hands and put on gloves.	5			
3. Explain the procedure to the patient.	5			
4. Load the lancet device with a sterile lancet.	5			
5. Examine the patient's index and ring fingers and pick a puncture site.	5			
6. Cleanse the chosen puncture site with alcohol and allow the site to air dry.	5			
7. Puncture the site and wipe away the first drop of blood with a sterile gauze square.	5			
8. Give the patient a clean gauze square and ask the patient to apply pressure to the puncture site.	5			
9. Remove a cholesterol testing strip from the container and close the container immediately	5			

Steps	Possible Points	First Attempt	Second Attempt	Third Attempt
10. Remove the foil protecting the test area of the strip and place the strip on a dry, hard, flat surface.	5			
11. Attach the capillary tube filled with blood to the pipettor.	5			
12. Squeeze the plunger of the pipettor completely to allow a drop of blood to form at the end of the capillary tube.	5			
13. Allow the drop of blood to fall onto the center of the red mesh application zone. Make sure that the tip of the capillary tube does not touch the test strip and that all blood is dispensed.	5			
14. Allow the sample to soak into the red mesh for 3 to 15 seconds.	5			
15. Insert the cholesterol strip into the test port. The ProAct device will count down approximately 160 seconds.	5			
16. Remove the capillary tube from the pipettor and discard it in a biohazard container.	5			
17. When the measurement time is completed, REMOVE STRIP will appear in the LED display window. Remove the used test strip and the test result will appear on the display.	5			
18. Examine the test area of the used testing strip for uneven color development before discarding it into the biohazard waste container.	5			
19. Discard all biohazard testing waste in appropriate containers, clean the testing area, remove gloves, and wash your hands.	5			
20. Record the test results in the patient's medical record.	5			

Documentation in the Medical Record

____

____

____

____

Comments:

Total Points Earned ________ Divided by ________ Total Possible Points = ________ % Score

Instructor's Signature ______________________

Student Name ______________________ Date ____________ Score ____________

Procedure 52-1 Preparing a Direct Smear or Culture Smear for Staining

Task: To prepare a smear for staining from a clinical specimen or from a culture medium.

Equipment and Supplies:
- Clean glass slides
- Permanent marker
- Incinerator
- Normal saline solution
- Specimen collected on a smear
- 24 hour culture on agar

Standards: Complete the procedure and all critical steps in ____________ minutes with a minimum score of ____________ % within three attempts.

Scoring: Divide points earned by total possible points. Failure to perform a critical step that is indicated with an asterisk (*), will result in an unsatisfactory overall score.

Time began ____________ **Time ended** ____________

Steps	Possible Points	First Attempt	Second Attempt	Third Attempt
1. Wash and dry your hands. Glove and put on face protection.	5			
2. Label the slide with a permanent marking pen.	5			
Direct Smear				
3. Prepare a thin smear by rolling the swab on the slide. Make certain that all areas of the swab touch the slide.	10			
4. Allow the smear to air dry. Do not wave it or heat-dry it.	10			
5. Hold the slide with the smear up. Heat-fix the slide using an incinerator. Check the heating process by touching the slide to the back of the hand. The slide should feel warm, not hot. Check it often by touching the back of the slide to the back of the hand. Cool the slide.	10			
Culture Smear				
6. Identify the colonies to be stained by circling them on the back of the plate and numbering them with a permanent marker. Label the slide accordingly.	10			

Steps	Possible Points	First Attempt	Second Attempt	Third Attempt
7. Apply a small drop of saline solution to the slide, using a loop.	10			
8. Touch, with a sterile loop, only the top of the colony chosen. Transfer the material picked up to the appropriate area of the slide, and spread it in a circular motion to the size of a dime. Repeat for each colony chosen using a separate slide.	10			
9. Allow the smear to air dry.	10			
10. Heat-fix the smear.	10			
Both Methods				
11. Properly dispose of all biohazard materials and clean the work area.	5			
12. Remove gloves and wash your hands.	5			

Documentation in the Medical Record

____

____

____

____

Comments:

Total Points Earned ________ Divided by ________ Total Possible Points = ________ % Score

Instructor's Signature ____________________

Student Name ______________________ Date ____________ Score ________

Procedure 52-2 Staining a Smear with Gram Stain

Task: To stain a slide, using the Gram stain, so that the organisms present are colored appropriately.

Equipment and Supplies:
- Gram stain reagents
- Staining rack
- Forceps
- Wash bottle of water
- Prepared smear for staining
- Absorbent paper

Standards: Complete the procedure and all critical steps in ____________ minutes with a minimum score of ____________ % within three attempts.

Scoring: Divide points earned by total possible points. Failure to perform a critical step that is indicated with an asterisk (*), will result in an unsatisfactory overall score.

Time began ____________ **Time ended** ____________

Steps	**Possible Points**	**First Attempt**	**Second Attempt**	**Third Attempt**
1. Wash and dry your hands.	5			
2. Place the slide face up on a level staining rack.	5			
3. Flood the slide with crystal violet. Time for 30 seconds.	10			
4. Flood the stain off with a sharp stream of water from the wash bottle. With forceps, tip the slide to remove the water.	10			
5. Flood the slide with Gram's iodine (mordant). Time for 30 seconds.	10			
6. Flood the iodine off with water. Grasp the slide with forceps, and hold it nearly vertical.	10			
7. Decolorize by running the decolorizer (alcohol) down the slide until the smear stops, giving off purple stain in all but the thickest portions (about 10 seconds).	10			
8. Rinse the slide with water, and return it to the staining rack.	5			
9. Flood the slide with safranin, and time for 30 seconds.				

Steps	Possible Points	First Attempt	Second Attempt	Third Attempt
10. Rinse the slide well with water.	5			
11. Wipe off the back of the slide with an alcohol tissue.	5			
12. Blot the slide dry between sheets of absorbent paper.	5			
13. Clean the work area. Remove gloves and wash your hands.	5			
14. Record the procedure in the patient's record.	5			

Documentation in the Medical Record

____

____

____

____

Comments:

Total Points Earned ________ Divided by ________ Total Possible Points = ________ % Score

Instructor's Signature ________________

Student Name ______________________ Date __________ Score __________

Procedure 52-3 Inoculating a Blood Agar Plate for Culture of *Streptococcus pyogens*

Task: To inoculate a blood agar plate for the detection of the etiologic agent of strep throat.

Equipment and Supplies:
- Blood agar plate
- Bacitracin disk or
- Blood agar plate
- Bacitracin disk or strep A disk
- Incinerator
- Inoculating loop
- Permanent marker
- Swab from patient's throat

Standards: Complete the procedure and all critical steps in __________ minutes with a minimum score of __________ % within three attempts.

Scoring: Divide points earned by total possible points. Failure to perform a critical step that is indicated with an asterisk (*), will result in an unsatisfactory overall score.

Time began __________ **Time ended** __________

Steps	Possible Points	First Attempt	Second Attempt	Third Attempt
1. Wash and dry your hands. Glove and apply face protection.	5			
2. Remove the swab from the container. Grasp the plate by the bottom (media side), and lift the cover, or lift the cover while the plate is on the table.	10			
3. Roll the swab down the middle of the top half of the plate, then use the swab to streak the same half of the plate. Dispose of the swab properly.	10			
4. Sterilize the loop in the Bacti-cinerator, and allow it to cool.	10			
5. Streak for isolation of colonies in the third and fourth quadrants, using the loop. Use the loop to make three slices in the agar in the area of heavy inoculum. Sterilize the loop.	10			
6. Sterilize the forceps and remove one disk from the vial. Place the disk on the agar in the first quadrant. Sterilize the forceps.	10			

Steps	Possible Points	First Attempt	Second Attempt	Third Attempt
7. Label with permanent marker the agar side of the plate with the patient's name and identification number and the date.	**10**			
8. Place the plate in the incubator, with the agar side of the plate on the top.	**10**			
9. Record all information in the patient's medical record.	**10**			
10. Incubate for 24 hours and then examine. Incubate negative cultures for an additional 24 hours.	**10**			
11. Clean the work area and properly dispose of all biohazard waste. Remove your gloves and wash your hands.	**5**			

Documentation in the Medical Record

____

____

____

____

Comments:

Total Points Earned ________ Divided by ________ Total Possible Points = ________ % Score

Instructor's Signature ____________________

Student Name ______________________________ Date ______________ Score ______________

Procedure 52-4 Performing a Rapid Strep Test

Task: To perform a rapid strep test to assist in the diagnosis of strep throat.

Equipment and Supplies:
- Directigen Strep A test kit
- Timer or wristwatch with sweep second hand
- Throat swab specimen

Standards: Complete the procedure and all critical steps in ______________ minutes with a minimum score of ______________ % within three attempts.

Scoring: Divide points earned by total possible points. Failure to perform a critical step that is indicated with an asterisk (*), will result in an unsatisfactory overall score.

Time began ______________ **Time ended** ______________

Steps	Possible Points	First Attempt	Second Attempt	Third Attempt
1. Collect all supplies and equipment needed to perform the test. Bring all reagents and reaction disks to room temperature (minimum of 30 minutes).	5			
2. Wash and dry your hands. Put on gloves and face protection.	5			
3. Position all bottles vertically, and dispense reagents slowly as free-falling drops. Avoid reagent contact with your eyes because the reagent is an irritant.	5			
4. Add 3 drops of reagent 1 to an extraction tube. This solution is pink.	10			
5. Add 3 drops of reagent 2 to the same tube. The solution should turn yellow.	10			
6. Place the specimen swab in the tube, twirling the swab in the mix.	5			
7. Let stand for exactly 1 minute.	5			
8. Add 3 drops of reagent 3 to the same tube, again twirling the swab in the tube to mix. This solution should be pink.	10			
9. Express the liquid from the swab by squeezing the tube with the thumb and forefinger and rotating the swab as it is withdrawn. The liquid must be thoroughly removed from the swab. Best results are achieved when the liquid reaches or exceeds the line on the tube.	10			

Steps	Possible Points	First Attempt	Second Attempt	Third Attempt
10. Discard the swab in a biohazard waste container.	5			
11. Remove the reaction disk from the pouch and place it on a dry, flat surface.	5			
12. Pour the entire contents of the tube into the reaction disk.	5			
13. Read the test results when the entire end of assay window turns red (5 to 10 minutes).	5			
14. Properly dispose of all contaminated waste.	5			
15. Clean work area, remove gloves, and wash your hands.	5			
16. Record the test results in the patient's medical record.	5			

Documentation in the Medical Record

____

____

____

____

Comments:

Total Points Earned ________ Divided by ________ Total Possible Points = ________ % Score

Instructor's Signature ________________

Student Name ________________ Date ________ Score ________

Procedure 52-5 The Urine Culture

Task: To include three plates with one microliter of urine in order to quantitate the number of bacteria and aid in the diagnosis of a urinary tract infection.

Equipment and Supplies:
- Urine specimen, collected CCMS in a sterile container
- Bacti-cinerator
- Microliter calibrated inoculating loop
- Blood agar plate, MacConkey agar plate, and Columbia nutrient agar plate

Standards: Complete the procedure and all critical steps in ________ minutes with a minimum score of ________ % within three attempts.

Scoring: Divide points earned by total possible points. Failure to perform a critical step that is indicated with an asterisk (*), will result in an unsatisfactory overall score.

Time began ________ **Time ended** ________

Steps	Possible Points	First Attempt	Second Attempt	Third Attempt
1. Wash and dry your hands. Glove and apply face protection.	5			
2. With the screw cap lid in place, mix the urine specimen thoroughly by swirling.	5			
3. Sterilize the calibrated loop, cool, and dip the tip into the specimen.	10			
4. Deposit the specimen on the plate.	10			
5. Inoculate the second and third plates in the same manner.	10			
6. Label the bottom of the plates with the patient's name and identification number and the date.	10			
7. Record all information in the patient's medical record.	10			
8. Place the plates in the incubator, with the agar sides of the plates facing up.	10			
9. Incubate for 24 hours, then count the colonies on the all-purpose medium.	10			

Steps	Possible Points	First Attempt	Second Attempt	Third Attempt
10. Interpret the count • >100 colonies = >100,000 colony forming units (cfu)/ ml of urine indicates a urinary tract infection • 10–100 colonies = 10,000 to 100,000 cfu/ml of urine indicates suspicion. The urine may have been allowed to stand at room temperature which facilitated overgrowth of bacteria or the patient may have a subclinical infection. Recollection of the specimen is recommended. • (10 colonies = 10,000 cfu/ml of urine and indicates normal urethral microbiota)	**10**			
11. Clean the work area, dispose of all biohazard waste, remove gloves, and wash your hands.	**5**			
12. Record procedure in patient's medical record.	**5**			

Documentation in the Medical Record

____

____

____

____

Comments:

Total Points Earned ________ Divided by ________ Total Possible Points = ________ % Score

Instructor's Signature ____________________

Student Name ______________________ Date ____________ Score ________

Procedure 52-6 Performing a Cellulose Tape Collection for Pinworms

Task: To obtain a rectal sample using cellulose tape for the purpose of testing for pinworm eggs.

Equipment and Supplies:
- Glass slide
- Clear cellulose tape
- Wooden tongue depressor
- Toluene
- Microscope
- Gauze or cotton balls

Standards: Complete the procedure and all critical steps in ____________ minutes with a minimum score of ____________ % within three attempts.

Scoring: Divide points earned by total possible points. Failure to perform a critical step that is indicated with an asterisk (*), will result in an unsatisfactory overall score.

Time began ____________ **Time ended** ____________

Steps	Possible Points	First Attempt	Second Attempt	Third Attempt
1. Gather and prepare supplies and equipment needed for obtaining the specimen.	5			
2. Place a strip of cellulose tape on a glass slide, starting 1/2 inch from one end and running toward the same end. Continuing around this end lengthwise. Tear off the strip so that it is even with the other end. Note: Do not use Magic transparent tape; use regular clear cellulose tape.	10			
3. Place a strip of paper measuring 1/2 × 1 inch between the slide and the tape at the end where the tape is torn flush. This will be the specimen labeling area.	10			
4. Wash hands, glove, and apply face protection.	10			
5. Remove the clothing and diaper from the child and lay the child in a prone position, over the parent's lap, with the buttocks in a superior plane.	10			
6. To obtain the perianal sample, first peel back the tape on the slide by gripping the label. With the tape looped (adhesive side outward) over a wooden tongue depressor that is held against the slide and extended about 1 inch beyond it, press the tape firmly against the right and left anal folds.	10			

Steps	Possible Points	First Attempt	Second Attempt	Third Attempt
7. Spread the tape back on the slide, adhesive side down.	5			
8. Smooth the tape using a cotton ball or gauze square.	5			
9. Write the patient's name and date on the slide label.	5			
10. Advise the parent that the child can be dressed or assist with dressing the child if needed.	5			
Testing the Sample				
11. Lift one side of the tape and apply 1 drop of toluene before pressing the tape back down on the glass slide.	10			
12. Place the prepared slide under the microscope's low-power objective and examine it under low illumination.	5			
13. Report and record your findings in the patient's record as a positive result if pinworm eggs were visualized and a negative result if no eggs were seen.	5			
14. Dispose of all biohazard waste, clean the work area, remove gloves, and wash your hands.	5			

Documentation in the Medical Record

____

____

____

____

Comments:

Total Points Earned ________ Divided by ________ Total Possible Points = ________ % Score

Instructor's Signature ____________________

Student Name ______________________ Date __________ Score __________

Procedure 53-1 Identifying Surgical Instruments

Task: To identify, correctly spell, and determine the use(s) of standard office instruments or those selected by your instructor.

Equipment and Supplies:
- Curved hemostat
- Straight hemostat
- Dressing (thumb) forceps
- Paper and pencil
- Scalpel and blade
- Dissecting scissors
- Towel clamp
- Vaginal speculum
- Bandage scissors
- Allis tissue forceps

Standards: Complete the procedure and all critical steps in __________ minutes with a minimum score of __________ % within three attempts.

Scoring: Divide points earned by total possible points. Failure to perform a critical step that is indicated with an asterisk (*), will result in an unsatisfactory overall score.

Time began __________ **Time ended** __________

Steps	Possible Points	First Attempt	Second Attempt	Third Attempt
1. Look for the following parts that determine usage: box-lock, serrations, finger rings, cutting edge, noncutting edge, thumb type, teeth ratchets, and electric attachments.	10			
2. Consider the general classification of the instrument: cutting and dissection, grasping and clamping, retracting, or probing and dilating.	10			
3. Carefully examine the teeth and serrations.	10			
4. Look at the length of the instrument to determine the area of the body for which it is used.	10			
5. Try to remember whether the instrument was named for a famous physician, university, or clinic.	10			
6. If the instrument is a pair of scissors, look at the points and determine whether the tips are sharp-sharp, sharp-blunt, or blunt-blunt.	10			
7. Carefully compare the instrument with similar instruments that you know, to determine whether it is in the same category or has the same name.	10			
8. Write, with correct spelling, the complete name of each instrument, including its category and usage.	30			

Documentation in the Medical Record

____

____

____

____

Comments:

Total Points Earned ________ Divided by ________ Total Possible Points = ________ % Score

Instructor's Signature ____________________

Student Name ______________________ Date ____________ Score ________

Procedure 54-1 Wrapping Instruments and Supplies for Steam Sterilization in an Autoclave

Task: To place dry, checked, sanitized supplies and instruments inside appropriate wrapping materials for sterilization and storage without contamination.

Equipment and Supplies:
- Dry, checked, sanitized items
- Assorted wrapping materials
- Autoclave tape
- Indicator tape
- A waterproof felt-tipped pen

Standards: Complete the procedure and all critical steps in ____________ minutes with a minimum score of ____________ % within three attempts.

Scoring: Divide points earned by total possible points. Failure to perform a critical step that is indicated with an asterisk (*), will result in an unsatisfactory overall score.

Time began ____________ **Time ended** ____________

Steps	Possible Points	First Attempt	Second Attempt	Third Attempt
1. Collect and assemble items to be wrapped.	5			
2. Place the wrapper to be used on a clean flat surface.	5			
3. Place the item(s) diagonally at the approximate center of the wrapping material. Make sure the size of the square is large enough for the items.	10			
4. With the squares that are cloth fabric, use two pieces if the cloth is single-layered, or follow the manufacturer's recommendation when using commercial autoclave wrapping paper.	10			
5. Open slightly any hinged instruments. If the instrument is sharp, its teeth or tip should be shielded with cotton or gauze.	10			
6. If the package is to contain several items, place a commercial sterilization indicator inside the package at the approximate center.	10			
7. Bring up the bottom corner of the wrap and fold back a portion of it.	10			
8. Fold over the right corner and turn back a portion of it. Fold over the left corner and turn back a portion of it.	10			

Steps	Possible Points	First Attempt	Second Attempt	Third Attempt
9. Fold the last flap over.	10			
10. Secure with autoclave tape.	10			
11. Secure with autoclave tape and label package with the date including year, contents, and your initials.	10			

Documentation in the Medical Record

Comments:

Total Points Earned ________ Divided by ________ Total Possible Points = ________ % Score

Instructor's Signature ____________________

Student Name ______________________ Date __________ Score __________

Procedure 54-2 Operating the Autoclave

Task: To sterilize properly prepared supplies and instruments by using the autoclave.

Equipment and Supplies:
- An autoclave
- Wrapped items ready to be sterilized

Standards: Complete the procedure and all critical steps in __________ minutes with a minimum score of __________ % within three attempts.

Scoring: Divide points earned by total possible points. Failure to perform a critical step that is indicated with an asterisk (*), will result in an unsatisfactory overall score.

Time began __________ **Time ended** __________

Steps	Possible Points	First Attempt	Second Attempt	Third Attempt
1. Check the water level in the reservoir and add distilled water as necessary.	5			
2. Turn the control to "fill" to allow water to flow into the chamber. The water will flow until you turn the control to its next position. Do not let the water overflow.	5			
3. Load the chamber with wrapped items, then space them for maximum circulation and penetration.	5			
4. Close and seal the door.	5			
5. Turn the control setting to "on" or "autoclave" to start the cycle.	5			
6. Watch the gauges until the temperature gauge reaches at least 250°F (121°C) and the pressure gauge reaches 15 pounds of pressure.	10			
7. Set the timer for the desired time.	10			
8. At the end of the timed cycle, turn the control setting to "vent."	10			
9. Wait for the pressure gauge to reach zero.	10			
10. Open the chamber door a fourth of an inch.	10			
11. Leave the autoclave control at "vent" to continue producing heat.	10			
12. Allow complete drying of all items.	5			

Steps	Possible Points	First Attempt	Second Attempt	Third Attempt
13. Using heat-resistant gloves or pads, remove the items from the chamber and place the sterilized packages on dry, covered shelves, or open door and allow items to cool.	5			
14. Turn the control knob to "off" and keep the door slightly ajar.	5			

Documentation in the Medical Record

Comments:

Total Points Earned ________ Divided by ________ Total Possible Points = ________ % Score

Instructor's Signature ________________

Student Name ______________________ Date __________ Score __________

Procedure 54-3 Performing Surgical Hand Scrub

Task: To scrub your hands with surgical soap, using friction, running water, and a sterile brush to sanitize your skin before assisting with any procedure that requires surgical asepsis

Equipment and Supplies:
- Sink with foot or arm control for running water
- Surgical soap in a dispenser
- Towels
- Nail file or orange stick
- Sterile brush

Standards: Complete the procedure and all critical steps in __________ minutes with a minimum score of __________ % within three attempts.

Scoring: Divide points earned by total possible points. Failure to perform a critical step that is indicated with an asterisk (*), will result in an unsatisfactory overall score.

Time began __________ **Time ended** __________

Steps	Possible Points	First Attempt	Second Attempt	Third Attempt
1. Remove all jewelry.	5			
2. Inspect your fingernails for length and your hands for skin breaks.	5			
3. Turn on the faucet and regulate the water to a comfortable temperature.	5			
4. Keep your hands upright and held at or above waist level.	5			
5. Clean your fingernails with a file, discard it, and rinse your hands under the faucet without touching the faucet or the insides of the sink basin.	5			
6. Allow water to run over your hands, apply acceptable solution, lather while holding your fingertips upward, and remember to rub between the fingers.	5			
7. Wash wrists and forearms while holding your hands above waist level. Rinse arms and forearms without touching the faucet or the insides of the sink basin.	10			
8. Apply more solution and repeat the scrub on the other side, remembering to wash and use friction between each finger with a firm, circular motion.	10			

Steps	Possible Points	First Attempt	Second Attempt	Third Attempt
9. Scrub all surfaces with a brush, being careful not to abrade your skin. The second washing process should take at least 3 minutes.	**10**			
10. Rinse thoroughly, keeping your hands up and above waist level. Discard scrub brush.	**10**			
11. Turn off the faucet with the foot or forearm lever, if available.	**10**			
12. Dry one hand with a sterile towel; use the opposite end of the towel for the other hand.	**10**			
13. Using a patting motion, continue to dry the forearms. Discard the towel and keep your hands up and above waist level.	**10**			

Comments:

Total Points Earned ________ Divided by ________ Total Possible Points = ________ % Score

Instructor's Signature ____________________

Student Name ________________ Date ________ Score ________

Procedure 54-4 Putting on Sterile Gloves

Task: To apply your own sterile gloves before performing sterile procedures.

Equipment and Supplies:
- A pair of packaged sterile gloves in your size

Standards: Complete the procedure and all critical steps in ________ minutes with a minimum score of ________ % within three attempts.

Scoring: Divide points earned by total possible points. Failure to perform a critical step that is indicated with an asterisk (*), will result in an unsatisfactory overall score.

Time began ________ **Time ended** ________

Steps	Possible Points	First Attempt	Second Attempt	Third Attempt
1. Open your glove pack. Remember, a 1-inch area around the perimeter of the glove wrapper is considered not sterile.	5			
2. Perform the surgical hand scrub.	5			
3. Dry your hands well.	5			
4. Glove your dominant hand first.	5			
5. With your nondominant hand, pick up the glove for your dominant hand with your thumb and forefinger, grabbing the top of the folded cuff, which is the inside of the glove.	10			
6. Lift the glove up and away from the sterile package.	10			
7. Hold your hands away from you and slide your dominant hand into the glove.	10			
8. Leave the cuff folded.	5			
9. With your gloved dominant hand, pick up the second glove by slipping your gloved fingers under the cuff so that your gloved hand only touches the outside of the second glove.	10			
10. Slide your nondominant hand into the glove, without touching the exterior of the glove or any part of your hand.	10			

Steps	Possible Points	First Attempt	Second Attempt	Third Attempt
11. Still holding your hands away from you, unroll the cuff by slipping the fingers up and out. Stay away from your bare arm.	10			
12. Now, slip your gloved fingers up under the first cuff and unroll it, using the same technique.	5			

Comments:

Total Points Earned ________ Divided by ________ Total Possible Points = ________ % Score

Instructor's Signature ____________________

Student Name ________________________ Date ____________ Score ________

Procedure 54-5 Donning a Sterile Gown

Task: To don a sterile gown before assisting with a surgical procedure.

Equipment and Supplies:
- terile gown and gloves (opened on a counter or Mayo stand, in an open area to dress)

Note: A mask and goggles and hair cover are also worn.

Standards: Complete the procedure and all critical steps in ____________ minutes with a minimum score of ____________ % within three attempts.

Scoring: Divide points earned by total possible points. Failure to perform a critical step that is indicated with an asterisk (*), will result in an unsatisfactory overall score.

Time began ____________ **Time ended** ____________

Steps	**Possible Points**	**First Attempt**	**Second Attempt**	**Third Attempt**
1. Scrub, using aseptic technique. Remember to keep hands up and above waist level.	**10**			
2. Grasp the sterile gown by the collar and gently lift it from the sterile gown wrapper.	**20**			
3. Hold the gown away from your body. Allow it to gently unfold, grasping only the inside of the gown.	**20**			
4. Slip your hands into the sleeve openings. Remember to touch only the inside of the gown.	**20**			
5. The hands and forearms are advanced only to the edge of the gown cuff.	**10**			
6. The circulating assistant touches only the inside of the gown, pulling the gown over the scrub assistant's shoulders.	**10**			
7. The waistline and neck ties are tied.	**10**			

Comments:

Total Points Earned ________ Divided by ________ Total Possible Points = ________ % Score

Instructor's Signature ________________________

Student Name ____________ Date ____________ Score ____________

Procedure 54-6 Gloving with a Sterile Gown On

Task: To apply sterile gloves while dressed in a sterile gown before assisting with a surgical procedure.

Equipment and Supplies:
- Sterile gloves, opened on a sterile field

Note: A mask, goggles, hair cover, and a sterile gown are worn. The gloves are applied with the hands covered by the sterile gown to avoid contamination.

Standards: Complete the procedure and all critical steps in ____________ minutes with a minimum score of ____________ % within three attempts.

Scoring: Divide points earned by total possible points. Failure to perform a critical step that is indicated with an asterisk (*), will result in an unsatisfactory overall score.

Time began ____________ **Time ended** ____________

Steps	**Possible Points**	**First Attempt**	**Second Attempt**	**Third Attempt**
1. Glove your nondominant hand first.	5			
2. Lift the glove with your dominant hand and use your thumb and forefinger to grasp the top of the folded cuff. Remember, your hands are covered with the sterile gown sleeves.	10			
3. Place the glove in the palm of your nondominant hand, with glove fingers pointing to elbows.	10			
4. Grasp the inside of the cuff with your fingers and gently stretch the glove cuff.	10			
5. Pull the glove over your hand as you push your arm through the gown cuff.	10			
6. Gently slide your fingers in the glove.	10			
7. With your nondominant gloved hand, slip your fingers under the cuff of the second glove.	10			
8. Follow steps 3, 4, 5, and 6 for the second glove.	10			
9. The cuffs may now be adjusted.	10			

Steps	Possible Points	First Attempt	Second Attempt	Third Attempt
10. The outside sterile gown ties may now be tied with the circulator's assistance.	**10**	______	______	______
11. The circulator grasps the red part of the tag by the corner.	**5**	______	______	______

Comments:

Total Points Earned ________ Divided by ________ Total Possible Points = ________ % Score

Instructor's Signature ____________________

Student Name ______________________ Date ____________ Score ____________

Procedure 54-7 Removal of Contaminated Gloves

Task: To properly remove and dispose of contaminated gloves after a procedure has been completed.

Equipment and Supplies:
- Contaminated gloved (sterile or nonsterile) hands
- (Note: The following procedure is written for someone who is right-handed. If you are left-handed, simply reverse each one of the hand designations for this procedure.)

Standards: Complete the procedure and all critical steps in ____________ minutes with a minimum score of ____________ % within three attempts.

Scoring: Divide points earned by total possible points. Failure to perform a critical step that is indicated with an asterisk (*), will result in an unsatisfactory overall score.

Time began ____________ **Time ended** ____________

Steps	Possible Points	First Attempt	Second Attempt	Third Attempt
1. Using your right hand, grasp the outside of the cuff of the glove on the left hand. Be careful not to touch the left arm during this step.	20			
2. Take the glove completely off of the left hand by pulling it away from the fingers and pulling it inside out.	20			
3. Now the contaminated left glove is inside out in the right hand. Using only the right hand, ball this dirty glove in the palm of the hand.	20			
4. Now use your left hand to carefully grasp the cuff of the right glove and pull it off over the hand (and the other glove), turning it inside out as this is done.	20			
5. Dispose of the gloves in the proper disposal receptacle or a biohazard bag if they are contaminated with blood or body fluids.	10			
6. Wash your hands.	10			

Comments:

Total Points Earned ________ Divided by ________ Total Possible Points = ________ % Score

Instructor's Signature ________________________

Student Name ______________________ Date ____________ Score ____________

Procedure 54-8 Skin Preparation for Surgery

Task: To prepare the patient's skin for a surgical procedure to reduce the risk of wound contamination.

Equipment and Supplies:
- Gauze sponges
- Cotton-tipped applicators
- Antiseptic soap
- Sterile gloves
- Two small stainless-steel bowls
- Antiseptic
- Optional: cotton balls, nail pick, scrub brush
- A waste receptacle

Standards: Complete the procedure and all critical steps in ____________ minutes with a minimum score of ____________ % within three attempts.

Scoring: Divide points earned by total possible points. Failure to perform a critical step that is indicated with an asterisk (*), will result in an unsatisfactory overall score.

Time began ____________ **Time ended** ____________

Steps	Possible Points	First Attempt	Second Attempt	Third Attempt
1. Wash your hands and dry them carefully. Follow standard precautions.	5			
2. Open your skin preparation pack.	5			
3. Arrange the items with sterile gloved hands.	5			
4. Add the surgical soap and antiseptic solutions to the two bowls.	5			
5. Explain the scrub procedure to the patient.	5			
6. Expose the site. Use a light if necessary.	5			
7. Don gloves using aseptic technique.	5			
8. Place two sterile towels at the edges of the area to be scrubbed.	5			
9. Start at the incision site, and begin washing with the antiseptic soap on a gauze sponge in a circular motion, moving from the center to the edges of the area to be scrubbed.	10			
10. After one complete wipe, discard the sponge, and begin again with a new sponge soaked in the antiseptic solution.	10			

Steps	Possible Points	First Attempt	Second Attempt	Third Attempt
11. Repeat the process using sufficient friction for 5 minutes (or follow office policy for the length of time required for a particular preparation).	10			
12. Dry the area using the same circular technique with dry sponges. The area may be dried by blotting with a third sterile towel.	10			
13. Check that no solutions are pooling under the patient.	10			
14. Paint on the antiseptic with the cotton-tipped applicators or gauze sponges, using the same circular technique, and never returning to an area that has already been painted.	10			

Comments:

Total Points Earned ________ Divided by ________ Total Possible Points = ________ % Score

Instructor's Signature ____________________

Student Name ______________________ Date ____________ Score ____________

Procedure 54-9 Opening a Sterile Pack and Creating a Sterile Field

Task: To open a sterile pack that contains a table drape with correct aseptic technique.

Equipment and Supplies:
- A sterile pack (autoclaved linen or disposable) that will serve as a sterile table drape or field
- A Mayo stand or countertop
- Disinfectant and gauze sponges

Standards: Complete the procedure and all critical steps in ____________ minutes with a minimum score of ____________ % within three attempts.

Scoring: Divide points earned by total possible points. Failure to perform a critical step that is indicated with an asterisk (*), will result in an unsatisfactory overall score.

Time began ____________ **Time ended** ____________

Steps	Possible Points	First Attempt	Second Attempt	Third Attempt
1. Check that the Mayo stand or countertop is dust-free and clean. If it is not, clean with 70% alcohol or another disinfectant and towel.	10			
2. Wash your hands and dry them carefully.	10			
3. Place the sterile pack on the Mayo stand or countertop and read the label.	10			
4. Check the expiration date. If using an autoclaved pack, check the indicator tape for color change.	10			
5. Position the package so that the outer envelope flap is face up and at the top as you look at the package.	10			
6. Open the first flap away from yourself.				
7. Pull away the two side flaps, one at a time. Be careful to lift each flap by reaching under the small folded-back tab without touching the inner surface of the pack or its contents.	20			
8. Pull the last flap toward you by its tab, exposing the towel.	10			
9. You now have a sterile drape to be used as a sterile work field and for the distribution of additional sterile supplies and instruments.	10			

Comments:

Total Points Earned ________ Divided by ________ Total Possible Points = ________ % Score

Instructor's Signature ________________________

Student Name ______________________ Date ____________ Score ____________

Procedure 54-10 Using Transfer Forceps

Task: To move sterile items on a sterile field or transfer sterile items to a gloved team member.

Equipment and Supplies:
- A sterile item to move or transfer
- A pair of packaged sterile gloves
- A pair of sterile wrapped transfer forceps
- A Mayo stand set-up with a sterile field and sterile instruments

Standards: Complete the procedure and all critical steps in ____________ minutes with a minimum score of ____________ % within three attempts.

Scoring: Divide points earned by total possible points. Failure to perform a critical step that is indicated with an asterisk (*), will result in an unsatisfactory overall score.

Time began ____________ **Time ended** ____________

Steps	**Possible Points**	**First Attempt**	**Second Attempt**	**Third Attempt**
1. Wash your hands and dry them carefully.	10			
2. Put on sterile gloves or open a package containing a pair of sterile transfer forceps.	10			
3. Using aseptic technique, handle sterile forceps by ring handle only. Always point forceps' tips down.	20			
4. Grasp an item on the sterile field with your sterile gloved hand or the sterile forceps, points down, and move it to its proper position for the procedure.	20			
5. Or transfer an instrument from the autoclave to the sterile field.	20			
6. Remove the transfer forceps after one-time use.	20			

Comments:

Total Points Earned ________ Divided by ________ Total Possible Points = ________ % Score

Instructor's Signature ________________________

Student Name ____________ Date ________ Score ________

Procedure 54-11 Pouring Solutions onto a Sterile Field(s)

Task: As a circulating assistant, pour a sterile solution into a stainless-steel bowl or medicine glass that is sitting at the edge of a sterile field.

Equipment and Supplies:
- A bottle of sterile solution
- A stainless-steel bowl or medicine glass
- A sterile field
- A sink or waste receptable

Note: A medicine glass or bowl on the sterile field should be near one edge of the field and the perimeter of the 1-inch barrier.

Standards: Complete the procedure and all critical steps in ________ minutes with a minimum score of ________ % within three attempts.

Scoring: Divide points earned by total possible points. Failure to perform a critical step that is indicated with an asterisk (*), will result in an unsatisfactory overall score.

Time began ________ **Time ended** ________

Steps	Possible Points	First Attempt	Second Attempt	Third Attempt
1. Wash your hands and dry them carefully.	10			
2. Read the label.	10			
3. Place your hand over the label and lift the bottle. Note: If the container has a double cap, set the outer cap on the counter inside up, then proceed.	10			
4. Lift the lid of the bottle straight up, and then slightly to one side, and hold the lid in your nondominant hand facing downward.	10			
5. Pour away from the label.	10			
6. If the container does not have a double cap, pour off a small amount of the solution into a waste receptacle.	10			
7. Pour away from the label, into the bowl, without allowing any part of the bottle to touch the bowl.	10			
8. Tilt the bottle up to stop the pouring while it is still over the bowl.	10			
9. Remove the bottle from over the sterile field.	10			
10. Replace the cap(s) off to the side, away from the sterile field.	10			

Comments:

Total Points Earned ________ Divided by ________ Total Possible Points = ________ % Score

Instructor's Signature ________________________

Student Name ______________________ Date ____________ Score ____________

Procedure 54-12 Assisting with Minor Surgery

Task: To maintain the sterile field and to pass instruments in a prescribed sequence during a surgical procedure that involves the creation of a surgical incision and the removal of a growth.

Equipment and Supplies:
- An open patient drape pack on the side counter
- A Mayo stand covered with a sterile drape
- Packaged sterile gloves (two pairs)
- A needle and syringe for anesthesia medication
- A vial of local anesthetic medication
- One medicine glass or small bowl
- A scalpel handle and a No. 15 blade
- A pair of Allis tissue forceps
- One skin retractor
- Three hemostats
- A supply of gauze sponges
- A waste receptacle

Standards: Complete the procedure and all critical steps in ____________ minutes with a minimum score of ____________ % within three attempts.

Scoring: Divide points earned by total possible points. Failure to perform a critical step that is indicated with an asterisk (*), will result in an unsatisfactory overall score.

Time began ____________ **Time ended** ____________

Steps	Possible Points	First Attempt	Second Attempt	Third Attempt
1. Wash your hands. Dry thoroughly.	2.5			
2. Don gloves using aseptic technique. Set up the sterile field, with instruments and supplies arranged in the sequence to be used.	2.5			
3. Remove your gloves. Read the label of the local anesthetic medication and pour the medication into a medicine glass.	5			
4. Don gloves using aseptic technique, and prepare the patient's skin with surgical soap and antiseptic solution. Explain the prep procedure to the patient.	5			
5. Scrub, using the surgical hand wash procedure. Follow standard precautions.	5			
6. Dry your hands thoroughly.	2.5			
7. Don gloves using aseptic technique.	5			

Steps	Possible Points	First Attempt	Second Attempt	Third Attempt
8. Position the Mayo stand near the patient and the operative site.	5			
9. Lift the patient drape from the open pack without touching the drape to any of the pack edges.	5			
10. Grasp the patient drape by holding one edge or corner in each hand.	5			
11. Drape the surgical site without touching any part of the patient or the operating area with your gloved hands.	5			
12. The surgeon injects the local anesthetic, after looking at the empty vial on the counter and confirming the type, strength, and expiration date. Note: The surgeon may drape the patient while you don gloves.	5			
13. Position yourself across from the surgeon. Arrange the sterile field. Check instrument placement condition.	5			
14. Place two sponges on the patient, next to the site where the incision will be made.	5			
15. Grasp the scalpel blade with a hemostat and mount the scalpel blade onto the scalpel handle. Keep all sharp equipment conspicuously placed on the sterile field.	5			
16. Pass the scalpel, blade down, to the surgeon or allow the surgeon to reach for it himself or herself. The surgeon will take the scalpel with the thumb and forefinger in the position ready for use.	5			
17. Grasp a pair of Allis tissue forceps by the tips, and pass it to the surgeon to grasp a piece of the tissue to be excised.	5			
18. Pass the forceps' handles into the surgeon's open palm with a firm and purposeful motion. A gentle "snap" is heard as the instrument makes contact with the surgeon's gloved hand.	5			
19. Dispose of soiled sponges, using the waste receptacle.	5			
20. Hold clean sponges in your hand to be passed to the surgeon, or to sponge the wound, as necessary.	5			
21. Safely position the specimen (if any) where it will not be disturbed on the sterile field.	5			

Steps	Possible Points	First Attempt	Second Attempt	Third Attempt
22. If there is a bleeding vessel or if a hemostat is requested, pass the hemostat in the manner described in steps 17 and 18.	**5**			
23. Receive instruments and place them on the sterile field.	**5**			
24. Continue to sponge blood from the wound site.	**5**			
25. Retract the wound edge, as needed, with a skin retractor.	**5**			
26. Continue to monitor the sterile field and assist the surgeon as necessary.	**2.5**			
27. Pass the suture to the surgeon for closure of the wound.	**5**			

Comments:

Total Points Earned ________ Divided by ________ Total Possible Points = ________ % Score

Instructor's Signature ____________________

Student Name ______________________________ Date ______________ Score __________

Procedure 54-13 Assisting with Suturing

Task: To assist the surgeon in wound closure, using sterile technique.

Equipment and Supplies:
- A sterile field on a Mayo stand
- Surgical scissors
- Suture material
- Sterile gloves
- Needle holder
- Gauze sponges

Note: This procedure may be a continuation of Procedure 54-12. If this procedure is done independently, you must perform the surgical scrub and glove before beginning step 1.

Standards: Complete the procedure and all critical steps in ______________ minutes with a minimum score of ______________ % within three attempts.

Scoring: Divide points earned by total possible points. Failure to perform a critical step that is indicated with an asterisk (*), will result in an unsatisfactory overall score.

Time began ______________ **Time ended** ______________

Steps	Possible Points	First Attempt	Second Attempt	Third Attempt
1. Hold the curved needle point in your nondominant hand, 4 to 5 inches over the sterile field.	**10**			
2. Always work over a sterile field.	**10**			
3. With your dominant hand, hold the needle holder halfway down its shaft, at the box-lock, with the suture needle point up.	**10**			
4. With your nondominant hand, hold the suture strand, and pass the needle holder into the surgeon's hand.	**10**			
5. Pick up the surgical scissors with your dominant hand and a gauze sponge with your nondominant hand.	**20**			
6. After the surgeon has placed a closure suture and knotted it, he or she will hold the two strands taut. Cut both suture strands in one motion. Cut between the knot and the surgeon, at the length requested, about 1/8 inch.	**20**			
7. Gently blot the closure once with the gauze sponge in your nondominant hand.	**10**			
8. If additional strands of suture are needed, repeat the process.	**10**			

Comments:

Total Points Earned ________ Divided by ________ Total Possible Points = ________ % Score

Instructor's Signature ________________________

Student Name ______________________ Date ____________ Score ____________

Procedure 54-14 Suture Removal

Task: To remove sutures from a healed incision with sterile technique and without injury to the closed wound.

Equipment and Supplies:
- ture removal scissors
- Gauze sponges
- Thumb forceps
- Steri-Strips or Band-Aids
- Skin antiseptic

Standards: Complete the procedure and all critical steps in ____________ minutes with a minimum score of ____________ % within three attempts.

Scoring: Divide points earned by total possible points. Failure to perform a critical step that is indicated with an asterisk (*), will result in an unsatisfactory overall score.

Time began ____________ **Time ended** ____________

Steps	Possible Points	First Attempt	Second Attempt	Third Attempt
1. Assemble necessary supplies.	5			
2. Wash and dry your hands. Follow standard precautions.	5			
3. Open the suture removal pack.	5			
4. Explain the procedure to the patient and instruct patient to lie or sit still during procedure.	5			
5. Place dry towels under the area from which sutures will be removed.	5			
6. Position patient comfortably and support the area.	5			
7. Place a gauze sponge next to the wound site.	5			
8. Grasp the knot of the suture with the dressing forceps, without pulling.	15			
9. Cut the suture at skin level.	15			
10. Lift—do not pull—the suture toward the incision and out with the dressing forceps.	5			
11. Place the suture on the gauze sponge, and check that the entire suture strand has been removed.	5			

Steps	Possible Points	First Attempt	Second Attempt	Third Attempt
12. If there is any bleeding, blot the area with a new gauze sponge before continuing.	5			
13. Continue in the same manner until all the other sutures have been removed.	5			
14. Remove the gauze sponge with the sutures on it.	5			
15. The surgeon may apply a Steri-Strip or Band-Aid for added support, strength, and protection.	5			
16. The patient is instructed to keep the wound edges clean and dry and not place excessive strain on the area.	5			

Documentation in the Medical Record

____

____

____

____

Comments:

Total Points Earned ________ Divided by ________ Total Possible Points = ________ % Score

Instructor's Signature ________________

Student Name ______________ Date ________ Score ________

Procedure 54-15 Applying/Changing a Dressing

Task: To properly apply a dressing at the completion of a surgical procedure.

Equipment and Supplies:
- Sterile dressing material or Telfa

Standards: Complete the procedure and all critical steps in ________ minutes with a minimum score of ________ % within three attempts.

Scoring: Divide points earned by total possible points. Failure to perform a critical step that is indicated with an asterisk (*), will result in an unsatisfactory overall score.

Time began ________ **Time ended** ________

Steps	**Possible Points**	**First Attempt**	**Second Attempt**	**Third Attempt**
1. Before the sterile drape is removed from the patient, pick up the dressing from the sterile field, place it on the wound, and hold it there.	**25**			
2. Remove the drape while switching hands to hold the dressing in place.	**25**			
3. Secure the dressing with paper tape and/or an appropriate bandage.	**25**			
4. Document the procedure in the patient's medical record.	**25**			

Documentation in the Medical Record

Comments:

Total Points Earned ________ Divided by ________ Total Possible Points = ________ % Score

Instructor's Signature ________________

Student Name ______________________ Date ____________ Score ____________

Procedure 54-16 Bandaging with Gauze and Elastic Dressings

Task: To apply an elastic bandage to the forearm.

Equipment and Supplies:
- One 3- or 4-inch elastic bandage

Standards: Complete the procedure and all critical steps in ____________ minutes with a minimum score of ____________ % within three attempts.

Scoring: Divide points earned by total possible points. Failure to perform a critical step that is indicated with an asterisk (*), will result in an unsatisfactory overall score.

Time began ____________ **Time ended** ____________

Steps	**Possible Points**	**First Attempt**	**Second Attempt**	**Third Attempt**
1. Choose the proper size bandage for the size of the arm you are bandaging.	**10**			
2. Start at the distal point and hold the roll so the bandage can be rolled away from you.	**10**			
3. Keep the roll close to the patient and keep it facing upward.	**10**			
4. Maintain even tension and spacing as you continue to apply the bandage up the forearm.	**10**			
5. When crossing a joint, slightly flex the joint.	**10**			
6. Fasten the end of the bandage with clips or tape.	**10**			
7. Check the patient's nail beds for cyanosis.	**10**			
8. Check the radial pulse.	**10**			
9. Have the patient move his or her fingers.	**10**			
10. Document the procedure in the patient's medical record.	**10**			

Documentation in the Medical Record

____

____

____

____

Comments:

Total Points Earned ________ Divided by ________ Total Possible Points = ________ % Score

Instructor's Signature ____________________

Student Name ______________________ Date ____________ Score ________

Procedure 55-1 Preparing a Resumé

Task: To write an effective resume for use as a tool in gaining employment.

Equipment and Supplies:
- Scratch paper
- Pen or pencil
- Former job descriptions, if available
- List of addresses of former employers, schools, and names of supervisors
- Computer or word processor
- Quality stationary and envelopes

Standards: Complete the procedure and all critical steps in ____________ minutes with a minimum score of ____________ % within three attempts.

Scoring: Divide points earned by total possible points. Failure to perform a critical step that is indicated with an asterisk (*), will result in an unsatisfactory overall score.

Time began ____________ **Time ended** ____________

Steps	Possible Points	First Attempt	Second Attempt	Third Attempt
1. Perform a self-evaluation by making notes about your strengths as a medical assistant. Consider job skills, self-management skills, and transferable skills.	10			
2. Explore formatting and decide on a professional resume appearance that best highlights your skills and experience. Use the templates available in word processing software or design your own.	10			
3. Place your name, address, and two telephone numbers where you can be contacted at the top of the resume.	10			
4. Write a job objective that specifies your employment goals.	10			
5. Provide details about your educational experience. List degrees and/or certifications obtained.	10			
6. Provide details about your work experience. Include all contact information and names of supervisors. Do not include salary expectations or reasons for leaving former jobs.	10			
7. Prepare a cover letter and a list of references. Send the references with the resume only when requested.	10			

Steps	Possible Points	First Attempt	Second Attempt	Third Attempt
8. Type the resume carefully and make certain that there are no errors on the document.	10			
9. Proofread the resume. Allow another person to read it as well and look for missed errors.*	5			
10. Print the resume on quality paper. Review the resume again for errors and to assure that it looks attractive on the printed page.	5			
11. Target each resume to a specific person or position. Do not send generic resumes to each prospective employer.	5			
12. Follow up on all resumes that are distributed with a phone call to arrange an interview.	5			

Documentation in the Medical Record

____

____

____

____

Comments:

Total Points Earned ________ Divided by ________ Total Possible Points = ________ % Score

Instructor's Signature ____________________

English-Spanish Terms for the Medical Assistant

abscess Localized collection of pus that causes tissue destruction and may be either under the skin or deep within the body.
absceso Cantidad de pus localizada en un lugar que puede estar bajo la piel o a más profundidad en el interior del cuerpo y causa la destrucción de los tejidos.

academic degree A title conferred by a college, university, or professional school after completion of a program of study.
grado académico Título concedido por una, universidad o escuela profesional, tras completar un programa de estudios.

accommodation Adjustment of the eye for seeing various sizes of objects at different distances.
acomodación Ajuste del ojo para ver distintos tamaños de objetos a distancias diferentes.

account A statement of transactions during a fiscal period and the resulting balance.
cuenta Estado de transacciones durante un periodo fiscal y el saldo resultante.

account balance The amount owed or on hand in an account.
saldo de la cuenta Suma que se debe o que está en una cuenta.

accounts receivable ledger A record of the income and payments due from creditors on an account.
libro mayor de cuentas por cobrar Registro de cargos y pagos asentados en una cuenta.

accreditation The process by which an organization is recognized for adhering to a group of standards that meet or exceed expectations of the accrediting agency.
acreditación Proceso por el cual se reconoce a una organización por su cumplimiento de ciertos estándares en un grado que cumple o sobrepasa las expectativas de la agencia que la acredita.

act The formal product of a legislative body; a decision or determination by a sovereign, a legislative council, or a court of justice.
ley Producto formal de un cuerpo legislativo; decisión o determinación por un soberano, un consejo legislativo o un tribunal de justicia.

acute Having a rapid onset and severe symptoms.
agudo Que tiene un comienzo rápido y síntomas serios.

adage A saying, often in metaphorical form, that embodies a common observation.
refrán Dicho, con frecuencia metafórico, que refleja una observación común.

adhesions Bands of scar tissue that bind together two anatomic surfaces that are normally separate.
adhesiones Bandas de tejido de una cicatriz que unen dos superficies anatómicas que están normalmente separadas.

adrenocorticotropic hormone (ACTH) A hormone, released by the anterior pituitary gland, that stimulates the production and secretion of glucocorticoids.
hormona adrenocorticotropina (ACTH) Hormona, liberada por la glándula pituitaria anterior, que estimula la producción y secreción de glucocorticoides.

advent A coming into being or use.
advenimiento Próximo a ser o a usarse.

advocate One who pleads the cause of another; one who defends or maintains a cause or proposal.
abogado Persona que defiende la causa de otro; aqel que defiende o apoya una causa o propuesta.

affable Being pleasant and at ease in talking to others; characterized by ease and friendliness.
afable Que es agradable y tiene un trato fácil con los demás; caracterizado por su trato fácil y amistoso.

agenda A list or outline of things to be considered or done.
agenda Lista o resumen de cosas a considerar o a hacer.

aggression A forceful action or procedure intended to dominate; hostile, injurious or destructive behavior, especially when caused by frustration.
agresión Acción o procedimiento forzado, con la intención de dominar; comportamiento hostil, injurioso o destructivo, en especial cuando es causado por frustración.

albuminuria Abnormal presence of albumin in the urine.
albuminuria Presencia anómala de albúmina en la orina.

aliquot A portion of a well-mixed sample removed for testing.
alícuota Porción de una muestra bien mezclada, separada para ser analizada.

allegation A statement of what a party to a legal action undertakes to prove.
alegación Declaración por una de las partes implicadas en un proceso legal para apoyar lo que dicha parte intenta probar.

allied health fields Areas of healthcare delivery or related services in which professionals assist physicians with the diagnosis, treatment, and care of patients in many different specialty areas.
campos relacionados con la salud Áreas del cuidado de la salud y servicios relacionados en los cuales profesionales ayudan a los médicos en el diagnóstico, tratamiento y atención de los pacientes en muchas áreas diferentes.

allocating Apportioning for a specific purpose or to particular persons or things.
distribuir Asignar a un fin específico o a personas o cosas en particular.

allopathy A method of treating a disease by introducing a condition that is intended to cause a pathologic reaction, which will be antagonistic to the condition being treated.
alopatía Método de tratar una enfermedad provocando una afección con el fin de causar una reacción patológica, la cual será opuesta a la enfermedad que se está tratando.

allowed charge The maximum amount of money that many third-party payors will pay for a specific procedure or service. Often based on the UCR fee.
cargo permitido Cantidad máxima de dinero que muchos pagadores intermediarios pagan por una práctica o servicio especifico; con frecuencia se basa en el cargo UCR.

alopecia Partial or complete lack of hair.
alopecia Pérdida de cabello, parcial o total.

alphabetic filing Any system that arranges names or topics according to the sequence of the letters in the alphabet.
archivo alfabético Cualquier sistema que ordena los nombres o temas siguiendo la secuencia de las letras del alfabeto.

alphanumeric Systems made up of combinations of letters and numbers.
alfanumérico Sistema constituido por combinaciones de letras y números.

ambiguous Capable of being understood in two or more possible senses or ways; unclear.
ambiguo Que puede entenderse de dos o más maneras; que no es claro.

amblyopia Reduction or dimness of vision with no apparent organic cause; often referred to as lazy eye syndrome.
ambliopía Reducción o disminución de la visión sin causa orgánica aparente; con frecuencia se conoce como síndrome del ojo vago.

ambulatory Able to walk about and not be bedridden.
ambulatorio Capaz de caminar y no tiene que estar postrado en la cama.

amenity Something conducive to comfort, convenience, or enjoyment.
amenidad Algo que proporciona confort, comodidad o placer.

amino acids Organic compounds that form the chief constituents of protein and are used by the body to build and repair tissues.
aminoácidos Compuestos orgánicos que son los constituyentes principales de la proteína y son usados por el cuerpo para formar y reparar tejidos.

amorphous Lacking a defined shape.
amorfo Que carece de forma definida.

analyte The substance or chemical being analyzed or detected in a specimen.
analito La sustancia o producto químico que se analiza o que se detecta en una muestra.

anaphylaxis Exaggerated hypersensitivity reaction that, in severe cases, leads to vascular collapse, bronchospasm, and shock.
anafilaxia Reacción de hipersensibilidad exagerada, la cual, en casos graves, conduce a colapso vascular, broncospasmo y choque.

anastomosis The surgical joining together of two normally distinct organs.
anastomosis Unión quirúrgica de dos órganos normalmente diferentes.

ancillary diagnostic services Services that support patient diagnoses (e.g., laboratory or x-ray)
servicios de diagnóstico auxiliares Servicios que apoyan el diagnóstico del paciente (como laboratorio o rayos x).

ancillary Subordinate; auxiliary.
auxiliar Subordinado, complementario.

"and" In the context of ICD-9-CM, the word "and" should be interpreted as "and/or."
"y" En el contexto de ICD-9-CM, la palabra "y" debe interpretarse como "y/o".

anemia A condition marked by deficiency of red blood cells.
anemia Enfermedad caracterizada por una deficiencia de glóbulos rojos en la sangre.

angiocardiography Radiography of the heart and great vessels using an iodine contrast medium.
angiocardiografía Radiografía del corazón y los vasos sanguíneos mayores usando un medio de contraste yodado.

angiography Radiography of blood vessels using an iodine contrast medium.
angiografía Radiografía de los vasos sanguíneos usando un medio de contraste yodado.

angioplasty Interventional technique using a catheter to open or widen a blood vessel to improve circulation
angioplastia Técnica quirúrgica que usa un catéter para abrir o hacer más ancho un vaso sanguíneo a fin de mejorar la circulación.

animate Full of life; to give spirit and support to expressions.
animar Dar vida; dar ánimo y apoyo a las manifestaciones.

annotating To furnish with notes, which are usually critical or explanatory.
anotar Añadir notas, por lo general, críticas o explicatorias.

annotation A note added by way of comment or explanation.
anotación Nota añadida a modo de comentario o explicación.

anomalies Faulty development of the fetus resulting in deformities or deviations from normal.
anomalías Desarrollo defectuoso del feto que tiene como resultado deformidades o desviaciones de lo normal.

anorexia Lack or loss of appetite for food.
anorexia Falta o pérdida del apetito.

anoxia Absence of oxygen in the tissues.
anoxia Ausencia de oxígeno en los tejidos.

anteroposterior (AP) Frontal projection in which the patient is supine or facing the x-ray tube.
anteroposterior (AP) Proyección frontal en la cual el paciente está en posición supina o frente al tubo de rayos X.

antibody Immunoglobulin produced by the immune system in response to bacteria, viruses, or other antigenic substances.
anticuerpo Inmunoglobulina producida por el sistema inmunológico en respuesta a bacterias, virus u otras substancias antigénicas.

anticoagulant A chemical added to the blood after collection to prevent clotting.
anticoagulante Producto químico que se añade a la sangre después de extraerla para que no forme coágulos.

antidiuretic hormone (ADH) A hormone secreted at the posterior pituitary gland; causes water retention in the kidneys; and an elevation of blood pressure also known as vasopressin.
hormona antidiurética (ADH) Hormona secretada por la glándula pituitaria posterior y que provoca retención de agua en los riñones y aumento de la presión sanguínea. Es conocida también como vasopresina.

antigen Foreign substance that causes the production of a specific antibody.
antígeno Substancia extraña que provoca la producción de un anticuerpo específico.

antimicrobial agent A drug that is used to treat infection.
agente antimicrobiano Substancia que se usa para tratar infecciones.

antiseptic Pertaining to substances that inhibit the growth of microorganisms such as alcohol and betadine.
antiséptico Perteneciente o relativo a las substancias que inhiben el crecimiento de microorganismos como el alcohol y la betadina.

antiseptic substance that kills **microorganisms.**
antiséptico Substancia que mata **microorganismos.**

antiseptic An agent that inhibits bacterial growth and that can be used on human tissue.
antiséptico Agente que inhibe el crecimiento bacteriano y que puede usarse en los tejidos humanos.

aortagram Radiography of the aorta using an iodine contrast medium.
aortograma Radiografía de la aorta usando un medio de contraste yodado.

apnea Absence or cessation of breathing.
apnea Ausencia o cese de la respiración.

appeal A legal proceeding by which a case is brought before a higher court for review of the decision of a lower court.
apelación Procedimiento legal por el cual un caso se lleva ante un tribunal superior para obtener una revisión de la decisión de un tribunal inferior.

appellate Having the power to review the judgment of another tribunal or body of jurisdiction, such as an appellate court.
de apelación Que tiene el poder de revisar el veredicto de otro tribunal o cuerpo jurídico, como una corte de apelación.

applications Software programs designed to perform specific tasks.
aplicaciones Programas informáticos diseñados para realizar tareas específicas.

appraisal To give an expert judgment of the value or merit of; judging as to quality.
evaluación Acción de emitir un juicio experto sobre el valor o mérito de algo; juzgar la calidad de algo; evaluar el rendimiento en el trabajo.

arbitration The hearing and determination of a cause in controversy by a person or persons either chosen by the parties involved or appointed under statutory authority.
arbitraje Vista y resolución de una causa en conflicto por una persona o personas elegida/s por las partes implicadas o designadas por la autoridad establecida por ley.

arbitrator A neutral person chosen to settle differences between two parties in a controversy.
árbitro Persona neutral seleccionada para poner fin a las diferencias entre dos partes involucradas en un conflicto.

archaic Of, relating to, or characteristic of an earlier or more primitive time.
arcaico Perteneciente o relativo a una época anterior o más primitiva; que tiene las características de dicha época.

archived To file or collect records or documents in or as if in an archive.
archivar Guardar o recoger informes o documentos en un archivo o de manera similar.

arrhythmia Abnormality or irregularity in the heart rhythm.
arritmia Anomalía o irregularidad en el ritmo cardiaco.

arteriography Radiography of arteries using an iodine contrast medium.
arteriografía Radiografía de las arterias usando un medio de contraste yodado.

arthritis Inflammation of a joint.
artritis Inflamación de una articulación.

arthrogram Fluoroscopic examination of the soft tissue components of joints with direct injection of a contrast medium into the joint capsule.
artrografía Examen fluoroscópico de los componentes de los tejidos blandos de las articulaciones con una inyección directa de un medio de contraste en la cápsula de la articulación.

articular Pertaining to a joint.
articulatorio Perteneciente o relativo a una articulación.

artificial intelligence The aspect of computer science that deals with computers taking on the attributes of humans. One such example is an expert system, which is capable of making decisions, like software that is designed to help a physician diagnose a patient, given a set of symptoms. Game-playing programming and programs designed to recognize human language are other examples of artificial intelligence.
inteligencia artificial Parte de la informática que se ocupa de la incorporación de atributos humanos a las computadoras. Un ejemplo de esto es un sistema práctico capaz de tomar decisiones, como los programas informáticos diseñados para ayudar a los médicos a diagnosticar a un paciente dado un conjunto de síntomas. Los programas de juegos y otros programas diseñados para reconocer el lenguaje humano son otros ejemplos.

ASCII American Standard Code for Information Interchange, a code representing English characters as numbers where each is given a number from 0 to 127.
ASCII Estándar Americano de Codificación para el Intercambio de Información; un código que representa carácteres ingleses como números, en el cual a cada uno se le asigna un número de 0 a 127.

asepsis Being free from infection or infectious materials.
asepsia Que está libre del infecciones.

assault An intentional, unlawful attempt to do bodily injury to another by force.
asalto Intento ilícito de causar daño físico a otro usando la fuerza.

assent To agree to something, especially after thoughtful consideration.
asentir Aceptar algo, especialmente cuando se hace tras una detenida reflexión.

asystole The absence of a heartbeat.
asistolia Ausencia de latidos del corazón.

ataxia Failure or irregularity of muscle actions and coordination.
ataxia Fallo o irregularidad del movimiento y coordinación musculare.

atherosclerosis A form of arteriosclerosis distinguished by fatty deposits within the inner layers of larger arterial walls.
aterosclerosis Forma de arteriosclerosis que se distingue por la presencia de depósitos de grasa en las capas internas de las paredes de las arterias mayores.

atria The two upper chambers of the heart.
aurículas Las dos cavidades superiores del corazón.

atrioventricular (AV) node Part of the cardiac conduction system located between the atria and the ventricles
nódulo aurioventricular (AV) Parte del sistema cardiaco que se encuentra entre las aurículas y los ventrílculos.

atrophy Decrease in the size of a normally developed organ.
atrofia Disminución del tamaño de un órgano desarrollado de forma normal.

atrophy Wasting away, decreasing size.
atrofia Desgastado, disminuido en tamaño.

attenuated Weakened, or change in virulence of, a pathogenic microorganism.
atenuado Cambio o debilitación en la virulencia de un microorganismo.

audiologist An allied health care professional specializing in evaluation of hearing function, detection of hearing impairment, and determination of the anatomic site of impairment.
audiólogo Profesional del cuidado de la salud que se especializa en evaluar la función auditiva, detectar las dificultades auditivas y determinar el lugar físico en el que se produce el problema auditivo.

audit A formal examination of an organization's or individual's accounts or financial situation; a methodical examination and review.
auditoría Análisis formal de las cuentas o estado financiero de una organización o un individuo; examen y revisión sistemáticos.

augment To make greater, more numerous, larger, or more intense.
aumentar Hacer mayor, más numeroso, más grande o más intenso.

aura Peculiar sensation preceding the appearance of more definite disturbance.
aura Sensación peculiar que precede a la aparición de un trastorno definido.

authorization A term used by managed care for an approved referral.
autorización Término usado en el cuido administrado para referirse a la aprobación de la referencia de un paciente de un médico a otro profesional del cuidod o de la salud.

autoimmune Disturbance in the immune system in which the body reacts against its own tissue. Examples of autoimmune disorders include Multiple Sclerosis, Rheumatoid Arthritis, and Systemic Lupus Erythematosus.
autoinmune Trastorno del sistema inmunológico en el cual el cuerpo reacciona contra sus propios tejidos. Algunos ejemplos de trastornos autoinmunes incluyen la esclerosis múltiple, la artritis reumatoide y el lupus eritematoso sistémico.

autoimmune Development of an immune response to one's own tissues; act against own cells to cause localized and systemic reactions.
autoinmune Desarrollo de una respuesta inmunológica a los propios tejidos; actuar contra sus propias células para originar reacciones sistémicas localizadas.

axial projection Radiograph taken with a longitudinal angulation of the x-ray beam; sometimes referred to as a semi-axial projection.
proyección axial Radiografía que se toma con un ángulo longitudinal del haz de rayos X; a veces se llama proyección semi-axial.

azotemia Retention in the blood of excessive amounts of nitrogenous wastes.
azotemia Retención en la sangre de cantidades de desperdicios nitrogenados.

back-up Any type of storage of files to prevent their loss in the event of hard disk failure.
copia de seguridad Cualquier tipo de almacenamiento de archivos para evitar que se pierdan en caso de que ocurrra un fallo en el disco duro.

bailiff An officer of some U.S. courts, usually serving as a messenger or usher, who keeps order at the request of the judge.
alguacil Funcionario de algunos tribunales estadounidenses que suele servir como mensajero o ujier y que se ocupa de mantener el orden a petición del juez.

bank reconciliation The process of proving that a bank statement and checkbook balance are in agreement
reconciliación bancaria Proceso por el cual se prueba que un estado bancario y un saldo de una libreta de cheques concuerdan.

banners Banners, or banner ads, are advertisements often found on a webpage, which can be animated and attract the user's attention in hopes that he or she will click on the ad and be redirected to the advertiser's home page, and hence purchase from the site or gain information from the site.
viñetas Viñetas o anuncios de viñetas; anuncios, a **veces** animados, que se hallan, con frecuencia en las páginas web; su fin es atraer la atención del usuario con la esperanza de que éste haga clic en el anuncio, y así sea llevado a la página principal del anunciante para que compre algo en ese sitio o para que obtenga información sobre el mismo.

battery A willful and unlawful use of force or violence upon the person of another. An offensive touching or use of force on a person without that person's consent
golpiza Uso de la fuerza o violencia en contra de la persona de otro, de manera intencional e ilegítima. Tocar de manera ofensiva a una persona o usar la fuerza en contra de ella sin su consentimiento.

beneficence The act of doing or producing good, especially performing acts of charity or kindness.
beneficencia Acción de hacer o producir el bien, en especial llevando a cabo obras caritativas o bondadosas.

beneficiary The person receiving the benefits of an insurance policy. The "insured" person on a Medicare claim.
beneficiario Persona que recibe los beneficios de una póliza de seguro. La persona "asegurada" en una reclamación de Medicare.

benefits A service or payment provided under a health plan, employee plan, or some other agreement, including programs such as health insurance, pensions, retirement planning, and many other options that may be offered to employees of a company or organization.
beneficios Servicio o pago proporcionado bajo un plan de salud, un plan de empleados o algún otro acuerdo, incluyendo programas como seguros de salud, pensiones, planes de retiro y muchas otras opciones que pueden ser ofrecidas a los empleados de una compañía u organización.

benefits The amount payable by the insurance company for a monetary loss to an individual insured by that company, under each coverage.
beneficios Suma que ha de pagar la compañía aseguradora por una pérdida monetaria a un individuo asegurado por dicha compañía, bajo cada cobertura.

benign Not cancerous and not recurring.
benigno No canceroso y no recurrente.

bevel Angled tip of a needle.
bisel Punta de aguja en ángulo.

bifurcate Divide from one into two branches.
bifurcar Dividir una unidad en dos ramas.

bifurcation The point of forking or separating into two branches
bifurcación Lugar en el que se separan dos ramas.

bilirubin Orange-colored pigment in bile, which, when it accumulates, leads to jaundice
bilirrubina Pigmento de color naranja que se encuentra en la bilis; cuando se acumula produce ictericia.

bilirubinuria Presence of bilirubin in the urine.
bilirrubinuria Presencia de bilirrubina en la orina.

biophysical Pertaining to the science dealing with the application of physical methods and theories to biologic problems.
biofísico Perteneciente o relativo a la ciencia que trata de la aplicación de métodos y teorías físicas a los problemas biológicos.

birthday rule When an individual is covered under two insurance policies, the insurance plan of the policyholder whose birthday comes first in the calendar year (month and day—not year) becomes primary.
regla del cumpleaños Cuando un individuo está cubierto bajo dos pólizas de seguro, el plan de seguro del titular de la póliza cuya fecha de cumpleaños esté antes en el año civil (mes y día, no año) se convierte en el plan primario.

blatant Completely obvious, conspicuous, or obtrusive, especially in a crass or offensive manner; brazen.
flagrante Completamente obvio, notorio o inoportuno, en especial de una manera torpe u ofensiva; desvergonzado.

bond A durable, formal paper used for documents.
obligación Papel duradero y formal usado para documentos.

bounding pulse Pulse that feels full because of increased power of cardiac contractions or due to increased blood volume.
pulso saltón Pulso que se siente lleno debido a un aumento de potencia en las contracciones cardiacas o debido a un aumento del volumen de la sangre.

bradycardia A slow heartbeat; a pulse below 60 beats per minute.
bradicardia Latido lento; pulso por debajo de 60 pulsaciones por minuto.

bradypnea Respirations that are regular in rhythm but slower than normal in rate.
bradipnea Respiración que tiene un ritmo regular pero es más lenta de lo normal.

broad-spectrum antimicrobial agent A drug used to treat a broad range of infections.
agente antimicrobiano de amplio espectro Sustancia que se usa para tratar una amplia gama de infecciones.

bronchiectasis Dilation of the bronchi and bronchioles associated with secondary infection or ciliary.
broncoectasia Dilatación de los bronquios y bronquiolos asociada con una infección secundaria o ciliar.

bronchoconstriction Narrowing of the bronchiole tubes.
broncoconstricción Estrechamiento de los bronquiolos.

bruit Abnormal sound or murmur heard on auscultation of an organ, vessel, or gland.
ruido Sonido o murmullo anómalo que se oye al auscultar un órgano, vaso sanguíneo o glándula.

bucky Moving grid device that prevents scatter radiation from fogging the film.
bucky Dispositivo de rejilla móvil que evita que la difusión de la radiación empañe la película.

bundle of His Fibers that conduct electrical impulses from AV node to ventricular myocardium.
haz de His Fibras que conducen impulsos eléctricos del nódulo aurioventricular al miocardio ventricular.

burnout Exhaustion of physical or emotional strength or motivation, usually as a result of prolonged stress or frustration.
agotamiento Llegar al fin de la fortaleza o motivación física o emocional, por lo general como resultado un prolongado estado de estrés o frustración.

bursa A fluid-filled sac-like membrane that provides for cushioning and frictionless motion between two tissues.
bursa Membrana con forma de saco llena de fluido que proporciona amortiguación y movimiento sin fricción entre dos tejidos.

byte A unit of data that contains eight binary digits.
byte Unidad de información que contiene ocho dígitos binarios.

C&S–culture and sensitivity A procedure performed in the microbiology laboratory through which a specimen is cultured on artifical media to detect bacterial or fungal growth, followed by appropriate screening for antibiotic sensitivity.
C&S–cultivo y sensibilidad Procedimiento llevado a cabo en el laboratorio de microbiología en el cual se cultiva un espécimen en un medio artificial para detectar el crecimiento de bacterias u hongos y después investigar su sensibilidad los antibióticos.

cache A special high-speed storage, which can be either part of the computer's main memory or a separate storage device. One function of cache is to store Web sites visited in the computer memory for faster recall the next time the Web site is requested.
caché Almacenamiento especial de alta velocidad que puede formar parte de la memoria principal de la computadora o puede ser un dispositivo de almacenamiento separado. Una función del caché es almacenar las páginas Web visitadas en la memoria de la computadora para llegar a ellas con mayor rapidez la próxima vez que desee ver la página.

candidiasis Infection caused by a yeast-like fungus which typically effects the vaginal mucosa and skin.
candidiasis Infección causada por una levadura (una especie de hongo) que típicamente afecta la mucosa y la piel vaginal.

cannula Rigid tube that surrounds a blunt trocar or a sharp, pointed trocar inserted into the body; when it is withdrawn, fluid may escape from the body through the cannula, depending on where it is inserted.
cánula Tubo rígido que envuelve un trocar romo o un trocar de punta afilada que se inserta en el cuerpo; cuando se saca, puede salir fluido corporal a través de la cánula, según en donde haya sido insertada.

caption A heading, title, or subtitle under which records are filed.
leyenda Encabezamiento, título o subtítulo bajo el cual se archivan los informes.

carbohydrates Chemical substances, including sugars, glycogen, starches, dextrins, and celluloses, that contain only carbon, oxygen, and hydrogen.
carbohidratos Sustancias químicas, en las que se incluyen azúcares, glucógenos, almidones, dextrinas y celulosas, y están formadas sólo por carbono, oxígeno e hidrógeno.

carcinogenic A substance that is known to cause cancer.
cancerígeno Sustancia que se sabe que produce cáncer.

carcinogens Substances or agents that cause the development of or increase the incidence of cancer.
carcinógeno Sustancia o agente que origina el desarrollo de cáncer o aumenta su incidencia.

cardiac arrest Cardiac contractions completely stop.
paro cardiaco Detención completa de las contracciones cardiacas.

cardiac arrhythmias Irregular heartbeat resulting from a malfunction of the electrical system of the heart.
arritmias cardiacas Pulso irregular que es resultado de un mal funcionamiento del sistema eléctrico del corazón.

cardioversion Utilizing an electroshock to convert an abnormal cardiac rhythm to a normal one.
cardioversión Utilización de un electrochoque para normalizar un ritmo cardiaco anómalo.

cartilage Rubbery, smooth, somewhat elastic connective tissue covering the ends of bones.
cartílago Tejido de unión similar a la goma, suave y un tanto elástico, que cubre los extremos de los huesos.

case management The process of assessing and planning patient care, including referral and follow-up to ensure continuity of care and quality management.
administración de casos Proceso de evaluación y planificación de la atención al paciente, incluyendo envío de pacientes a especialistas y seguimiento del caso para asegurar la continuidad del tratamiento y la calidad de la administración.

cash on delivery (COD) Method of payment used when an article or item is delivered, and payment is expected before it is released.
contra reembolso (COD) Método de pago usado cuando se entrega un artículo u objeto y el destinatario ha de pagar antes de recibirlo.

casts Fibrous or protein material molded to the shape of the part in which it has accumulated and thrown off into the urine in kidney disease.
cálculos Materiales fibrosos o proteínicos que han tomado la forma de la parte del cuerpo en la que han sido acumulados y que se expulsan a través de la orina en los casos de enfermedades renales.

categorically Placed in a specific division of a system of classification.
categorizado Colocado en un lugar específico dentro de una división de un sistema de clasificación.

caustic A remark or phrase dripping with sarcasm.
cáustico Comentario o frase dicha con sarcasmo.

caustic A substance that burns or destroys tissue by chemical action.
cáustico Substancia que quema o destruye tejidos por acción química.

CD Burner A CD writer that is capable of writing data onto a blank CD, or copying data from a CD to another blank CD.
grabador de CD Dispositivo que puede escribir datos en un CD en blanco o copiar datos de un CD a otro CD en blanco.

centrifuge An apparatus consisting essentially of a compartment spun about a central axis to separate contained materials of different specific gravities, or to separate colloidal particles suspended in a liquid.
centrifugadora Aparato que consiste básicamente de un compartimiento que gira alrededor de un eje central para separar materiales con diferentes pesos específicos, o para separar partículas coloidales suspendidas en un líquido.

cerebrospinal fluid Fluid within the subarachnoid space, the central canal of the spinal cord, and the four ventricles of the brain.
fluido cerebroespinal Fluido del interior del espacio subaracnoideo, el canal central de la médula espinal y los cuatro ventrículos del cerebro.

certification Attested as being true, as represented, or as meeting a standard; to have been tested, usually by a third party, and awarded a certificate based on proven knowledge.
certificación Atestiguar que algo es verdadero en cuanto a lo que representa, o al cumplimiento de un estándar; que ha sido examinado, por lo general por una tercera parte, y que se le ha concedido un certificado basándose en el conocimiento del que ha dado prueba.

cerumen A waxy secretion in the ear canal, commonly called *ear wax*.
cerumen Secreción cerosa del canal del oído, comúnmente se conoce como *cera de los oídos*.

cervical Neck region containing seven cervical vertebrae.
cervical Región del cuello en la que hay siete vértebras cervicales.

chain of command A series of executive positions in order of authority.
cadena de mando Serie de puestos ejecutivos en orden de autoridad.

channels A means of communication or expression; a way, course, or direction of thought.
canales Medios de comunicación o de expresión; vía, curso o dirección del pensamiento.

characteristic A distinguishing trait, quality, or property.
característica Rasgo, cualidad o propiedad distintiva.

chief complaint Reason for patient seeking medical care.
problema principal Razón por la cual un paciente solicita atención médica.

chiropractic A medical discipline in which a chiropractic physician focuses on the nervous system and manually and painlessly adjusts the vertebral column in order to affect the nervous system, resulting in healthier patients.
quiropráctica Disciplina médica en la que los médicos quiroprácticos se centran en el sistema nervioso y ajustan la columna vertebral manualmente y sin dolor, para lograr un efecto sobre el sistema nervioso, dando como resultado pacientes más sanos.

cholesterol Substance produced by the liver, found in plant and animal fats, that can produce fatty deposits or atherosclerotic plaques in the blood vessels.
colesterol Sustancia que produce el hígado y que se halla en las grasas animales y vegetales, y que puede producir depósitos grasos o placas **ateroscleróticas** en los vasos sanguíneos.

chronic Persisting for a prolonged period of time.
crónico Que persiste por largo tiempo.

chronic bronchitis Recurrent inflammation of the membranes lining the bronchial tubes.
bronquitis crónica Inflamación recurrente de las membranas que recubren los tubos bronquiales.

chronologic order Of, relating to, or arranged in or according to the order of time.
orden cronológico Perteneciente o relativo al orden en el tiempo; organizado según el orden en el tiempo.

circumvention To manage to avoid something, especially by ingenuity or stratagem.
circunvenir Lograr evitar algo usando ingeniosidad o estratagemas.

cite To quote by way of example, authority, or proof, or to mention formally in commendation or praise.
cita Que se nombra para servir de ejemplo, autoridad o prueba o para hacer una mención formal como recomendación o alabanza.

claims clearinghouse A centralized facility (sometimes called a third-party administrator or TPA) to whom insurance claims are transmitted, and who checks and redistributes claims electronically to various insurance carriers.
centro de reclamaciones Establecimiento centralizado (algunas veces conocido como administrador mediador o TPA) al cual se transmiten las reclamaciones de seguros y que se encarga de verificar y redistribuir las reclamaciones electrónicamente a varias compañías de seguros.

clarity The quality or state of being clear.
claridad Calidad o estado de claro.

clauses A group of words containing a subject and predicate and functioning as a member of a complex or compound sentence.
cláusulas Conjunto de palabras que incluye un sujeto y un predicado y que funciona como miembro de una oración compuesta.

clean claim An insurance claim form that has been completed correctly (with no errors or omissions) and can be processed and paid promptly.
reclamación limpia Formulario de reclamación de seguro que ha sido llenado correctamente (sin errores ni omisiones) y que puede procesarse y pagarse prontamente.

clearinghouses Networks of banks that exchange checks with each other.
sistema de compensación Redes bancarias que intercambian cheques entres sí.

clinical trials A research study that tests how well new medical treatments or other interventions work in the subjects, usually human beings.
ensayos clínicos Estudio de investigación que prueba cómo actúan los nuevos tratamientos médicos u otras intervenciones en los sujetos, normalmente en los seres humanos.

clitoris Small, elongated erectile body situated above the urinary meatus at the superior point of the labia minora.
clítoris Órgano eréctil pequeño y alargado situado sobre el meato urinario a la altura de los labios menores.

clubbing Abnormal enlargement of the distal phalanges (fingers and toes), associated with cyanotic heart disease or advanced chronic pulmonary disease.
hipocratismo digital (dedos en palillo de tambor) Engrosamiento anómalo de las falanges distales (en los dedos de las manos y de los pies), relacionado con una enfermedad cardiaca cianótica o una enfermedad pulmonar crónica avanzada.

coagulate Capable of being formed into clots.
coagular Formar coágulos.

"code also" When more than one code is necessary to fully identify a given condition, "code also" of "use additional code" is used.
"código adicional" Cuando se necesita más de un código para identificar por completo una afección (enfermedad) determinado, se usa "código adicional" o "usar código adicional".

Code of Federal Regulations (CFR) The Code of Federal Regulations (CFR) is a coded delineation of the rules and regulations published in the Federal Register by the various departments and agencies of the federal government. The CFR is divided into 50 Titles, which represent broad subject areas, and further into chapters, which provide specific detail.
Código de Regulaciones Federales (CFR) El Código de Regulaciones Federales (CFR) es un resumen codificado de las normas y regulaciones publicadas en el Registro Federal por los diferentes departamentos y agencias del gobierno federal. El CFR se divide en 50 Títulos que representan amplias áreas temáticas, los cuales, a su vez, se subdividen en capítulos que proporcionan detalles específicos.

cognitive Pertaining to the operation of the mind process by which we become aware of perceiving, thinking, and remembering.
cognitivo Perteneciente o relativo a la operación del proceso mental por el cual nos damos cuenta de cómo, percibimos, pensamos y recordamos.

cohesive The state of sticking together tightly; exhibiting or producing the cohesion.
cohesivo El estado de estar estrechamente unidos; mostrar o producir cohesión.

coitus Sexual union between male and female; also known as intercourse.
coito Unión sexual entre un macho y una hembra.

collagen Protein that forms the inelastic fibers of tendons, ligaments, and fascia.
colágeno Proteína que forma las fibras no elásticas de los tendones, los ligamentos y la fascia.

collodion Preparation of cellulose nitrate that, when applied to the skin, dries to a strong, thin, protective, transparent film.
colodión Preparación de nitrato de celulosa que, cuando se aplica a la piel, se seca formando una película fina resistente, protectora y transparente.

colloidal Pertaining to a gluelike substance.
coloidal Perteneciente o relativo a una substancia parecida a la cola.

colostrum Thin, yellow, milky fluid secreted by the mammary glands a few days before and after delivery.
calostro Fluido lácteo poco espeso y amarillo que segregan las glándulas mamarias unos días antes y después del parto.

coma An unconscious state from which the patient cannot be aroused.
coma Estado inconsciente del cual el paciente no puede ser despertado.

comfort zone A place in the mind where an individual feels safe and confident.
zona de bienestar Un lugar en la mente en el que un individuo se siente seguro y confiado.

commensurate Corresponding in size, amount, extent, or degree; equal in measure.
equiparable Que es equivalente en tamaño, cantidad o grado; de igual medida.

commercial insurance Plans (sometimes called private insurance) that reimburse the insured (or his or her dependents) for monetary losses due to illness or injury according to a specific schedule as outlined in the insurance policy and on a fee-for-service basis. Individuals insured under these plans are normally not limited to any one physician and can usually see the health care provider of their choice.
seguro comercial Planes (a veces llamados seguros privados) que reembolsan al asegurado (o a sus dependendientes) por pérdidas monetarias debidas a enfermedad o lesión siguiendo una escala específica que se explica en la póliza de seguro y cobrando un cargo por cada servicio. Los individuos asegurados bajo estos planes, por lo general, no están limitados a un solo médico y suelen poder acudir al proveedor del cuidado de la salud que elijan.

comorbidities Preexisting conditions that will, because of their presence with a specific principal diagnosis, cause an increase in length of stay by at least 1 day in approximately 75 percent of cases.
patologías coexistentes Enfermedades preexistentes que, debido a su presencia junto al diagnóstico principal, causan un aumento en la duración de la estadía de al menos un día en aproximadamente 75 por ciento de los casos.

competence The quality or state of being competent; having adequate or requisite capabilities.
competencia Capacidad o aptitud de quien es competente en algo; tener las capacidades necesarias o cumplir con los requisitos necesarios para hacer algo.

competent Having adequate abilities or qualities; having the capacity to function or perform in a certain way.
competente Que tiene ciertas capacidades o cualidades; que tiene la capacidad de funcionar o actuar de un modo determinado.

complications Conditions that arise during the hospital stay that prolong the length of stay by at least 1 day in approximately 75 percent of the cases.
complicaciones Condiciones que surgen durante la permanencia en el hospital que prolongan el tiempo de la estadía en al menos un día en aproximadamente 75 por ciento de los casos.

compression The state of being pressed together.
compresión Condición de estar apretado.

computed tomography (CT) Computerized x-ray imaging modality providing axial and three-dimensional scans.
tomografía asistida por computadora (TAC) Modalidad de formación computarizada de imágenes de rayos X que proporciona imágenes de escáner axiales y tridimensionales.

computer A machine that is designed to accept, store, process, and give out information.
computadora (u ordenador) Máquina diseñada para aceptar, almacenar, procesar y emitir información.

concise Expressing much in brief form.
conciso Que expresa mucho en forma breve.

concurrently Occurring at the same time.
concurrente Que ocurre al mismo tiempo.

cones Structures found in the retina that make the perception of color posible.
conos Estructuras que se encuentran en la retina y que hacen posible la percepción del color.

congruence The verbal expression of the message matches the sender's nonverbal body language.
congruencia Expresión verbal del mensaje que corresponde al lenguaje corporal no verbal del emisor.

congruent Being in agreement, harmony, or correspondence; conforming to the circumstances or requirements of a situation.
congruente Que está en acuerdo, armonía o correspondencia; conforme a las circunstancias o requisitos de una situación.

connotation An implication; something suggested by a word or thing.
connotación Implicación; lo que sugiere una palabra o una cosa.

contaminated Soiled with pathogens or infectious material; nonsterile.
contaminado Manchado con materiales patógenos o infecciosos; no estéril.

contamination Becoming unsterile by contact with any nonsterile material.
contaminación Pasar al estado de no estéril por contacto con cualquier material no estéril.

contamination To make impure or unclean; to make unfit for use by the introduction of unwholesome or undesirable elements.
contaminación Volver impuro o sucio; hacer que algo sea inadecuado para el uso por la introducción de elementos insalubres o indeseables.

continuation pages The second and following pages of a letter.
paginas de continuación En una carta, la segunda página y las siguientes.

continuing education credits (CEUs) Credits for courses, classes, or seminars related to an individual's profession, designed to promote education and to keep the professional up-to-date on current procedures and trends in his or her field; often required for licensing.
créditos de educación continua (CEU) Créditos por cursos, clases o seminarios relacionados con la profesión de un individuo y que tienen la finalidad de promocionar la educación y mantener al profesional al corriente de los procedimientos y tendencias actuales en su campo; con frecuencia son obligatorios para obtener una licencia.

continuity of care Care that continues smoothly from one provider to another so that the patient receives the most benefit and no interruption in care.
continuidad de la atención Atención que continúa sin interrupciones de un proveedor a otro, de manera que el paciente recibe los máximos beneficios sin que haya una interrupción de la atención sanitaria.

contralateral Pertaining to the opposite side of the body.
colateral Perteneciente o relativo a la parte opuesta del cuerpo.

contrast media Substances used to enhance visualization of soft tissues in imaging studies.
medios de contraste Substancias usadas para mejorar la visualización de los tejidos blandos en estudios de formación de imágenes.

contributory negligence Statutes in some states that may prevent a party from recovering damages if he or she contributed in any way to the injury or condition.
negligencia concurrente Estatutos existentes en algunos estados que impiden que una parte sea recompensada por daños si esta parte ha contribuido en algún modo a provocar la lesión o enfermedad.

cookies A message that is sent to the Web browser from the Web server, which identifies users and can prepare custom Web pages for them, possibly displaying their name upon return to the site.
cookies Mensaje que se envía al navegador de la red desde el servidor, el cual identifica a los usuarios y puede preparar páginas web especiales para ellos, posiblemente, mostrando su nombre la próxima vez que visiten el sitio.

coordination of benefits The mechanism used in group health insurance to designate the order in which multiple carriers are to pay benefits to prevent duplicate payments.
coordinación de beneficios Mecanismo usado en seguros de enfermedad de grupo para designar el orden en el que varias compañías de seguros tienen que pagar los beneficios para evitar pagos dobles.

copayment A copayment (or coinsurance) is a policy provision frequently found in medical insurance, whereby the policyholder and the insurance company share the cost of *covered* losses in a specified ratio (i.e., 80/20–80 percent by the insurer and 20 percent by the insured).
co-pago Un co-pago (o co-seguro) es una provisión frecuente de la póliza en los seguros médicos, por la que el titular de la póliza y la compañía aseguradora comparten el costo de las pérdidas *cubiertas* en una proporción determinada (ej.: 80/20–80 por ciento por parte del asegurador y 20 por ciento por parte del asegurado).

COPD chronic obstructive pulmonary disease A progressive and irreversible lung condition that results in diminished lung capacity.
COPD enfermedad pulmonar obstructiva crónica Enfermedad pulmonar progresiva e irreversible que conlleva una reducción de la capacidad pulmonar.

copulation Sexual intercourse.
copulación Cópula sexual.

coronal plane Plane that divides the body into anterior and posterior parts.
plano coronal Plano que divide el cuerpo en una anterior y una posterior.

corticosteroids Anti-inflammatory hormones, natural or synthetic.
corticosteroides Hormonas antiinflamatorias, naturales o sintéticas.

costal Pertaining to the ribs.
costal Perteneciente o relativo a las costillas.

coulombs per kilogram (C/kg) International unit of radiation exposure.
culombios por kilogramo (C/kg) Unidad internacional de exposición a la radiación.

counteroffer A return offer made by one who has rejected an offer or job.
contraoferta Oferta-respuesta hecha por quien ha rechazado una oferta o trabajo.

creatinine Nitrogenous waste from muscle metabolism excreted in urine.
creatinina Residuo nitrogenado del metabolismo muscular que se excreta en la orina.

credentialing The act of extending professional or medical privileges to an individual; the process of verifying and evaluating that person's credentials.
concesión de credenciales Acción de conceder privilegios profesionales o médicos a un individuo; proceso de verificar y evaluar los credenciales de esa persona.

credibility The quality or power of inspiring belief.
credibilidad Calidad de creíble; facilidad para ser creído.

credit An entry on an account constituting an addition to a revenue, net worth, or liability account; the balance in a person's favor in an account.
crédito Dato que se entra en una cuenta y que constituye una adición a los ingresos, ganancia neta o cuenta de pasivo; saldo a favor de una persona en una cuenta.

crenate Forming notches or leaflike scalloped edges on an object.
crenar Formar muescas o bordes en forma de concha o de hoja en un objeto.

crepitation Dry, crackling sound or sensation.
crepitación Sonido o sensación seca y crujiente.

critical thinking The constant practice of considering all aspects of a situation when deciding what to believe or what to do.
razonamiento crítico Práctica constante de considerar todos los aspectos de una situación al decidir qué creer o qué hacer.

cross-training Training in more than one area so that a multitude of duties may be performed by one person, or so that substitutions of personnel may be made when necessary or in emergencies.
entrenamiento cruzado Entrenamiento en más de un área, de modo que una persona pueda desempeñar varias labores o que se puedan realizar sustituciones de personal cuando sea necesario o en caso de emergencia.

cryosurgery Technique of exposing tissue to extreme cold to produce a well-defined area of cell destruction.
criocirugía Técnica que consiste en exponer los tejidos a un frío extremo para producir una destrucción de células en un área bien definida.

cryptogenic Hidden origin.
criptogénico De origen oculto.

cultivate To foster the growth of; to improve by labor, care, or study.
cultivar Promover el desarrollo; mejorar algo por medio de trabajo, cuidado o estudio.

curettage Act of scraping a body cavity with a surgical instrument such as a curette.
curetaje Acción de raspar una cavidad corporal con un instrumento quirúrgico, como una cureta o cucharilla cortante.

cursor A symbol appearing on the monitor that shows where the next character to be typed will appear.
cursor Símbolo que aparece en el monitor y que muestra el lugar donde aparecerá el próximo carácter que se escriba.

curt Marked by rude or peremptory shortness.
cortante Caracterizado por una interrupción ruda o perentoria.

cyanosis Blue color of the mucous membranes and body extremities caused by lack of oxygen.
cianosis Color azul de las membranas mucosas y las extremidades provocado por una falta de oxígeno.

cyberspace A word used to describe the non-physical space of the online world of computer networks.
ciberespacio Palabra que se usa para describir el espacio no-físico del mundo en linea de las redes informáticas.

cyst A small capsule-like sac that encloses certain organisms in their dormant or larval stage.
quiste Pequeño saco en forma de cápsula que encierra ciertos organismos en estado letárgico o larval.

damages Loss or harm resulting from injury to person, property, or reputation; compensation in money imposed by law for losses or injuries.
daños Pérdidas o perjuicios que resultan de injuriar a una persona, atentar contra una propiedad o una reputación; compensación monetaria impuesta por ley en casos de pérdidas o injurias.

database A collection of related files that serves as a foundation for retrieving information.
base de datos Conjunto de archivos relacionados que sirven de base para la recuperación de información.

debit An entry on an account constituting an addition to an expense or asset balance, or a deduction from a revenue, net worth, or liability balance.
débito Dato que se entra en una cuenta y que constituye una adición a los gastos o a una cuenta de activo o una deducción de un ingreso, ganancia neta o cuenta de pasivo.

debit card A card similar to a credit card by which money may be withdrawn or the cost of purchases paid directly from the holder's bank account without the payment of interest.
tarjeta de débito Tarjeta similar a la de crédito pero con la cual se puede retirar dinero o pagar compras directamente de la cuenta bancaria del titular sin tener que pagar intereses.

debridement Removal of foreign material and dead, damaged tissue from a wound.
desbridamiento Eliminación de materiales extraños y tejidos muertos y deteriorados de una herida.

decedent A legal term used to represent a deceased person.
difunto Término legal usado para referirse a una persona muerta.

decode To convert, as in a message, into intelligible form; to recognize and interpret.
decodificar Convertir la información, como en un mensaje, de modo que sea inteligible; reconocer e interpretar.

decubitus ulcer A sore or ulcer over a bony prominence that is due to ischemia from prolonged pressure; a bed sore.
úlcera por decúbito Llaga o úlcera sobre una prominencia ósea debida a una isquemia por presión prolongada; escara.

deductible A specific amount of money a patient must pay out-of-pocket, up front before the insurance carrier begins paying. Often this amount is in the range of from $100 to $1000. This deductible amount must be met on a yearly or per incident basis.
deducible Cantidad de dinero específica que un paciente debe pagar de su bolsillo antes de que la compañía de seguros comience a pagar. Con frecuencia esta suma está entre 100 y 1000 dólares. Esta cantidad deducible ha de satisfacerse anualmente o por caso.

default A failure to pay financial debts, especially a student loan.
incumplimiento Dejar de pagar deudas financieras, especialmente en un préstamo de estudiante.

defense mechanisms Psychological methods of dealing with stressful situations that are encountered in day-to-day living.
mecanismos de defensa Métodos psicológicos de hacer frente a situaciones tensas que surgen en la vida diaria.

deferment A postponement, especially of a student loan.
aplazamiento Postergación de un pago, especialmente en un préstamo de estudiante.

defibrillator Machine used to deliver electroshock to the heart through electrodes placed on the chest wall.
desfibrilador Máquina usada para dar un electrochoque al corazón por medio de electrodos colocados en la pared torácica.

deficiencies Conditions caused by a below-normal intake of a particular substance.
deficiencias Estados causados por un consumo menor del normal de una sustancia específica.

demeanor Behavior toward others; outward manner.
conducta Comportamiento hacia los demás; comportamiento que se exterioriza.

demographic The statistical characteristics of human populations (as in age or income), used especially to identify markets.
dato demográfico Característica estadística de la población humana (como edad o ingresos), que se usa sobre todo para identificar mercados.

detrimental Obviously harmful or damaging.
perjudicial Que es obvio que causa daño o perjuicio.

device driver The program or commands given to a device connected to a computer, which enable the device to function. For instance, a printer may come equipped with a software program that must be loaded onto the computer first, so that the printer will work.
controlador de dispositivo Programa que controla un dispositivo conectado a una computadora y que hace que dicho dispositivo pueda funcionar. Por ejemplo, una impresora puede estar equipada con un programa que primero ha de cargarse en la computadora para que ésta funcione.

diabetes mellitus type 2 Inability to utilize glucose for energy due to either a lack of insulin production in the pancreas or resistance to insulin on the cellular level.
diabetes mellitus tipo 2 Incapacidad de utilizar la glucosa para producir energía, debido a una falta de producción de insulina en el páncreas o a una resistencia a la insulina en el nivel celular.

diagnosis Concise technical description of the cause, nature, or manifestations of a condition or problem. *Initial:* Physician's temporary impression, sometimes called a *working diagnosis. Differentiated diagnosis:* comparison of two or more diseases with similar signs and symptoms. *Final:* Conclusion physician reaches after evaluating all findings, including laboratory and other test results.
diagnóstico Descripción técnica y concisa de la causa, naturaleza o manifestaciones de una enfermedad o problema. *Inicial:* Impresión momentánea del médico, a veces se llama *diagnóstico de trabajo. Diagnóstico diferenciado:* comparación de dos o más enfermedades con signos y síntomas similares. *Final:* Conclusión médica a la que se llega tras evaluar todos los datos, incluyendo los resultados de análisis de laboratorio y otras pruebas.

"diagnosis" The determination of the nature of a disease, injury, or congenital defect.
"diagnóstico" Determinación del origen de una enfermedad, lesión o defecto congénito.

diaphoresis The profuse excretion of sweat.
diaforesis Excreción profusa de sudor.

diaphysis Middle portion of a long bone containing the medullary cavity.
diafisis Parte intermedia de un hueso largo en la que está la cavidad medular.

dictation The act or manner of uttering words to be transcribed.
dictado Acción de pronunciar palabras para que sean transcritas.

diction The choice of words, especially with regard to clearness, correctness, and effectiveness.
dicción Acción de elegir las palabras, especialmente para lograr claridad, corrección y eficacia en el discurso.

digestion Process of converting food into chemical substances that can be used by the body.
digestión Proceso de transformar alimentos en sustancias químicas que pueden ser usadas por el cuerpo.

Digital Subscriber Lines (DSL) High speed, sophisticated modulation schemes that operate over existing copper telephone wiring systems; often referred to as "last-mile technologies" because DSL is used for connections from a telephone switching station to a home or office, and not between switching stations.
Línea de Abonado Digital (DSL) Sofisticado sistema de modulación de alta velocidad que opera en sistemas de cableado telefónicos de cobre ya existentes; con frecuencia se habla del DSL como "tecnología de las últimas millas" porque se utiliza para conexiones entre un centro de conmutación telefónica y un hogar u oficina, y no entre centros de conmutación.

Digital Versatile Disk (DVD) The DVD is an optical disk that holds approximately 28 times more information than a CD, and is most commonly used to hold full length movies. Compared to a CD which holds approximately 600 megabytes, a DVD has the capacity to hold approximately 4.7 gigabytes.
Disco Digital Versátil (DVD) El DVD es un disco óptico con capacidad para almacenar unas

28 veces más información que un CD; su uso más común es para guardar películas de larga duración. Mientras que un CD puede almacenar unos 600 megabytes, un DVD tiene una capacidad aproximada de almacenamiento de 4.7 gigabytes.

dilatation Opening or widening the circumference of a body orifice with a dilating instrument.
dilatación Proceso de abrir o ensanchar un orificio corporal con un instrumento dilatador.

dilation The opening of the cervix through the process of labor; measured as 0 to 10 centimeters dilated.
dilatación Ensanchamiento del cuello del útero durante el proceso del parto; se mide en centímetros, de 0 a 10.

dilation & curettage The widening of the cervix and scraping of the endometrial wall of the uterus.
dilatación y curetaje Proceso de hacer más ancho el cuello del útero y raspar su pared endometrial.

diluent A liquid used to dilute a specimen or reagent.
diluyente Líquido usado para diluir un espécimen o un reactivo.

dingy claim A claim that is put on hold because it lacks certain adjunction that allows it to be processed, often due to system changes.
reclamación oscura Reclamación en espera de ser procesada debido a que se necesita alguna información o elemento adicional, con frecuencia, debido a cambios en el sistema.

diplopia Double vision.
diplopía Visión doble.

direct filing system A filing system in which materials can be located without consulting an intermediary source of reference.
sistema directo de archivo Sistema de archivo en el cual los materiales pueden ser localizados sin consultar una fuente de referencia intermedia.

dirty claim Claims that contain errors or omissions that cannot be processed or that must be processed by hand due to OCR scanner rejection.
reclamación sucia Reclamación con errores u omisiones que no puede procesarse o que debe procesarse manualmente debido a que el escáner OCR la rechaza.

disbursements Funds paid out.
desembolsos Dinero o fondos que se pagan.

discretion The quality of being discrete; having or showing good judgment or conduct, especially in speech.
discreción Calidad de discreto; tener sensatez o tacto al obrar, especialmente al hablar.

disease Pathologic process having a descriptive set of signs and symptoms.
enfermedad Proceso patológico que tiene una serie descriptiva de signos y síntomas.

disinfection Destruction of **pathogens** by physical or chemical means.
desinfección Destrucción de **agentes patógenos** con medios físicos o químicos.

disk A magnetic surface that is capable of storing computer programs.
disco Superficie magnética capaz de almacenar programas de computadora.

disk drives Devices that load a program or data stored on a disk into the computer.
unidades de discos Dispositivos que cargan en la computadora un programa o datos almacenados en un disco.

disorder A disruption of normal system functions.
trastorno Interrupción de las funciones normales de un sistema.

disparaging Speaking slightingly about something or someone, with a negative or degrading tone.
menospreciar Hablar con desdén de algo o alguien, con un tono negativo o degradante.

disposition The tendency of something or someone to act in a certain manner under given circumstances.
disposición Tendencia de algo o alguien a actuar de un modo específico en determinadas circunstancias.

disruption A breaking down, or throwing into disorder.
disrupción Interrupción o creación de un estado de trastorno.

dissect To cut or separate tissue with a cutting instrument or scissors.
diseccionar Cortar o separar tejidos con tijeras u otro instrumento cortante.

dissection To separate into pieces and expose parts for scientific examination.
disección Separar en piezas y dejar las partes a la vista para realizar un estudio científico.

disseminate To disperse throughout.
diseminar Dispersar, esparcir.

disseminate To disburse; to spread around.
diseminado Suelto, esparcido.

diurnal rhythm Patterns of activity or behavior that follow day-night cycles.
ritmo diurno Patrones de actividad o comportamiento que siguen a los ciclos nocturnos.

docket A formal record of judicial proceedings; a list of legal causes to be tried.
orden del día Registro formal de procesos judiciales; lista de causas legales a juzgar.

domestic mail Mail that is sent within the boundaries of the United States and its territories.
correo nacional Correo que se envía dentro de los límites de Estados Unidos y sus territorios.

dosimeter Badge for monitoring exposure to radiation of personnel.
dosímetro Placa para controlar la exposición a la radiación del personal.

drawee Bank or facility on whom a check is drawn or written.
librado Banco o entidad contra la que se gira o emite un cheque.

due process A fundamental, constitutional guarantee that all legal proceedings will be fair, that one will be given notice of the proceedings and an opportunity to be heard before the government acts to take away life, liberty, or property; a constitutional guarantee that a law will not be unreasonable or arbitrary.
proceso debido Garantía fundamental constitucional de que todos los procesos legales serán justos, que las partes implicadas serán notificadas de los procedimientos y que se les dará la oportunidad de ser escuchados **rantes** que el gobierno les quite su vida, libertad o propiedad; garantía constitucional de que la ley no irá en contra de la razón ni será arbitraria.

duty Obligatory tasks, conduct, service, or functions that arise from one's position, as in life or in a group.
deber Tareas, conducta, servicio o funciones de carácter obligatorio que conlleva el ocupar un puesto, en la vida o como miembro de un grupo.

dyspnea Difficult or painful breathing.
disnea Respiración difícil o dolorosa.

e-banking Electronic banking via computer modem or over the Internet.
banca electrónica Operaciones bancarias a través del módem de una computadora o en Internet.

ecchymosis A hemorrhagic skin discoloration, commonly called bruising.
equimosis Descoloramient o hemorrágico de la piel comúnmente conocido como magulladura.

eCommerce A term used to describe the sale and purchase of goods and services over the Internet; doing business over the Internet; an abbreviation for "electric commerce."
comercio electrónico Expresión que se usa para describir la compra y venta de bienes y servicios a través de Internet; hacer negocios a través de Internet. Se conoce también con la abreviatura de comercio-e.

edema Abnormal accumulation of fluid in the interstitial spaces of tissue; swelling between layers of tissue.
edema Acumulación anómala de fluido en los espacios intersticiales de los tejidos; inflamación entre capas de tejidos.

effacement The thinning of the cervix during labor, measured in percentages from 0 to 100 percent effaced.
borramiento Adelgazamiento del cuello del útero durante el parto. Se mide en porcentaje, borrado de 0 a 100 por ciento.

elastic pulse Pulse with regular alterations of weak and strong beats, without changes in cycle.
pulso elástico Pulso con alteraciones regulares de latidos fuertes y débiles sin cambios en el ciclo.

elastin Essential part of elastic connective tissue that, when moist, is flexible and elastic.
elastina Parte esencial del tejido conectivo elástico que cuando está húmedo es flexible y elástico.

electrodesiccation Destructive drying of cells and tissue by means of short, high-frequency electrical sparks.
electrodesecación Secado destructivo de células y tejidos por medio de cortas descargas eléctricas de alta frecuencia.

electrolytes Small molecules that conduct an electrical charge. Electrolytes are necessary for proper functioning of muscle and nerve cells.
electrolitos Pequeñas moléculas que conducen una carga eléctrica. Los electrolitos son necesarios para un funcionamiento correcto de los músculos y las células nerviosas.

electronic claims Claims that are submitted to insurance processing facilities using a computerized medium such as direct data entry, direct wire, dial-in telephone digital fax, or personal computer download/upload.
reclamación electrónica Reclamaciones enviadas al lugar de procesamiento de la compañía aseguradora usando un sistema computarizado, tales como entrada de datos directa, cable directo, fax digital con marcado telefónico, o a través de una computadora personal.

e-mail Communications transmitted via computer using a modem.
correo electrónico Comunicaciones transmitidas a través de una computadora usando un módem.

emancipated minor A person under legal age who is self-supporting and living apart from parents or guardian.
menor emancipado Persona que no ha alcanzado la mayoría de edad legal y que se mantiene a sí misma y vive sin la custodia de padres o tutores.

embezzlement Stealing from an employer; appropriation without permission of goods, services, or funds for personal use.
desfalco Robo a un empleador; apropiación sin permiso de bienes, servicios o fondos para uso personal.

embolization Interventional technique using a catheter to block off a blood vessel to prevent hemorrhage.
embolización Técnica de intervención usando un catéter para bloquear un vaso sanguíneo y evitar una hemorragia.

embolus Foreign material blocking a blood vessel, frequently a blood clot that has broken away from some other part of the body.
émbolo Material extraño que bloquea un vaso sanguíneo, con frecuencia un coágulo de sangre procedente de otra parte del cuerpo.

emetic A substance that causes vomiting.
emético Sustancia que causa vómito.

emisor Person who writes a check.
emisor Persona que emite un cheque.

empathy Sensitivity to the individual needs and reactions of patients.
empatía Sensibilidad ante las necesidades y reacciones individuales de los pacientes.

emphysema Pathologic accumulation of air in the tissues or organs; in the lungs, the bronchioles become plugged with mucus and lose elasticity.
enfisema Acumulación patológica de aire en los tejidos u órganos; en los pulmones, los bronquiolos se obstruyen con mucosidade y pierden elasticidad.

emulsification Dispersement of ingested fats into small globules by bile.
emulsionamiento Dispersión (llevada a cabo por la bilis) en pequeños glóbulos de las grasas ingeridas.

encode To convert from one system of communication to another; to convert a message into code.
codificar Convertir de un sistema de comunicación a otro; convertir un mensaje en un código.

encounter Any contact between a healthcare provider and a patient that results in treatment or evaluation of the patient's condition, not limited to in-person contact.
encuentro Cualquier contacto entre un proveedor de atención sanitaria y un paciente que resulta en un tratamiento o evaluación del estado del paciente; no se limita a un contacto personal.

encroachments To advance beyond the usual or proper limits.
intrusiones Ir más allá de los límites habituales o apropiados.

endemic Disease or microorganism that is specific to a particular geographic area.
endémico Enfermedad o microorganismo que es específico de una zona geográfica en particular.

endocervical curettage The scraping of cells from the wall of the uterus.
curetaje endocervical Raspado de células de la pared uterina.

endorser Person who signs his or her name on the back of a check for the purpose of transferring title to another person.
endosante Persona que firma en la parte posterior de un cheque a fin de transferir la propiedad del mismo a otra persona.

enteric-coated An oral medication with a coating that resists the effects of stomach juices; designed so medicine is absorbed in the small intestine; drug formulation in which tablets are coated with a special compound that does not dissolve until the tablet is exposed to the fluids of the small intestine
cubierta entérica Capa exterior que se añade a un medicamento que se toma por vía oral, la cual es resistente a los efectos de los jugos gástricos; recubrimiento diseñado para que la medicina sea absorbida en el intestino delgado; formulación usada en medicinas en la cual las tabletas se recubren con un componente especial que no se disuelve hasta que la tableta es expuesta a los fluidos del intestino delgado.

enunciate To utter articulate sounds; the act of being very distinct in speech.
articular Pronunciar los sonidos de manera cuidada; hablar de una forma muy clara.

enunciation The utterane of articulate, clear sounds; the act of being very distinct in speech.
articulación Pronunciación cuidada, con sonidos claros.

enzymatic reaction Chemical reaction controlled by an enzyme.
reacción enzimática Reacción química controlada por una enzima.

enzyme Any of several complex proteins produced by cells that act as catalysts in specific biochemical reactions.
enzima Cualquiera de las varias proteínas complejas que producen las células y que actúan como catalíticos en reacciones bioquímicas específicas.

epiphysis End of a long bone.
epífisis Extremo de un hueso largo.

erythropoietin Substance released from the kidney and liver that promotes red blood cell formation.
eritropoyetina Sustancia liberada por los riñones y el hígado y que promueve la formación de glóbulos rojos.

essential hypertension Elevated blood pressure of unknown cause that develops for no apparent reason; sometimes called *primary hypertension.*
hipertensión esencial Presión sanguínea alta de causa desconocida que surge sin razón aparente; a veces se llama *hipertensión primaria.*

established patients Patients who are returning to the office and who have previously seen the physician.
pacientes establecidos Pacientes que regresan al consultorio médico que ya han sido atendidos por el médico con anterioridad.

etiology Classifying a claim according to the cause of the disorder.
etiología Clasificación de una reclamación según la causa del trastorno.

eukaryote A single-celled or multicellular organism whose cells contain a distinct membrane-bound nucleus.
eucariote Organismo unicelular o multicelular cuyas células tienen un núcleo diferenciado **rodeado** por una membrana.

euthanasia The act or practice of killing or permitting the death of hopelessly sick or injured individuals in a relatively painless way for reasons of mercy.
eutanasia Acción o práctica de matar o permitir la muerte de enfermos o heridos en estado terminal, de una forma relativamente sin dolor, por razones de piedad.

exacerbation An increase in the seriousness of a disease marked by greater intensity in the signs and symptoms. Worsening of disease symptoms.
exacerbación Aumento en la gravedad de una enfermedad, caracterizado por una mayor intensidad de los signos y síntomas. Empeoramiento de los síntomas de una enfermedad.

"excludes" Exclusion terms are always written in italics, and the word "Excludes" is enclosed in a box to draw particular attention to these instructions. Exclusion terms may apply to a chapter, a section, a category, or a subcategory.

The applicable code number usually follows the exclusion term.
"excluye" Las expresiones de exclusión siempre se escriben en cursiva y la palabra "Excluye" se encierra en una casilla para llamar la atención acerca de estas instrucciones. Los términos de exclusión pueden ser aplicables a un capítulo, una sección, una categoría o una subcategoría. El número de código correspondiente por lo general sigue al término de exclusión.

expediency A situation requiring haste or caution; a means of achieving a particular end.
prontitud Situación que requiere actuar con prisa o precaución; un medio de alcanzar un fin específico.

expert witness A person who provides testimony to a court as an expert in a certain field or subject to verify facts presented by one or both sides in a lawsuit, often compensated and used to refute or disprove the claims of one party.
testigo perito Persona que da testimonio ante un tribunal como perito o experto en cierto campo o tema para verificar los hechos presentados por una o ambas partes en litigio, a menudo, cobrando una retribución económica, y cu yo testimonio suele usarse para refutar o impugnar las demandas de una de las partes.

external noise Noise outside the brain that interferes with the communication process.
ruido externo Ruido producido fuera del cerebro y que interfiere con el proceso de comunicación.

externalization To attribute an event or occurrence to causes outside the self.
exteriorización Acción de atribuir a un suceso o acontecimiento causas externas al mismo.

externship/internship A training program that is part of a course of study of an educational institution and is taken in the actual business setting in that field of study; these terms are often interchanged in reference to medical assisting.
prácticas internas/externas Programa de entrenamiento que es parte de un curso de estudio de una institución educativa y se sigue en un lugar real de trabajo en el campo de estudio; estos términos se intercambian cuando se refieren a los asistentes médicos.

exudates Fluids with high concentration of protein and cellular debris that has escaped from the blood vessels and has been deposited in tissues or on tissue surfaces.
exudados Fluidos con una alta concentración de proteínas y restos celulares extravasados de los vasos sanguíneos y depositados en los tejidos o en sus superficies.

familial Occurring in or affecting members of a family more than would be expected by chance.
familiar Que sucede o afecta a miembros de una familia más de lo que podría esperarse por azar.

fascia Sheet or band of fibrous tissue located deep in the skin that covers muscles and body organs.
fascia Lámina o banda de tejido fibroso localizada bajo la piel y que cubre los músculos y los órganos.

fastidious Requiring specialized media or growth factors to grow.
exigente Que requiere un medio o factores especiales para crecer.

fat Stored as adipose tissue in the body and serving as a concentrated energy reserve.
grasa Sustancia que se almacena como tejido adiposo en el cuerpo y sirve como reserva de energía concentrada.

fax Abbreviation for facsimile; a document sent using a fax machine.
fax Abreviatura de facsímile; documento que se envía usando una máquina de fax.

febrile Pertaining to an elevated body temperature.
febril Perteneciente o relativo a una temperatura corporal elevada.

fecalith A hard, impacted mass of feces in the colon.
fecaloma Masa de heces endurecidas e impactadas en el colon.

fee profile A compilation or average of physician fees over a given period of time.
perfil de cargo s Recopilación o porcentaje de cargos médicos en un periodo de tiempo dado.

fee schedule A compilation of preestablished fee allowances for given services or procedures.
escala de cargos Recopilación de asignaciones de cargos preestablecidos para servicios o procedimientos dados.

feedback The transmission of evaluative or corrective information to the original or controlling source about an action, event, or process.
reacciones y comentarios Envío de información de evaluación o corrección a la fuente original o a la que ejerce el control sobre una acción, suceso o proceso.

felony A major crime, such as murder, rape, or burglary; punishable by a more stringent sentence than that given for a misdemeanor.
crimen Delito mayor, como asesinato, violación o robo; se penaliza con una sentencia más severa que un delito menor o falta.

fermentation An enzymatically controlled transformation of an organic compound.
fermentación Transformación de un compuesto orgánico controlada por enzimas.

fervent Exhibiting or marked by great intensity of feeling.
ferviente Que posee sentimientos de gran intensidad o que da muestra de ellos.

fibrillation Rapid, random, ineffective contractions of the Herat.
fibrilación Contracciones cardiacas rápidas, aleatorias e inefectivas.

fidelity Faithfulness to something to which one is bound by pledge or duty.
fidelidad Fe en algo a lo que se está unido por juramento o deber.

filtrate Fluid that remains after a liquid is passed through a membranous filter.
filtrado Fluido que queda después de pasar un líquido a través de un filtro membranoso.

fine A sum imposed as punishment for an offense; a forfeiture or penalty paid to an injured party or the government in a civil or criminal action.
multa Suma impuesta como penalización por un delito menor; suma que se paga a una parte a la que se ha perjudicado o dañado, o al gobierno, en un proceso civil o penal.

fiscal agent An organization or private plan under contract to the government to act as financial representatives in handling insurance claims from providers of health care; also referred to as fiscal intermediary.
agente fiscal Organización o plan privado bajo contrato con el gobierno para actuar como representantes financieros en la administración de reclamaciones de seguros por parte de proveedores de atención sanitaria; también se conoce como intermediario fiscal.

fiscal intermediary An organization that contracts with the government and other insuring entities to handle and mediate insurance claims from medical facilities.
intermediario fiscal Organización que establece un contrato con el gobierno y otras entidades aseguradoras para administrar reclamaciones de seguro provenientes de centros médicos y para mediar en ellas.

fissures Narrow slits or clefts in the abdominal wall.
fisuras Grietas o hendiduras estrechas en la pared abdominal.

fistulas Abnormal, tubelike passages within the body tissue, usually between two internal organs, or from an internal organ to the body surface.
fístulas Pasajes anómalos en forma de tubos entre los tejidos corporales, por lo general entre dos órganos internos, o de un órgano interno a la superficie del cuerpo.

flagged Marked in some way so as to remind or remember that specific action needs to be taken.
señalado Marcado de alguna forma para recordar que se necesita que se tomen medidas al respeto.

flash Animation technology often used on the opening page of a Web site used to draw attention, excite, and impress the user.
flash Tecnología de imágenes animadas que se usa con frecuencia en la página inicial de un sitio web para llamar la atención del usuario, entusiasmarlo e impresionarlo.

flatus Gas expelled through the anus.
flato Gas expulsado a través del ano.

fluoroscopy Direct observation of the x-ray image in motion.
fluoroscopía Observación directa de una imagen de rayos x en movimiento.

flush Directly abutting or immediately adjacent, as set even with an edge of a type page or column; having no indention.
alineado Directamente contiguo o inmediatamente adyacente, ordenado de forma regular en relación con un borde de una página o columna; sin sangría o espacios en blanco.

follicle-stimulating hormone (FSH) A hormone secreted by the anterior pituitary; stimulates oogenesis and spermatogenesis.
hormona foliculoestimulante (FSH) Hormona que segrega la pituitaria anterior y que estimula los procesos de formación y desarrollo de óvulos y de espermatozoides.

font A design, as in typesetting, for a set of characters.
fuente tipográfica Diseño similar al de la composición para un conjunto de caracteres.

format To magnetically create tracks on a disk where information will be stored, usually done by the manufacturer of the disk.
formatear Crear pistas magnéticas en un disco destinado a almacenar información; por lo general, el fabricante del disco es quien se encarga de hacerlo.

fovea centralis A small pit in the center of the retina that is considered the center of clearest vision.
fóvea central Pequeña concavidad en el centro de la retina que se cree que es el centro de visión más claro.

frontal projection Radiographic view in which the coronal plane of the body or body part is parallel to the film plane; AP or PA.
proyección frontal Vista radiográfica en la cual el plano coronal del cuerpo o de la parte del cuerpo está paralelo al plano de la película; AP o PA.

gait Manner or style of walking.
andares Forma o estilo de caminar.

gamete A mature male or female germ cell, usually possessing a haploid chromosome set and capable of initiating formation of a new diploid individual.
gameto Célula germinal madura, tanto masculina como femenina, que por lo general tiene un conjunto cromosómico haploide y es capaz de iniciar la formación de un nuevo individuo diploide.

gangrene Death of body tissue due to loss of nutritive supply and followed by bacteria invasion and putrefaction.
gangrena Muerte de tejido corporal debido a la pérdida de suministro de nutrientes por invasión bacteriana y putrefacción.

gantry Doughnut-shaped portion of a scanner than surrounds the patient and that functions, at least in part, to gather imaging data.
gantry Parte de un escáner con forma de rosquilla que rodea al paciente y funciona, al menos en parte, reuniendo datos de formación de imágenes.

generic Drugs that are not protected by trademark.
genéricas Medicinas que no están protegidas por una marca registrada.

genome The genetic material of an organism.
genoma El material genético de un organismo.

genuineness Expressing sincerity and honest feeling.
autenticidad Expresión de sentimientos sincera y honrada.

germicides Agents that destroy **pathogenic** organisms.
germicidas Agentes químicos que destruyen o matan organismos **patógenos**.

gigabyte Approximately one billion bytes.
gigabyte Aproximadamente, mil millones de bytes.

girth A measure around a body or item.
contorno Medida alrededor de un cuerpo o artículo.

glean To gather information or material bit by bit; to pick over in search of relevant material.
recopilar Reunir información o material pedazo a pedazo; examinar en busca de material pertinente.

glucagon A hormone produced by the alpha cells of the pancreatic islets; stimulates the liver to convert glycogen into glucose.
glucagón Hormona producida por las células alfa de los islotes pancreáticos; estimula al hígado para que convierta el glucógeno en glucosa.

glucosuria The abnormal presence of glucose in the urine.
glucosuria Presencia anómala de glucosa en la orina.

glycogen The sugar (starch) formed from glucose and stored mainly in the liver.
glucógeno Azúcar (almidón) formado a partir de la glucosa y almacenado principalmente en el hígado.

glycohemoglobin or hemoglobin A1c A type of hemoglobin that is made slowly during the 120-day life span of the red blood cell (RBC). Glycohemoglobin makes up 3 to 6 percent of hemoglobin in a normal RBC, in diabetes mellitus it makes up to 12 percent.
glucohemoglobina o hemoglobina A1c Tipo de hemoglobina que se produce lentamente durante el periodo de los 120 días de vida de los glóbulos rojos (RBC). La glucohemoglobina constituye de un 3 a un 6 por ciento de la hemoglobina en un RBC normal; en los casos de diabetes mellitus constituye hasta un 12 por ciento.

glycosuria Presence of glucose in the urine.
glucosuria Presencia de glucosa en la orina.

goniometer Instrument for measuring the degrees of motion in a joint.
goniómetro Instrumento para medir los grados de movimiento de una articulación.

government plan An insurance or health care plan that is sponsored and/or subsidized by the state or federal government, such as Medicaid and Medicare.
plan del gobierno Seguro o plan de atención sanitaria patrocinado y subvencionado por el gobierno estatal o federal, como Medicaid y Medicare.

grammar The study of the classes of words, their inflections, and their functions and relations in the sentence; a study of what is to be preferred and what avoided in inflection and syntax.
gramática Estudio de las clases de palabras, sus desinencias y sus funciones y relaciones en la oración; estudio del uso que se prefiere y de lo que hay que evitar en cuanto a desinencias y sintaxis.

gray (Gy) International unit of radiation dose.
gray (Gy) Unidad internacional de dosis de radiación.

grief An unfortunate outcome; a deep distress caused by bereavement.
pesar Resultado desafortunado; profunda aflicción causada por la pérdida de un ser querido.

group policy Insurance written under a policy that covers a number of people under a single master contract issued to their employer or to an association with which they are affiliated.
póliza de grupo Seguro contratado bajo una póliza que cubre a varias personas bajo un único contrato maestro establecido con su empleador o con una asociación a la que estén afiliados.

growth hormone (GH) Also called somatotropic hormone, stimulates tissue growth and restricts tissue glucose dependence when nutrients are not available.
hormona del crecimiento (GH) También llamada hormona somatotrópica, estimula el crecimiento de los tejidos y restringe la dependencia de la glucosa de los tejidos cuando no hay nutrientes disponibles.

guarantor A person who makes or gives a guarantee of payment for a bill.
garante Persona que paga una factura o que garantiza su pago.

guardian ad litem Legal representative for a minor.
tutor ad litem Representante legal de un menor.

hard copy The readable paper copy or printout of information.
copia impresa Copia impresa en papel o impresión de la información.

harmonious Marked by accord in sentiment or action; having the parts agreeably related.
armonioso Caracterizado por una armonía en los sentimientos o acciones; partes de un todo relacionadas de forma agradable.

health insurance Protection in return for periodic premiums, which provides reimbursement of monetary losses due to illness or injury. Included under this heading are various types of insurance such as accident insurance, disability income insurance, medical expense insurance, and accidental death and dismemberment insurance. Also known as accident and health insurance or disability income insurance.
seguro de enfermedad Cobertura a cambio del pago de primas periódicas, la cual proporciona el reembolso de las pérdidas monetarias debidas a enfermedad o lesión. Bajo este nombre se incluyen varios tipos de seguros como seguro de accidente, seguro de incapacidad, seguro de gastos médicos y seguro en caso de muerte y pérdida de extremidades. También se conoce como seguro de accidente y enfermedad o seguro de incapacidad.

hematemesis Vomiting of bright red blood, indicating rapid upper gastrointestinal bleeding, associated with esophageal varices or peptic ulcer.
hematemesis Vómito de sangre roja brillante que indica hemorragia rápida del sistema gastrointestinal superior, relacionado con varices esofágicas o úlcera péptica.

hematocrit The percentage by volume of packed red blood cells in a given sample of blood after centrifugation. Volume percentage of erythrocytes in whole blood.
hematocrito Porcentaje por volumen de glóbulos rojos en una muestra de sangre dada después de ser centrifugada. Porcentaje del volumen de eritrocitos en la sangre completa.

hematoma A sac filled with blood that may be the result of trauma.
hematoma Saco lleno de sangre que puede ser el resultado de una lesión.

hematuria Blood in the urine.
hematuria Sangre en la orina.

hemoconcentration A situation in which the concentration of blood cells is increased in proportion to the plasma.
hemoconcentración Situación en la cual la concentración de glóbulos rojos ha aumentado en proporción al plasma.

hemoglobin Protein found in erythrocytes that transports molecular oxygen in the blood.
hemoglobina Proteína que se encuentra en los eritrocitos que transportan el oxígeno en la sangre.

hemolysis The destruction or dissolution of red blood cells, with subsequent release of hemoglobin.
hemolisis Destrucción o disolución de los glóbulos rojos, con la subsiguiente liberación de hemoglobina.

hemolyzed A term used to describe a blood sample in which the red blood cells have ruptured.
hemolizado Término usado para describir una muestra de sangre en la cual los glóbulos rojos se han roto.

hepatomegaly Abnormal enlargement of the liver.
hepatomegalia Agrandamiento anómalo del hígado.

hereditary Pertaining to a characteristic, condition, or disease transmitted from parent to offspring on the DNA chain.
hereditario Perteneciente o relativo a una característica, estado o enfermedad transmitida de padres a hijos en la cadena de ADN.

hermetically sealed Sealed so no air is allowed to enter or escape.
herméticamente sellado Sellado de forma que el aire no pueda entrar o escapar.

HMO An organization that provides a wide range of comprehensive health care services for a specified group at a fixed periodic payment. HMOs can be sponsored by the government, medical schools, hospitals, employers, labor unions, consumer groups, insurance companies, and hospital-medical plans.
HMO Organización que proporciona una amplia gama de servicios completos de atención sanitaria para un grupo específico por un pago periódico fijado. Las HMO puedes estar patrocinadas por el gobierno, facultades de medicina, hospitales, patronos, sindicatos laborales, grupos de consumidores, compañías aseguradoras y planes médico-hospitalarios.

holder Person presenting a check for payment.
portador Persona que presenta un cheque para cobrarlo.

holistic Related to or concerned with all of the systems of the body, rather than breaking it down into parts.
holístico Relacionado con todos los sistemas corporales y no dividido en partes.

homeostasis Maintenance of constant internal ambient conditions compatible with life.
homeostasis Mantenimiento de unas condiciones ambientales internas constantes compatibles con la vida.

homeostatic Maintaining a constant internal environment.
homeostático Que mantiene un ambiente interno constante.

hormone A substance, usually a peptide or steroid, produced by one tissue and conveyed by the bloodstream to another to effect physiological activity such as growth or metabolism; a chemical transmitter produced by the body and transported to target tissue or organs by the bloodstream.
hormona Sustancia química transmisora, por lo general un péptido o un esteroide, que es producida por un tejido y transportada por la corriente sanguínea hasta el tejido u órgano objetivo para provocar un efecto en la actividad fisiológica, como el crecimiento o el metabolismo.

HTML Abbreviation for hypertext markup language, which is the language used to create documents for use on the Internet.
HTML Abreviatura de lenguaje de marcas de hipertexto, que es el lenguaje que se emplea para crear documentos destinados a usarse en Internet.

HTTP Abbreviation for hypertext transfer protocol, which defines how messages are defined and transmitted over the Internet; when a URL is entered into the computer, an HTTP command tells the Web server to retrieve the requested Web page.
HTTP Abreviatura de protocolo de transporte de hipertexto, que define cómo se interpretan y transmiten los mensajes en Internet; cuando un URL entra en la computadora, una orden de HTTP manda la señal al servidor web para que busque la página web que se solicita.

Hub A common connection point for devices in a network containing multiple ports, often used to connect segments of a LAN.
Nodo Punto de conexión común para dispositivos en una red de conexiones de varios puertos; suele usar se para conectar segmentos de una LAN (red de área local).

hydrocephaly Enlargement of the cranium caused by abnormal accumulation of cerebrospinal fluid within the cerebral system.
hidrocefalia Agrandamiento del cráneo causado por una acumulación anómala de fluido cerebroespinal en el interior del sistema cerebral.

hydrogenated Combined with, treated with, or exposed to hydrogen.
hidrogenado Combinado con hidrógeno, tratado con él o expuesto a él.

hyperlipidemia Excess of fats or lipids in the blood plasma.
hiperlipemia Exceso de grasas o lípidos en el plasma sanguíneo.

hyperplasia An increase in the number of cells.
hiperplasia Aumento del número de células.

hyperpnea Increase in the depth of breathing.
hiperpnea Aumento en la profundidad de la respiración.

hypertension High blood pressure (systolic pressure consistently above 140 mm Hg and diastolic pressure above 90 mm Hg).
hipertensión Presión sanguínea alta (presión sistólica continuamente por encima de 140 mm Hg y presión diastólica por encima de 90 mm Hg).

hyperventilation Abnormally prolonged and deep breathing, usually associated with acute anxiety or emotional tension.
hiperventilación Respiración profunda anómalamente prolongada, que suele estar asociada con una ansiedad aguda o con tensión emocional.

hypotension Blood pressure that is below normal (systolic pressure below 90 mm Hg and diastolic pressure below 50 mm Hg).
hipotensión Presión sanguínea que está por debajo de lo normal (presión sistólica por debajo de 90 mm Hg y presión diastólica por debajo de 50 mm Hg).

icon A picture, often on the desktop of a computer, which represents a program or object. By clicking on the icon, the user is directed to the program.
icono Dibujo, con frecuencia colocado en el escritorio de la computadora, que representa un programa o un objeto. Al hacer clic sobre el icono, el usuario es llevado a dicho programa.

idealism The practice of forming ideas or living under the influence of ideas.
idealismo Práctica de formarse ideas o vivir bajo la influencia de ideas.

idiopathic Unknown cause
idiopático Causa desconocida.

ileocecal valve Valve guarding the opening between the ileum and cecum; also called the ileocolic valve.
válvula ileocecal Válvula que controla la abertura entre el íleo y el intestino ciego; también se llama válvula ileocólica.

ileostomy Surgical formation of an opening of the ileum onto the surface of the abdomen through which fecal material is emptied.
ileostomía Formación quirúrgica de una abertura del íleo en la superficie del abdomen, a través de la cual se vacían los materiales fecales.

immigrant A person who comes to a country to take up permanent residence.
inmigrante Persona que va a un país para vivir allí de forma permanente.

immunotherapy Administering repeated injections of diluted extracts of the substance that causes an allergy; also called desensitization.
inmunoterapia Administración de repetidas inyecciones de extractos diluidos de la substancia que provoca una alergia; también se conoce como desensibilización.

impenetrable Incapable of being penetrated or pierced; not capable of being damaged or harmed.
impenetrable Que no puede ser penetrado o traspasado; que no puede ser dañado o perjudicado.

implied consent Presumed consent, such as when a patient offers an arm for a phlebotomy procedure.
consentimiento tácito Consentimiento que se supone que ha sido dado, como cuando un paciente presenta el brazo para que se le extraiga sangre.

in vitro Refers to conditions outside of a living body.
in vitro Expresión que se refiere a condiciones exteriores de un ser vivo.

incentive Something that incites or spurs to action; a reward or reason for performing a task.
incentivo Algo que incita o impulsa a actuar; recompensa o razón para llevar a cabo una tarea.

"includes" The appearance of this term under a subdivision such as a category (three-digit code) or two-digit procedure code, indicates that the code and title include these terms. Other terms also classified to that particular code and title are listed in the Alphabetic Indexes.
"incluye" La presencia de esta expresión, cuando aparece bajo una subdivisión, como una categoría (código de tres dígitos) o como un código de procedimiento de dos dígitos, indica que el código y el título incluyen estos términos. En los Índices alfabéticos se enumeran otros términos también clasificados para este código específico.

incontinence Inability to control excretory functions.
incontinencia Incapacidad de controlar las funciones excretoras.

indemnity plan Traditional health insurance plan that pays for all or a share of the cost of covered services, regardless of which doctor, hospital, or other licensed health care provider is used. Policyholders of indemnity plans and their dependents choose when and where to get health care services.
plan de indemnización Plan de seguro de enfermedad tradicional que paga todo o parte del costo de los servicios que cubre, sin importar a qué médico, hospital u otro proveedor de atención sanitaria licenciado se acuda. Los titulares de pólizas de planes de indemnización y las personas que dependen de estos titulares escogen cuándo y dónde recibir atención médica.

indicators An important point or group of statistical values that, when evaluated, indicate the quality of care provided in a healthcare institution.
indicadores Importante punto o grupo de valores estadísticos que al ser evaluados indican la calidad del servicio que se proporciona en una institución de atención sanitaria.

indicted To charge with a crime by the finding or presentment of a jury with due process of law.
acusado Que se le imputa con un cargo criminal por conclusión o acusación de un jurado con el proceso legal debido.

indigent Totally lacking in something of need.
indigente Que carece totalmente de algo necesario.

indirect filing system A filing system in which an intermediary source of reference, such as a card file, must be consulted to locate specific files.
sistema indirecto de archivo Sistema de archivo en el cual debe consultarse una fuente de referencia intermedia, como un fichero, para localizar documentos específicos.

individual policy An insurance policy designed specifically for the use of one person (and his or her dependents) not associated with the amenities of a group policy, namely higher premiums. Often referred to as "personal insurance."
póliza individual Póliza de seguros destinada específicamente a ser usada por una persona (y quienes dependan de ella) y que no conlleva los beneficios de una póliza de grupo y tiene primas más altas. Con frecuencia se le llama "seguro personal".

induration An abnormally hard, inflamed area.
induración Área anómalamente dura, inflamada.

infarction Area of tissue that has died due to lack of blood supply.
infarto Área de tejido que ha muerto debido a una falta de suministro de sangre.

infection Invasion of body tissues by **micro-organisms**, which then proliferate and damage tissues.
infección Invasión de los tejidos corporales por **microorganismos**, los cuales entonces proliferan y dañan los tejidos.

infertile Not fertile or productive; not capable of reproducing.
estéril Que no es fértil o productivo; que no tiene la capacidad de reproducirse.

inflammation Tissue reaction to trauma or disease that includes redness, heat, swelling, and pain.
inflamación Reacción de los tejidos ante una lesión o enfermedad que incluye enrojecimiento, calentamiento, hinchazón y dolor.

inflection A change in pitch or loudness of the voice.
inflexión Cambio en el tono o volumen de la voz.

informed consent A consent in which there is understanding of what treatment is to be undertaken and of the risks involved, why it should be done, and alternative methods of treatment available (including no treatment) and their attendant risks.
consentimiento informado Consentimiento que implica la comprensión del tratamiento al que se va a ser sometido y de los riesgos que conlleva, del porqué de dicho tratamiento, así como la comprensión de los tratamientos alternativos disponibles (incluyendo la ausencia de tratamiento) y los riesgos que conllevan.

infraction Breaking the law; a minor offense of the rules.
infracción Incumplimiento de la ley; delito menor contra las normas establecidas.

initiative The causing or facilitating of the beginning of; the initiation of something into happening.
iniciativa El causar o facilitar el comienzo de algo; el hacer que algo comience a ocurrir.

innate Existing in, belonging to, or determined by factors present in an individual since birth.
innato Que existe en un individuo, que le pertenece o que está determinado por factores existentes en ese individuo desde el momento de su nacimiento.

input Information entered into and used by the computer.
entrada Información introducida en una computadora y que la computadora utiliza.

instigate To goad or urge forward; provoke.
instigar Incitar, exhortar, provocar.

insubordination Disobedience to authority.
insubordinación Desobediencia a la autoridad.

insulin Hormone secreted by the beta cells of the pancreatic islets in response to increased levels of glucose in the blood.
insulina Hormona que segregan las células beta de los islotes pancreáticos en respuesta a la presencia de altos niveles de glucosa en la sangre.

insured A person or organization who is covered by an insurance policy, along with any other parties for whom protection is provided under the policy terms.
asegurado Persona u organización que está cubierta por una póliza de seguro junto con cualquier otro a quien se proporcione cobertura bajo los términos de la póliza.

intangible Incapable of being perceived, especially by touch; incapable of being precisely identified or realized by the mind.
intangible Que no se puede percibir, especialmente que no se puede tocar; que no puede ser identificado con precisión ni ser comprendido por la mente.

integral Essential; being an indispensable part of a whole.
integral Esencial; parte indispensable de un todo.

interaction A two-way communication; mutual or reciprocal action or influence
interacción Comunicación bidireccional; acción o influencia recíproca o mutua.

intercom A two-way communication system with a microphone and loudspeaker at each station for localized use.
intercomunicador Sistema de comunicación bidireccional con un micrófono y un altavoz en cada estación para uso local.

intermittent claudications Recurring cramping in the calves caused by poor circulation of blood to the muscles of the lower leg.
cojeras intermitentes Calambres recurrentes en las pantorrillas causados por una mala circulación de la sangre de los músculos de la parte inferior de la pierna.

intermittent Coming and going at intervals; not continuous
intermitente Que va y viene a intervalos; de forma no continua.

intermittent pulse Pulse in which beats are occasionally skipped.
pulso intermitente Pulso en el cual de vez en cuando se salta algún latido.

internal noise Noise inside the brain that interferes with the communication process.
ruido interno Ruido en el interior del cerebro que interfiere con el proceso de comunicación.

International Classification of Diseases, Ninth Revision, Clinical Modification (ICD-9-CM) System for classifying disease to facilitate collection of uniform and comparable health information for statistical purposes, and for indexing medical records for data storage and retrieval.
Clasificación Internacional de Enfermedades, Novena Revisión, Modificación clínica (ICD-9-CM) Sistema de clasificación de enfermedades para facilitar la recopilación de información médica uniforme, tanto para fines estadísticos como para indexar informes médicos a fin de almacenar y recuperar datos.

International Classification of Diseases, Tenth Revision (ICD-10) System containing the greatest number of changes in ICD's history. To allow more specific reporting of disease and newly recognized conditions, the ICD-10 contains approximately 5,500 more codes than ICD-9.
Clasificación Internacional de Enfermedades, Décima Revisión (ICD-10) Sistema que contiene el mayor número de cambios en la historia de la ICD. Para permitir elaborar informes más precisos de las enfermedades y de los estados patológicos que se conocen sólo recientemente, la ICD-10 incluye aproximadamente 5,500 códigos más que la ICD-9.

international mail Mail that is sent outside the boundaries of the United States and its territories.
correo internacional Correo que se envía fuera de los límites de Estados Unidos y sus territorios.

interval Space of time between events.
intervalo Espacio de tiempo entre dos sucesos.

intolerable Not tolerable or bearable.
intolerable Que no se puede tolerar o soportar.

intravenous urogram (IVU) Radiographic examination of the urinary tract using intravenous injection of an iodine contrast medium.
urograma intravenoso (IVU) Examen radiográfico del tracto urinario usando una inyección intravenosa de un medio de contraste yodado.

intrinsic Belonging to the essential nature or constitution of a thing; indwelling, inward.
intrínseco Que pertenece a la naturaleza o constitución básica de una cosa; inherente, interno.

introspection An inward, reflective examination of one's own thoughts and feelings.
introspección Examen de nuestros propios pensamientos y sentimientos.

invariably Consistently; without changing or being capable of change.
invariablemente De forma constante; que no cambia ni puede cambiar.

invasive Involving entry into the living body, as by incision or insertion of an instrument.
invasivo Que entra en un organismo vivo, como por incisión o inserción de un instrumento.

ipsilateral Pertaining to the same side of the body.
isolateral Perteneciente a la misma parte del cuerpo.

irregular pulse Pulse that varies in force and frequency.
pulso irregular Pulso que varía en fuerza y frecuencia.

ischemia Decreased blood flow to a body part or organ, caused by constriction or plugging of the supplying artery; temporary interruption in blood supply to a tissue or organ.
isquemia Disminución del flujo sanguíneo a una parte del cuerpo u órgano provocada por la constricción o atasco de la arteria suministradora; interrupción temporal del suministro de sangre a un tejido u órgano.

islets (of Langerhans) Cells of the pancreas that produce insulin (beta cells) and glucagon (alpha cells); also called pancreatic islets.
islotes (de Langerhans) Células del páncreas que producen insulina (células beta) y glucagón (células alfa); también llamados islotes pancreáticos

jargon The technical terminology or characteristic idiom of a particular group or special activity.
jerga Terminología técnica o lenguaje característico de un grupo específico o una actividad especial.

jaundice Yellowness of the skin and mucous membranes caused by deposition of bile pigment. It is not a disease, but a symptom of a number of diseases, especially liver disorders.
ictericia Coloración amarilla en la piel y las membranas mucosas causada por deposición del pigmento biliar. No es una enfermedad pero es un síntoma de muchas enfermedades, sobre todo de trastornos hepáticos.

java An object-oriented high-level programming language commonly used and well-suited for the Internet.
java Lenguaje de programación de alto nivel y orientado a objetos que es usado ampliamente y es muy adecuado para Internet.

judicial Of or relating to a judgment, the function of judging, the administration of justice, or the judiciary.
judicial Perteneciente o relativo al juicio, los procesos jurídicos, la administración de justicia o a la judicatura.

jurisdiction A power constitutionally conferred upon a judge or magistrate, to decide cases according to law and to carry sentence into execution. Jurisdiction is original when it is conferred on the court in the first instance (original jurisdiction); it is appellate when an appeal is given from the judgment of another court (apellate jurisdiction).
jurisdicción Poder constitucional otorgado a un juez o magistrado para resolver casos de acuerdo con la ley y hacer que se cumplan las sentencias. Es jurisdicción original cuando se otorga en un tribunal de primera instancia; es jurisdicción en apelación cuando existe una apelación al juicio de otro tribunal.

jurisprudence The science or philosophy of law; a system or body of law, or the course of court decisions.
jurisprudencia Ciencia o filosofía que trata sobre la ley; sistema o cuerpo legal; línea de decisiones de los tribunales.

keratin Very hard, tough protein found in hair, nails, and epidermal tissue.
queratina Proteína muy dura que se encuentra en el pelo, uñas y tejidos epidérmicos.

keratinocytes Any one of the skin cells that synthesize keratin.
queratinocitos Cualquiera de las células de la piel que sintetizan queratina.

ketosis Abnormal production of ketone bodies in the blood and tissues resulting from fat catabolism in cells. Ketones accumulate in large quantities when fat, instead of sugar, is used as fuel for energy in cells.
quetosis Producción anormal de cuerpos de quetosis en la sangre y tejidos como resultado de un catabolismo graso en las células. Los quetones se acumulan en grandes cantidades cuando se usa grasa, en lugar de azúcar, como combustible para las células.

kyphosis Abnormal convex curvature of the thoracic spine region.
cifosis Curvatura convexa anómala de la región espinal torácica.

lacrimation The secretion or discharge of tears.
lagrimeo Secreción o descarga de lágrimas.

language barrier Any type of interference that inhibits the communication process and is related to the difference in languages spoken by the people attempting to communicate.
barrera del idioma Cualquier tipo de interferencia que inhibe el proceso de comunicación y que está relacionado con la diferencia en los idiomas que hablan las personas que intentan comunicarse.

laryngoscopy Visual examination of the voice box area through an endoscope equipped with a light and mirrors for illumination.
laringoscopia Examen visual de la laringe por medio de un endoscopio equipado con una luz y espejos.

latent image Invisible changes in exposed film that will become a visible image when the film is processed.
imagen latente Cambios invisibles en la película que se convertirán en una imagen visible cuando se procese la película.

law A binding custom or practice of a community; a rule of conduct or action prescribed or formally recognized as binding or enforceable by a controlling authority.
ley Costumbre o práctica obligatoria de una comunidad; norma de comportamiento o proceder prescrita o reconocida formalmente como norma obligatoria o que se puede hacer cumplir por una autoridad encargada.

learning style The way that an individual perceives and processes information in order to learn new material.
estilo de aprendizaje Forma en la que un individuo percibe y procesa la información para aprender cosas nuevas.

leukoderma White patches on the skin.
leucodermia Manchas blancas en la piel.

liable Obligated according to law or equity; responsible for an act or circumstance.
responsable Que tiene alguna obligación según la ley o el derecho lato; responsable de un acto o circunstancia.

libel A written defamatory statement or representation that conveys an unjustly unfavorable impression.
libelo Escrito difamatorio que produce una impresión desfavorable injusta.

ligament A tough connective tissue band that holds joints together by attaching to the bones on either side of the joint.
ligamento Banda de tejido conectivo resistente que sostiene las articulaciones uniendo los huesos de cada lado de la articulación.

ligation The process of tying off something to close it—for example, a blood vessel during surgery—with a tie called a ligature.
ligado Proceso de atar algo, por ejemplo, un vaso sanguíneo durante una cirugía, con una atadura llamada ligadura.

limited radiography A limited-scope radiography practice, usually in an outpatient setting, that does not require the same credentials needed for professional radiologic technology; also called practical radiography.
radiografía limitada Práctica radiográfica de alcance limitado que se suele usar con pacientes externos y que no requiere las mismas credenciales que se necesitan para la tecnología radiográfica profesional. También se llama radiografía práctica.

lithotripsy A procedure for eliminating a stone (as in the bladder) by crushing or dissolving it in situ through the use of high-intensity sound waves.
litotripsia Procedimiento para eliminar una piedra rompiéndola o disolviéndola in situ por medio del uso de ondas sonoras de alta intensidad.

litigious Prone to engage in lawsuits.
litigioso Propenso a iniciar pleitos y litigios.

loading dose A double dose of medication administered as the first dose. It is usually done with antibiotic therapy to reach therapeutic blood levels quickly.
dosis de ataque Dosis doble de una medicación ladministrada como primera dosis. Suele hacerse con terapia antibiótica para alcanzar rápidamente los niveles terapéuticos en sangre.

lordosis Abnormal concave curvature of the cervical and lumbar spine regions.
lordosis Curvatura cóncava anómala de la espina cervical y lumbar.

lower GI series Fluoroscopic examination of the colon, usually employing rectal administration of barium sulfate (also called barium enema) as a contrast medium.
serie GI inferior Examen fluoroscópico del colon, por lo general usando una administración rectal de sulfato de bario (también llamado enema de bario) como medio de contraste.

lumbar The lower back region, containing five lumbar vertebrae.
lumbar Región posterior inferior en la que hay cinco vértebras lumbares.

lumen An open space, such as within a blood vessel, the intestine, a needle, a tube, or an examining instrument.
lumen Espacio abierto, como en el interior de un vaso sanguíneo, el intestino, una aguja, un tubo o un instrumento para examinar.

luteinizing hormone (LH) A hormone produced by the pituitary gland that promotes ovulation.
hormona luteinizante (LH) Hormona que produce la glándula pituitaria y que promueve la ovulación.

luxation Dislocation of a bone from its normal anatomical location.
luxación Dislocación de un hueso de su ubicación anatómica normal.

lymphadenopathy Any disorder of the lymph nodes or lymph vessels.
linfadenopatía Cualquier trastorno de los nódulos o de los vasos linfáticos.

macromolecules The molecules needed for metabolism: carbohydrates, lipids, proteins, and nucleic acids.
macromoléculas Moléculas que se necesitan para el metabolismo: carbohidratos, lípidos, proteínas y ácidos nucleicos.

magnetic resonance imaging (MRI) An imaging modality that uses a magnetic field and radiofrequency pulses to create computer images of both bones and soft tissues, in multiple planes.
formación de imágenes por resonancia magnética (MRI) Modalidad de formación de imágenes en la que se usa un campo magnético y pulsos de radiofrecuencia para crear imágenes computarizadas, tanto de huesos como de tejidos blandos, en planos múltiples.

major diagnostic categories (MDCs) Broad clinical categories differentiated from all others on the basis of body system involvement and disease etiology.
categorías de diagnosis principales (MDCs) Amplias categorías clínicas que se diferencian de todas las demás en base a la inclusión del sistema corporal y la etiología de la enfermedad.

maker (of a check) Any individual, corporation, or legal party who signs a check or any type of negotiable instrument.
signatario (de un cheque) Cualquier individuo, corporación o parte legal que firma un cheque o cualquier tipo de instrumento negociable.

malignant Cancerous.
maligno Canceroso.

managed care An umbrella term for all health care plans that provide health care in return for preset monthly payments and offer coordinated care through a defined network of primary care physicians and hospitals.
atención administrada Término que engloba todos los planes de atención sanitaria que proporcionan atención médica a cambio de pagos mensuales preestablecidos y atención coordinada a través de una red definida de médicos de cabecera y hospitales.

mandated Required by an authority or law.
obligatorio Que lo exige una autoridad o la ley.

mandatory Containing or constituting a command.
obligatorio Que contiene una orden o que es una orden en sí mismo.

manifestation Something that is easily understood or recognized by the mind.
manifestación Algo que puede ser comprendido o reconocido por la mente con facilidad.

manipulation Moving or exercising a body part by an externally applied force.
manipulación Mover o ejercitar una parte del cuerpo por medio de la aplicación de una fuerza externa.

mastectomy Surgical removal of the breast that usually includes excision of lymph nodes in the axillary region.
mastectomía Eliminación quirúrgica del seno que por lo general incluye la escisión de los nódulos linfáticos de la región axilar.

matrix Something in which a thing originates, develops, takes shape, or is contained; a base upon which to build.
matriz Algo donde las cosas se originan, desarrollan, toman forma o están contenidas; base sobre la cual construir.

m-banking Banking through the use of wireless devices, such as cellular phones and wireless internet services.
banca-m Operaciones bancarias a través de dispositivos inalámbricos, como teléfonos celulares y servicios de comunicaciones inalámbricas.

media The term applied to agencies of mass communication, such as newspapers, magazines, and telecommunications.
medios de comunicación Término que se aplica a las agencias de noticias o de comunicación de masas, como periódicos, revistas y telecomunicaciones.

mediastinum The space in the center of the chest, under the sternum.
mediastino Espacio en el centro del pecho, bajo el esternón.

medical savings account A tax-deferred bank or savings account combined with a low-premium/high-deductible insurance policy, designed for individuals or families who choose to fund their own health care expenses and medical insurance.
cuenta de ahorros para gastos médicos Cuenta bancaria o de ahorros de impuestos diferidos combinada con una póliza de seguro con primas bajas y deducibles altos destinada a individuos o familias que eligen financiar ellos mismos sus gastos de atención sanitaria y su seguro médico.

medically indigent An individual who can afford to pay for his or her normal daily living expenses but cannot afford adequate health care.
médicamente indigente Individuo que puede pagar sus gastos normales de la vida cotidiana pero que no puede abordar el pago de un servicio de atención sanitaria adecuado.

medically necessary Criteria used by third-party payors to decide whether a patient's symptoms and diagnosis justify specific medical services or procedures; also known as medical necessity.
médicamente necesario Criterio usado por pagadores intermediarios para decidir si los síntomas y el diagnóstico de un paciente justifican el uso de procedimientos o servicios médicos específicos; también se conoce como necesidad médica.

medigap A term sometimes applied to private insurance products that supplement Medicare insurance benefits.
medigap Término que se aplica algunas veces a seguros privados que complementan los beneficios del seguro Medicare.

medullary cavity The inner portion of the diaphysis, containing bone marrow.
cavidad medular Porción interna de la diafisis que contiene la médula ósea.

megabyte Approximately one million bytes.
megabyte Aproximadamente, un millón de bytes.

megahertz A measuring unit for microprocessors, abbreviated MHz. A megahertz is a million cycles of electromagnetic current alternation per second and is used as a unit of measure for the clock speed of computer microprocessors. The hertz is a unit of measure named after Heinrich Hertz, a German physicist.
megahercio Unidad de medida para microprocesadores, abreviada MHz. Un megahercio es un millón de ciclos de alternancia de corriente electromagnética por segundo y se usa como unidad de medida para la velocidad de los microprocesadores de computadoras. El hercio recibe su nombre de Heinrich Hertz, un físico alemán.

melena Black, tarry stool containing digested blood and usually the result of bleeding in the upper GI tract.
melena Deposición negra y alquitranada que contiene sangre digerida y por lo general es le resultado de una hemorragia en el tracto gastrointestinal superior.

mentor A trusted counselor or guide.
mentor Consejero o guía de confianza.

metabolite A substance produced by metabolism.
metabolito Sustancia producida por el metabolismo.

meticulous Marked by extreme or excessive care in the consideration or treatment of details.
meticuloso Caracterizado por una atención exagerada o excesiva a los detalles.

microcephaly Small size of the head in relation to the rest of the body.
microcefalia Tamaño pequeño de la cabeza en relación con el resto del cuerpo.

microfilm A film bearing a photographic record of printed or other graphic matter on a reduced scale.
microfilm Película que contiene una fotografía de un documento impreso u otro elemento gráfico a escala reducida.

microorganism An organism of microscopic or submicroscopic size.
microorganismo Organismo de tamaño microscópico o sub-microscópico.

MIDI The abbreviation for musical instrument digital interface. A MIDI interface allows computers to record and manipulate sound.
MIDI Abreviatura para interfaz digital para instrumentos musicales. Una interfaz MIDI permite a las computadoras grabar y manipular sonido.

miotic Any substance or medication that causes contraction of the pupil.
miótico Cualquier sustancia o medicamento que produce una contracción de la pupila.

misdemeanor A minor crime, as opposed to a felony, punishable by fine or imprisonment in a city or county jail rather than in a penitentiary.
falta Delito menor, por oposición a delito mayor, se penaliza con multa o prisión en una cárcel de una ciudad o condado más bien que con prisión en una penitenciaría.

mock To imitate or practice.
simular Imitar o practicar.

modem The acronym for modulator demodulator; a device that allows information to be transmitted over phone lines, at speeds measured in bits per second (bps).
módem Abreviatura para modulador desmodulador, un dispositivo que permite transmitir información a través de las líneas telefónicas a velocidades que se miden en bits por segundos (bps).

molecule A group of like or different atoms held together by chemical forces.
molécula Grupo de átomos iguales o diferentes que se mantiene unido por fuerzas químicas.

monochromatic Having or consisting of one color or hue.
monocromático Que tiene un solo color o tonalidad.

mononuclear white blood cell A leukocyte having an unsegmented nucleus; monocytes and lymphocytes in particular.
glóbulo blanco mononuclear Leucocito que tiene un núcleo sin segmentar; en particular los monocitos y linfocitos.

mons pubis The fat pad that covers the symphysis pubis.
monte del pubis Almohadilla de grasa que cubre la sínfisis púbica.

morale The mental and emotional condition (such as enthusiasm, confidence, or loyalty) of an individual or group with regard to the function or tasks at hand.
moral Estado mental y emocional (como entusiasmo, lealtad o confianza) de un individuo o grupo en cuanto al puesto que desempeña o el trabajo que realiza.

motivation The process of inciting a person to some action or behavior.
motivación Proceso de incitar a una persona a hacer algo o a comportarse de una forma determinada.

multimedia The presentation of graphics, animation, video, sound, and text on a computer in an integrated way, or all at once. CD-ROMs are the most effective multimedia devices.
multimedia Presentación de gráficos, imágenes animadas, video, sonido y texto en una computadora de forma integrada o simultánea. Los CD ROM son los dispositivos de multimedia más eficaces.

multiparous Pertaining to women who have had two or more pregnancies.
multípara Perteneciente o relativo a la mujer que ha tenido dos o más embarazos.

multi-tasking Performing multiple tasks at one time.
multitarea Realización de varias tareas diferentes al mismo tiempo.

municipal court A court that sits in some cities and larger towns and that usually has civil and criminal jurisdiction over cases arising within the municipality.
Municipal corte Se aplica al juzgado con sede en algunas ciudades y pueblos grandes y que suele tener jurisdicción civil y penal sobre casos que surgen dentro de la municipalidad.

murmur An abnormal sound heard when auscultating the heart. It may or may not be pathologic.
murmullo Sonido anómalo que se escucha al auscultar el corazón y que puede ser patológico o no.

myelography Fluoroscopic examination of the spinal canal with spinal injection of an iodine contrast medium.
mielografía Examen fluoroscópico del canal espinal con una inyección espinal de un medio de contraste yodado.

myelomeningocele A herniation of a portion of the spinal cord and its meninges that protrudes through a congenital opening in the vertebral column.
mielomeningocele Hernia de una parte de la médula espinal y sus meninges que sale hacia fuera a través de una abertura congénita en la columna vertebral.

myocardial Pertaining to the heart muscle.
miocárdico Perteneciente o relativo al músculo cardiaco.

myocardium The heart muscle.
miocardio Músculo cardiaco.

myoglobinuria Abnormal presence in the urine of a hemoglobin-like chemical of muscle tissue, which is the result of muscle deterioration.
mioglobinuria Presencia anómala en la orina de una susbtancia química del tejido muscular parecida a la hemoglobina; es el resultado de una deterioración muscular.

mysticism The experience of seeming to have direct communication with God or ultimate reality.
misticismo Experiencia de parecer tener comunicación directa con Dios o una realidad superior.

nanometer One billionth (10^{-9}) of a meter.
nanómetro Una mil millonésima parte (10^{-9}) de metro.

naturopathy An alternative to conventional medicine in which holistic methods are used, as well as herbs and natural supplements, with the belief that the body will heal itself. Naturopathic physicians can currently be licensed in twelve states.
naturopatía Alternativa a la medicina convencional en la que se usan métodos holísticos, así como hierbas y suplementos naturales, con la creencia de que el cuerpo sanará por sí mismo. En la actualidad, los médicos naturópatas pueden obtener la licencia en doce estados.

necrosis Pertaining to the death of cells or tissue.
necrosis Perteneciente o relativo a la muerte de células o tejidos.

negative feedback mechanism A homeostatic mechanism that responds as a regulator to counteract a change.
mecanismo de respuesta negativ a Mecanismo homeostático que responde como regulador para contrarrestar un cambio.

negligence Failure to exercise the care that a prudent person usually exercises; implied inattention to one's duty or business; implied want of due or necessary diligence or care.
negligencia Falta de cuidado en algo que se hace; falta implicita de atención en el deber o trabajo; deseo implicito de una diligencia o cuidado necesario o merecido.

negotiable Legally transferable to another party.
negociable Que se puede transferir legalmente a otra parte.

networking The exchange of information or services among individuals, groups, or institutions; meeting and getting to know individuals in the same or similar career fields, and sharing information about available opportunities.
interconexión Intercambio de información o servicios entre individuos, grupos o instituciones; conocer a individuos del mismo campo profesional o de campos similares y compartir información acerca de oportunidades de empleo.

neural tube defect Any of a group of congenital anomalies involving the brain and spinal column that are caused by the failure of the neural tube to close during embryonic development.
defecto del tubo neural Cualquiera de las anomalías congénitas que afectan al cerebro y a la médula espinal y que tienen su origen en que el tubo neural no logró cerrarse durante el desarrollo embrionario.

nodule A small lump, lesion, or swelling felt when palpating the skin.
nódulo Pequeña protuberancia, herida o hinchazón que se siente al tocar la piel.

nomogram A graph on which variables are plotted so that a particular value can be read on the appropriate line.
nomograma Gráfica en la que las variables están presentadas de tal manera que se puede leer un valor específico en la línea adecuada.

nonmaleficence Refraining from the act of harming or committing evil.
ausencia de maleficencia No hacer el mal.

no-show A person who fails to keep an appointment without giving advance notice.
no-acudió Persona que no acude a una cita médica sin dar previo aviso.

nosocomial infection Infection acquired during hospitalization or in a healthcare setting. It is often due to *E. coli*, hepatitis viruses, *pseudomonas*, and staphylocci microorganisms.
infección nosocomial Infección adquirida en un establecimiento de atención sanitaria o durante una hospitalización. Con frecuencia se debe a *E. coli*, virus de hepatitis, *pseudomonas* y estafilococos.

nosocomial Pertaining to or originating in the hospital, said of an infection not present or incubating prior to admission to the hospital.
nosocomial Perteneciente o relativo al hospital, incubado en el hospital, dícese de la infección que no estaba presente ni en estado de incubación antes de ser ingresado al hospital.

"note" Notes are found in both the Alphabetic Index and the Tabular List as instructions or guides in classification assignments, defining category content or the use of subdivision codes.
"nota" Las notas se encuentran tanto en los Índices alfabéticos como en las instrucciones o guías en las Asignaciones de clasificación, para definir el contenido de la categoría o el uso de los códigos de subdivisión.

NSAIDs Non-steroidal antiinflammatory drugs.
NSAID Medicamentos antiinflamatorios no esterioides.

nuclear medicine An imaging modality that uses radioactive materials injected or ingested into the body to provide information about the function of organs and tissues.
medicina nuclear Modalidad de la formación de imágenes que usa materiales radioactivos inyectados en el cuerpo o ingeridos para obtener información acerca del funcionamiento de órganos y tejidos.

obesity An excessive accumulation of body fat (usually defined as more than 20 percent above the recommended body weight).
obesidad Acumulación excesiva de grasa en el cuerpo (se suele definir como más del 20 por ciento del peso recomendado).

objective information Information that is gathered by watching or observating a patient.
información objetiva Información que se recoge vigilando u observando a un paciente.

oblique projection Radiographic view in which the body or part is rotated so that the projection is neither frontal nor lateral.
proyección oblicua Vista radiográfica en la cual que cuerpo o parte del cuerpo se gira de forma que la proyección no es frontal ni lateral.

obliteration Making something indecipherable or imperceptible by obscuring or wearing away.
obliterar Hacer algo indescifrable o imperceptible oscureciéndolo o desgastándolo.

obturator A disk or plate that closes an opening.
obturador Disco o placa que cierra una abertura.

obturator A metal rod with a smooth rounded tip that is placed into hollow instruments to decrease destruction of the body tissues during insertion.
obturador Varilla de metal con un extremo redondeado que se coloca en el interior de instrumentos huecos para disminuir la destrucción de los tejidos corporales durante su inserción.

occlusion The complete blocking off of an opening.
oclusión Cierre completo de una abertura.

"omit code" This term is used primarily in Volume 3 when the procedure is the method of approach for an operation.
"omitir código" Esta expresión se usa sobre todo en el tomo 3 cuando el procedimiento es el método de acercamiento a una operación.

opaque Not translucent or transparent.
opaco Que no es translúcido ni transparente.

OPIM (other potentially infectious material) Substances or material other than blood (body fluids such as, urine, semen, etc., for example) which have the potential to carry infectious pathogens
OPIM (otras materias potencialmente peligrosas) Sustancias o materias además de la sangre (como, por ejemplo, los fluidos corporales, la orina, el semen, etc.).

opinion A formal expression of judgment or advice by an expert; the formal expression of the legal reasons and principles upon with a legal decision is based.
opinión Expresión formal de un juicio o consejo dado por un experto; expresión formal de las razones y principios legales sobre los que se basa una decisión legal.

opportunistic infection Infection caused by a normally nonpathogenic organism in a host whose resistance has been decreased.
infección oportunista Infección en una persona con una resistencia a las enfermedades más baja de lo normal, provocada por un organismo que en condiciones normales no resulta patógeno.

optic disc Region at the back of the eye where the optic nerve meets the retina. It is considered the blind spot of the eye because it contains only nerve fibers and no rods or cones, and thus is insensitive to light.
papila óptica Región en la parte posterior del ojo donde el nervio óptico se une con la retina. Se considera el punto ciego del ojo, ya que allí sólo hay fibras nerviosas y no bastoncillos ni conos, y por tanto es insensible a la luz.

optic nerve The second cranial nerve, which carries impulses for the sense of sight.
nervio óptico Segundo nervio del cráneo que transporta impulsos para el sentido de la vista.

optical character recognition (OCR) The electronic scanning of printed items as images, then using special software to recognize these images (or characters) as ASCII text.
reconocimiento óptico de caracteres (OCR) Proceso de escanear electrónicamente documentos impresos como si fueran imágenes y después, usando un programa de computadora especial, reconocer esas imágenes (o caracteres) como texto ASCII.

ordinance An authoritative decree or direction; a law set forth by a governmental authority, specifically a municipal regulation.
ordenanza Decreto u orden de la autoridad; ley definida por una autoridad gubernamental, específicamente, una regulación municipal.

organelle A differentiated structure within a cell, such as a mitochondrion, vacuole, or chloroplast, that performs a specific function.
organelo Estructura diferenciada dentro de una célula, como un mitocondrio, vacuola o cloroplasto que realiza una función específica.

orthopnea Difficulty breathing when in a supine position. The individual must sit or stand to breathe comfortably.
ortopnea Dificultad para respirar estando en posición supina. El individuo debe estar sentado o de pie para respirar con comodidad.

orthostatic (postural) hypotension A temporary fall in blood pressure when a person rapidly changes from a recumbent position to a standing position.
hipotensión ortostática (relacionada con la postura) Baja temporal de la presión sanguínea cuando una persona cambia con rapidez de una posición recostada a una posición en pie.

osteopathy A medical discipline based primarily on the manual diagnosis and holistic treatment of impaired function resulting from loss of movement in all kinds of tissues.
osteopatía Disciplina médica que se basa primordialmente en el diagnóstico manual y el tratamiento holístico de funciones deterioradas como resultado de la pérdida de movilidad en todo tipo de tejidos.

osteoporosis The loss of bone density. Lack of calcium intake is a major factor in its development.
osteoporosis Disminución de la densidad de los huesos. La falta de consumo de calcio es uno de los factores principales de su desarrollo.

otitis externa Inflammation or infection of the external auditory canal.
otitis externa Inflamación o infección del canal auditivo externo.

otosclerosis The formation of spongy bone in the labyrinth of the ear, often causing the auditory ossicles to become fixed and unable to vibrate when sound enters the ears.
otosclerosis Formación de huesos parecidos a esponjas en el laberinto del oído, a menudo causando que los huesecillos auditivos queden fijos y que no puedan vibrar cuando el sonido entra en los oídos.

ototoxic Pertaining to a substance or medication that damages the eighth cranial nerve or the organs of hearing and balance.
ototóxico Perteneciente o relativo a una sustancia o medicamento que daña el octavo nervio craneal o los órganos auditivos y del equilibrio.

OUTfolder A folder used to provide space for the temporary filing of materials.
Carpeta OUT Carpeta que se usa para proporcionar espacio para archivar materiales de forma temporal.

OUTguide A heavy guide that is used to replace a folder that has been temporarily moved from the filing space.
Guía OUT Guía grande que se usa para reemplazar una carpeta que ha sido retirada temporalmente del archivo.

Output Information that is processed by the computer and transmitted to a monitor, printer, or other device.
Salida Información procesada por la computadora y enviada a un monitor, impresora u otro dispositivo.

over-the-counter drugs Medications legally sold without a prescription.
medicinas de venta libre Medicinas que se venden sin receta legalmente.

oxytocin A hormone secreted by the posterior pituitary gland that stimulates smooth muscle contractions of the uterus or mammary glands.
oxitocina Hormona que segrega la glándula pituitaria posterior y que estimula las contracciones del útero o de las glándulas mamarias.

palliative An agent that relieves or alleviates symptoms without curing the disease; something that alleviates or eases a painful situation without curing it.
paliativo Agente que calma o alivia los síntomas sin curar la enfermedad; algo que alivia o hace más soportable una situación dolorosa sin curarla.

pandemic Affecting the majority of the people in a country or a number of countries.
pandémico Que afecta a la mayoría de la población de un país o de varios países.

paper claims Hard copies of insurance claims that have been completed and sent by surface mail.
reclamaciones de papel Copias impresas de reclamaciones de seguros que han sido completadas y enviadas por correo ordinario.

papilledema Bulging of the optic disk and dilated retinal veins seen by ophthalmoscopic examination of the retina. Papilledema is a sign of increased intracranial pressure.
edema papilar Abultamiento de la papila óptica y de las venas retinianas dilatadas que se ven en un examen oftalmoscópico de la retina. La emeda papilar es una señal de un aumento en la presión intracraneal.

paraphrased Pertaining to a text, passage, or work that has been restated to give the meaning in another form.
parafraseado Perteneciente o relativo a un texto, selección u obra que ha sido expresado nuevamente para dar su significado de otra forma.

paraphrasing Expressing an idea in different wording in an effort to enhance communication and clarify meaning.
parafrasear Expresar una idea con palabras diferentes para mejorar la comunicación y hacer más claro su significado.

parenteral Referring to injection or introduction of substances into the body through any route other than the digestive tract, such as subcutaneous, intravenous, or intramuscular administration.
parenteral Inyección o introducción de sustancias en el cuerpo a través de cualquier otra vía que no sea el tracto digestivo, como administración subcutánea, intravenosa o intramuscular.

paresthesia An abnormal sensation of burning, prickling, or stinging.
parestesia Sensación anómala de ardor, escozor o aguijoneo.

paroxysmal Pertaining to a sudden, recurrent spasm of symptoms.
paroxístico Perteneciente o relativo a espasmos repentinos recurrentes o a sus síntomas.

participating provider A physician or other health care provider who enters into a contract with a specific insurance company or program, and by doing so, agrees to abide by certain rules and regulations set forth by that particular third-party payor.
proveedor participante Médico u otro proveedor de atención sanitaria que establece un contrato con una compañía o programa de seguro específico, y al hacerlo acepta respetar ciertas normas y regulaciones establecidas por ese pagador intermediario.

parturition The act or process of giving birth to a child.
parto Acción o proceso de dar a luz un niño.

patency The condition of a body cavity or canal that is open or unobstructed.
abertura Estado abierto de un cuerpo, cavidad o canal.

pathogen An agent that causes disease, especially a living microorganism such as a bacterium or fungus; a **disease**-causing **microorganism.**
patógeno Agente que causa enfermedades, especialmente microorganismos vivos como bacterias u hongos; **microorganismos** causantes de **enfermedades**.

pathogenic Pertaining to disease-causing microorganisms.
patogénico Perteneciente o relativo a los microorganismos causantes de enfermedades.

pathophysiology The study of biological and physical manifestations of disease as they are related to system abnormalities and physiologic disturbances.
patofisiología Estudio de las manifestaciones biológicas y físicas de las enfermedades y cómo se relacionan con las anomalías del sistema y las alteraciones fisiológicas.

payables The balance due to a creditor on an account.
pendiente de pago Saldo que se le debe al acreedor en una cuenta.

payee The person named on a draft or check as the recipient of the amount shown.
beneficiario Persona que se nombra en una letra de cambio o en un cheque como receptor de la cantidad indicada.

payer The person who writes a check to be cashed by the payee.
pagador Persona que emite el cheque a ser cambiado por el beneficiario.

peer review organization A group of medical reviewers who are contracted by HCFA to ensure quality control and the medical necessity of services provided by a facility.
organizacione de revisión colegial Grupo de revisores médicos contrata dos por HCFA para garantizar el control de calidad y la necesidad médica de los servicios ofrecidos por un establecimiento.

pegboard system A method of tracking patient accounts that allows the figures to be proven accurate by using mathematical formulas; also called the "write-it-once" system.
sistema de tablero perforado Método de controlar las cuentas de los pacientes que permite la demostración de la exactitud de las cifras por medio de fórmulas matemáticas; también conocido como sistema "escríbelo una vez."

perceiving The process of an individual looking at information and seeing it as real.
percibir Proceso en el cual un individuo mira la información y la ve como real.

perception A quick, acute, and intuitive cognition; capacity for comprehension; an awareness of the elements of the environment.
percepción Conocimiento rápido, agudo e intuitivo; capacidad de comprensión; conocimiento de los elementos del medio ambiente.

pericardium The membranous sac that encloses the heart.
pericardio Saco membranoso que envuelve el corazón.

periosteum The thin, highly innervated, membranous covering of a bone.
periostio Membrana fina y sin nervios que recubre un hueso.

peristalsis The wavelike movement by which the gastrointestinal tract moves food downward.
peristalsis Movimiento ondulatorio por el cual el tracto gastrointestinal mueve la comida hacia abajo.

perjured testimony Testimony involving the voluntary violation of an oath or vow, either by swearing to what is untrue or by failing to do what has been promised under oath; false testimony.
perjuro Testimonio que comprende la violación voluntaria de un juramento o promesa, ya sea jurando algo que es falso o no cumpliendo lo que se ha prometido bajo juramento; falso testimonio.

perks Extra advantages or benefits from working in a specific job that may or may not be commonplace in that particular profession.
beneficios adicionales Ventajas o beneficios adicionales del trabajar en un puesto de trabajo específico que pueden ser o no comunes a esa profesión en particular.

permeable Allowing a substance to pass or soak through.
permeable Permite el paso o penetración de una sustancia.

persona An individual's social facade or front that reflects the role the individual is playing in life; the personality that a person projects in public.
persona Lo que vemos de un individuo, la imagen social que refleja el papel que dicho individuo tiene en la sociedad; la personalidad que una persona proyecta en público.

pertinent Having a clear, decisive relevance to the matter at hand.
pertinente Que tiene una importancia clara y decisiva en el asunto que se está tratando.

petechiae Small, purplish hemorrhagic spots on the skin.
petequia Pequeñas manchas en la piel, hemorrágicas y de color violeta.

phenylalanine An essential amino acid found in milk, eggs, and other foods.
fenilalanina Aminoácido esencial que se encuentra en la leche, los huevos y otros alimentos.

philanthropist An individual who makes an active effort to promote human welfare.
filántropo Individuo que se ocupa activamente de promover el bienestar humano.

philosopher A person who seeks wisdom or enlightenment; an expounder of a theory in a certain area of experience.
filósofo Persona que busca la sabiduría o el esclarecimiento; persona que expone una teoría en cierta área de experiencia.

phlebotomy The invasive procedure used to obtain a blood specimen for testing, experimentation, or diagnosis of disease.
flebotomía Procedimiento invasivo que se usa para obtener un espécimen de sangre para analizar, experimentar o diagnosticar una enfermedad.

phonetic Describing an alteration of ordinary spelling that better represents the spoken language, that employs only characters of the regular alphabet, and that is used in a context of conventional spelling.
escritura fonética Alteración de la escritura normal que representa mejor el lenguaje hablado, emplea sólo caracteres del alfabeto normal y se usa en un contexto de escritura convencional.

phosphors Fluorescent crystals that give off light when exposed to x-rays.
fósforos Cristales fluorescentes que alumbran cuando se exponen a los rayos X.

photometer An instrument for measuring the intensity of light, specifically to compare the relative intensities of different lights or their relative illuminating power.
fotómetro Instrumento para medir la intensidad de la luz, específicamente para comparar las intensidades relativas de luces diferentes o su poder de iluminación relativo.

photophobia Abnormal visual sensitivity to light.
fotofobia Sensibilidad visual anómala a la luz.

physiological noise Physiological interference with the communication process.
ruido fisiológico Interferencia fisiológica con el proceso de comunicación.

pipette A cylindrical glass or plastic tube used to deliver fluids.
pipeta Tubo cilíndrico de vidrio o plástico que se usa para distribuir fluidos.

pitch The property of a sound, especially a musical tone, that is determined by the frequency of the waves producing it; the highness or lowness of sound; the relative level, intensity, or extent of some quality or state.
tono Propiedad de un sonido, especialmente de un tono musical, que está determinada por la frecuencia de las ondas que lo producen; cualidad alta o baja de un sonido; nivel, intensidad o extensión relativos de alguna cualidad o estado.

plaque An abnormal accumulation of a fatty substance.
placa Acumulación anómala de una sustancia grasa.

plasma The liquid portion of whole blood that contains active clotting agents.
plasma Parte líquida de la sangre completa que contiene agentes coagulantes activos.

policyholder The person who pays a premium to an insurance company (and in whose name the policy is written) in exchange for the insurance protection provided by a policy of insurance.
titular de la póliza Persona que paga una prima a una compañía aseguradora (y a cuyo nombre se contrata la póliza) a cambio de la cobertura que proporciona una póliza de seguro.

polycythemia vera A condition marked by an abnormally large number of red blood cells in the circulatory system.
policitemia vera Afección que se caracteriza por una cantidad anómalamente elevada de glóbulos rojos en el sistema circulatorio.

polydipsia Excessive thirst.
polidipsia Sed excesiva.

polymorphonuclear white blood cells Leukocytes having a segmented nucleus; also known as PMN (polymorphonuclear neutrophils) or segmented neutrophils.
glóbulos blancos polimorfonucleares Leucocitos que tienen un núcleo segmentado; también se conocen como PMN (neutrófilos polimorfonucleares) o neutrófilos segmentados.

polyphagia Excessive appetite.
polifagia Aumento del apetito.

polyps Tumors on stems frequently found in or on mucous membranes and in the mucosal lining of the colon.
pólipos Tumores en racimos que se encuentran con frecuencia en las membranas mucosas y en el recubrimiento mucoso del colon.

polyuria Excessive urine production; excretion of an unusually large amount of urine.
poliuria Producción y excreción de orina excesivas.

portal hypertension Increased venous pressure in the portal circulation caused by cirrhosis or compression of the hepatic vascular system.
hipertensión portal Aumento de la presión venosa en la circulación portal causado por cirrosis o compresión del sistema vascular hepático.

portfolio A set of pictures, drawings, documents, or photographs either bound in book form or loose in a folder.
portafolio Conjunto de ilustraciones, dibujos, documentos o fotografías, organizadas ya sea archivadas en forma de libro, o sueltas en una carpeta.

posterioanterior (PA) Frontal projection in which the patient is prone or facing the x-ray film or image receptor.
posterioanterior (PA) Proyección frontal en la que el paciente está boca abajo o de frente a la película de rayos X o al receptor de imagen.

posting To transfer or carry from a book of original entry to a ledger; to enter figures in an accounting system.
asentar Transferir o traer desde un libro de entradas originales a un libro mayor; entrar cifras en un sistema de contabilidad.

postmortem Done, collected, or occurring after death.
postmortem Hecho, recogido o sucedido después de la muerte.

power of attorney A legal instrument authorizing a person to act as the attorney or agent of the grantor. The authority may be limited to the handling of specific procedures. The person authorized to act as the agent is known as the *attorney in fact.*
potestad legal Instrumento legal que autoriza a una persona a actuar como abogado o agente de la persona que le concede el poder. La autorización puede estar limitada al manejo de

procedimientos específicos. La persona autorizada a actuar como agente se conoce como *abogado de hecho*.

precedence Superiority in rank, dignity, or importance; the condition of being, going, or coming ahead or in front of.
precedencia Superioridad en rango, dignidad o importancia; condición de estar, ir o venir primero o antes.

precedent A person or thing that serves as a model; something done or said that may serve as an example or rule to authorize or justify a subsequent act of the same kind.
precedente Persona o cosa que sirve como modelo; algo hecho o dicho anteriormente y que puede servir como ejemplo o norma para autorizar o justificar un acto subsiguiente del mismo tipo.

preexisting condition A physical condition of an insured person that existed before the issuance of the insurance policy.
afección preexistente Afección física de una persona asegurada que ya existía antes de la emisión de la póliza de seguro.

premium The consideration paid for a contract of insurance; the periodic (monthly, quarterly, or annual) payment of a specific sum of money to an insurance company that, in return, agrees to provide certain benefits.
prima Pago por un contrato de seguro; pago periódico (mensual, trimestral o anual) de una suma específica de dinero a una compañía aseguradora, la cual, a cambio, acepta proporcionar ciertos beneficios.

preponderance A superiority or excess in number or quantity; majority.
preponderancia Superioridad o mayor número o cantidad; mayoría.

preponderance of the evidence Evidence that is of greater weight or more convincing than the evidence offered in opposition to it; evidence that, as a whole, shows that the fact sought to be proven is more probable than not.
preponderancia de evidencia Evidencia que tiene mayor peso o que es más convincente que la evidencia con la que se confronta; evidencia que, en conjunto, muestra que el hecho que se pretende probar es más posible que imposible.

prerequisite Something that is necessary to achieve a result or to carry out a function.
requisito previo Algo que es necesario para obtener un resultado o para desempeñar una función.

present illness The chief complaint, written in chronological sequence with dates of onset.
enfermedad actual Problema principal, descrito en secuencia cronológica con las fechas de cada acceso.

preservatives Substances added to a specimen to prevent deterioration of cells or chemicals.
preservativos Sustancias añadidas a un espécimen para prevenir el deterioro de células o sustancias químicas.

pressboard A strong, highly glazed composition board resembling vulcanized fiber; heavy card stock.
cartón prensado Cartón de composición resistente y muy satinado que se parece a la fibra vulcanizada; cartulina de gran resistencia.

primary diagnosis The condition or chief complaint for which a patient is treated in outpatient (physician's office or clinic) medical care.
diagnóstico primario Afección o problema principal por el cual se trata a un paciente con atención médica externa (en un consultorio médico o una clínica).

principal A capital sum of money due as a debt or used as a fund, for which interest is either charged or paid.
principal Capital o suma de dinero que se debe como deuda o que se usa como fondo, por el cual se cargan o se cobran intereses.

principal diagnosis A condition, established after study, that is chiefly responsible for the *admission* of a patient to the hospital. It is used in coding inpatient hospital insurance claims.
diagnóstico principal Enfermedad o lesión que, tras su estudio, se determina que es la causa principal por la que un paciente *ingresa* en el hospital. Es usado en la codificación de reclamaciones de seguros de pacientes hospitalizados.

privately owned laboratories (POLs) Laboratories owned by a private individual or corporation, such as a free-standing laboratory or the lab inside a physician's office.
laboratorios privados (POLs) Laboratorios cuyo propietario es un individuo o una corporación privada, como el laboratorio dentro de un consultorio médico o un laboratorio independiente.

processing How an individual internalizes new information and makes it his or her own.
procesar Forma en la que un individuo interioriza y asimila la información nueva.

procrastination Intentionally putting off the doing of something that should be done.
procrastinación Dejar a un lado o retrasar, de manera intencional, algo que debe hacerse.

professional behaviors Those actions that identify the Medical Assistant as a member of a healthcare profession, including dependability, respectful patient care, initiative, positive attitude, and teamwork.
comportamientos profesionales Características que identifican al asistente médico como profesional de la atención sanitaria, incluyendo confiabilidad, trato respetuoso a los pacientes, iniciativa, actitud positiva y disposición para trabajar en equipo.

professional courtesy Reduction or absence of a fee to professional associates.
cortesía profesional Reducción o supresión de un cargo para los asociados profesionales.

professionalism Characterizing or conforming to the technical or ethical standards of a profession; exhibiting a courteous, conscientious, and generally businesslike manner in the workplace.
profesionalismo Actitud que se caracteriza por cumplir o actuar de acuerdo con los estándares técnicos y éticos de una profesión; dar muestras de cortesía, meticulosidad y, en general, mostrar un comportamiento adecuado en el lugar de trabajo.

proficiency Competency as a result of training or practice.
pericia Estado de competencia en algo, que se alcanza por medio de entrenamiento o práctica.

profit sharing Offer of part of the company's profits to employees or other designated individuals or groups.
participación en los beneficios Oferta de parte de los beneficios de la compañía a los empleados u otros individuos o grupos designados.

progress notes Notes entered in the patient chart to track the progress and condition of the patient.
notas del progreso Notas escritas en historial médico del paciente para seguir el progreso y estado del mismo.

prokaryote A unicellular organism that lacks a membrane-bound nucleus
procaryota Organismo unicelular cuyo núcleo no está unido por una membrana.

prolactin (PRL) A hormone secreted by the anterior pituitary gland that stimulates the development of the mammary gland.
prolactina (PRL) Hormona que segrega la glándula pituitaria anterior y que estimula el desarrollo de la glándula mamaria.

proofread To read text and mark corrections.
corregir pruebas Leer un texto y marcar correcciones.

prosthesis The artificial replacement for a body part.
prótesis Pieza artificial para reemplazar una parte del cuerpo.

proteins Organic compounds, occurring in plants and animals, that contain the major elements carbon, hydrogen, oxygen, and nitrogen and the amino acids essential for life maintenance.
proteínas Compuestos orgánicos que existen en plantas y animales y que contienen los elementos principales: carbón, hidrógeno, oxígeno y nitrógeno y los aminoácidos esenciales para el mantenimiento de la vida.

provider An individual or company that provides medical care and services to patients or the public.
proveedor Individuo o compañía que proporciona atenciones y servicios médicos pacientes o al público.

provisional diagnosis A temporary diagnosis made prior to receiving all test results.
diagnóstico provisional Diagnóstico temporal llevado a cabo antes de recibir todos los resultados de las pruebas.

proxemics The study of the nature, degree, and effect of the spatial separation individuals naturally maintain.
proxemia Estudio de la naturaleza, grado y efecto de la separación espacial que los individuos mantienen de forma natural.

prudent Marked by wisdom or judiciousness; shrewd in the management of practical affairs.
prudente Caracterizado por poseer sabiduría o sensatez; hábil en el manejo de los asuntos prácticos.

psoriasis A usually chronic, recurrent skin disease marked by bright red patches covered with silvery scales.
psoriasis Enfermedad recurrente de la piel, por lo general crónica, caracterizada por manchas de color rojo brillante cubiertas por escamas plateadas.

psychosocial Pertaining to a combination of psychological and social factors.
psicosocial Perteneciente o relativo a una combinación de factores psicológicos y sociales.

public domain The realm embracing property rights that belong to the community at large, are unprotected by copyright or patent, and are subject to appropriation by anyone.
dominio público Campo que abarca los derechos de propiedad que pertenecen a la comunidad en general, que no están protegidos por leyes de derechos de autor ni por patentes y están sujetos a apropiación por parte de cualquiera.

pulmonary consolidation In pneumonia, the process by which the lungs become solidified as they fill with exudates.
solidificación pulmonar Proceso por el cual los pulmones se vuelven rígidos a medida que se llenan con exudados en los casos de pulmonía.

pulse deficit When the radial pulse is less than the apical pulse. It may indicate peripheral vascular abnormality.
déficit del pulso Cuando el pulso radial es menor que el apical. Puede indicar una anomalía vascular periférica.

pulse pressure The difference between the systolic and the diastolic blood pressures (less than 30 points or more than 50 points is considered normal)
presión del pulso Diferencia entre las presiones sanguíneas sistólica y diastólica (menos de 30 puntos o más de 50 puede considerarse normal).

pure culture A bacterial or fungal culture that contains a single organism.
cultivo puro Cultivo de bacterias u hongos que contiene un solo organismo.

putrefaction The decomposition of organic matter that results in a foul smell.
putrefacción Descomposición de materia orgánica que da como resultado un olor fétido.

pyemia The presence of pus-forming organisms in the blood.
piemia Presencia en la sangre de organismos formadores de pus.

quackery The pretense of curing disease.
curanderismo Práctica del que finge curar enfermedades.

quality control An aggregate of activities designed to ensure adequate quality, especially in manufactured products or in the service industries.
control de calidad Conjunto de actividades destinadas a garantizar la calidad adecuada, en especial en productos manufacturados o en las industrias de servicios.

queries Requests for information from a database.
consultas Peticions de información de una base de datos.

rad The conventional unit of absorbed radiation dose.
rad Unidad convencional de dosis de radiación absorbido.

radiograph An x-ray image.
radiografía Imagen obtenida con el uso de rayos X.

radiographer A person qualified to perform radiographic examinations.
técnico de radiología Persona cualificada para realizar exámenes radiológicos.

radiography Making diagnostic images using x-rays.
radiografía Proceso de diagnosticar imágenes usando rayos X.

radiologist A physician specialist in medical imaging and/or therapeutic applications of radiation.
médico radiólogo Médico especialista en formación de imágenes o en aplicaciones terapéuticas de la radiación.

radiolucent Describing a substance that is easily penetrated by x-rays; these substances appear dark on radiographs.
transparente a la radiación Término que se aplica a una substancia que puede ser penetrada con facilidad por los rayos X; estas substancias aparecen oscuras en las radiografías.

radiopaque Describing a substance that can be easily visualized on an x-ray image; describing a substance that is not easily penetrated by x-rays; these substances appear light on radiographs.
opaco a la radiación Sustancia que puede visualizarse con facilidad en la imagen de rayos X. Término que se aplica a una substancia que no puede ser penetrada con facilidad por los rayos X; estas substancias aparecen claras en las radiografías.

rales Abnormal or crackling breath sounds during inspiration.
estertores Sonidos respiratorios o crujidos anómalos durante la inspiración.

ramifications Consequences produced by a cause or following from a set of conditions.
ramificaciones Consecuencias producidas por una causa o que siguen a una serie de estados.

rapport A relationship of harmony and accord between the patient and the health care professional.
concordia Relación de armonía y acuerdo entre el paciente y el profesional de la atención sanitaria.

Raynaud's phenomenon Intermittent attacks of ischemia in the extremities resulting in cyanosis, numbness, tingling, and pain.
fenómeno de Raynaud Ataques intermitentes de isquemia en las extremidades, resultando en cianosis, entumecimiento, picazón y dolor.

RBRVS (resource-based relative value system) A fee schedule designed to provide national uniform payment of Medicare benefits after being adjusted to reflect the differences in practice costs across geographic areas.
RBRVS (sistema de valor relativo basado en recursos) Escala de cargos diseñada para proporcionar un pago de beneficios de Medicare uniforme a nivel nacional después de haber sido ajustado para reflejar las diferencias en los costos prácticos a través de áreas geográficas.

ream A quantity of paper consisting of 20 quires or variously 480, 500, or 516 sheets.
resma Una cantidad de papel que consiste de 20 manos o que varía entre 480, 500 o 516 hojas.

reasonable doubt Doubt based on reason and arising from evidence or lack of evidence; not doubt that is imagined or conjured up, but doubt that would cause reasonable persons to hesitate before acting in a manner important to themselves.
duda razonable Duda basada en la razón o que surge de evidencia o falta de evidencia; no es una duda imaginaria ni inventada, sino una duda que puede hacer que una persona razonable vacile antes de dar un paso importante.

receipts Amounts paid on patient accounts.
recibos Sumas pagadas en las cuentas de los pacientes.

recipient The receiver of some thing or item.
receptor El que recibe un artículo u objeto.

rectify To correct by removing errors.
rectificar Corregir eliminando errores.

reduction The return to correct anatomical position, as in the reduction of a fracture.
reducción Regreso a la posición anatómica correcta, como en el caso de reducción de una fractura.

referral (reference) laboratory A private or hospital-based laboratory that performs a wide variety of tests, many of them specialized. Physicians often send specimens collected in the office to referral laboratories for testing.
laboratorio de referencia Laboratorio privado o de un hospital que realiza una amplia gama de análisis, muchos de ellos especializados. Con frecuencia los médicos envían especímenes recogidos en la consulta a estos laboratorios para ser analizados.

reflection The process of considering new information and internalizing it to create new ways of examining information.
reflexión Proceso de estudiar información nueva e interiorizarla para crear formas nuevas de examinar información.

refractile Capable of causing light rays to bend thus thus altering or distorting an image.
refractante Capaz de provocar la refracción de la luz, desviación alterando o distorcionando una imagen.

registered dietitian (RD) A professionally certified person with a bachelor's degree in food and nutrition who is concerned with the maintenance and promotion of health and the treatment of diseases through proper diet.
dietista registrado (RD) Profesional certificado persona con titulación universitaria en alimentos y nutrición y que se preocupa del mantenimiento y la promoción de la salud y el tratamiento de las enfermedades a través de la dieta adecuado.

relapse The recurrence of disease symptoms after apparent recovery.
recaída Recurrencia de los síntomas de una enfermedad tras una aparente recuperación.

relevant Having significant and demonstrable bearing on the matter at hand.
pertinente Que tiene una relación importante y demostrable con el asunto que se está tratando.

rem The dose of ionizing radiation equivalent to one roentgen of x-ray exposure.
rem La dosis de radiación ionizante equivalente a un roentgen de exposición a rayos X.

remission A decrease in the severity of a disease or symptoms; the partial or complete disappearance of the clinical and subjective characteristics of a chronic or malignant disease.
remisión Disminución de la gravedad de una enfermedad o sus síntomas; desaparición parcial o total de las características clínicas y subjetivas de una enfermedad crónica o maligna.

remittent fever Fever in which temperature fluctuates greatly but never falls to the normal level.
fiebre remitente Fiebre en la cual la temperatura fluctúa mucho pero nunca baja al nivel normal.

renal threshold The level above which a substance cannot be reabsorbed by the renal tubules and is thus excreted in the urine
umbral renal Nivel por encima del cual una sustancia no puede ser reabsorbida por los túbulos renales y por lo tanto es excretada en la orina.

reparations The act of making amends, offering atonement, or giving satisfaction for a wrong or injury.
reparaciones Acción de enmendar u ofrecer compensaciones por un error o un daño.

reprimands Criticisms for a fault; a severe or formal reproof.
reprimendas Críticas por una falta; reprobación severa o formal.

reproach An expression of rebuke or disapproval; a cause or occasion of blame, discredit, or disgrace.
reproche Expresión de crítica o desaprobación; causa o motivo de culpa, descrédito u oprobio.

requisites Things considered essential or necessary.
requisitos Cosas que se consideran esenciales o necesarias.

resolution The ability of the eye to distinguish two objects that are very close together; the sharpness of an image.
resolución Capacidad del ojo para distinguir dos objetos que están muy cerca uno del otro; nitidez de una imagen.

retention schedule A method or plan for retaining or keeping track of medical records and their movement from active to inactive to closed filing.
plan de retención Método o plan para retener o guardar expedientes médicos, y el paso de los mismos del estado de expediente activo a pasivo y a cerrado.

retention Keeping something in possession or use; to keeping someone's pay or service.
retención El hecho de mantener en posesión o en uso; mantener a alguien a su servicio o como empleado.

retribution The giving or receiving of reward or punishment; something given or exacted in recompense.
retribución Acto de dar o recibir una recompensa o castigo; algo que se da o se cobra como recompensa.

rhinitis Inflammation of the mucous membranes of the nose.
rinitis Inflamación de las membranas mucosas de la nariz.

rhonchi Abnormal rumbling sounds during expiration that indicate airway obstruction caused by thick secretions or spasms; continuous dry rattling in the throat or bronchial tube due to partial obstruction.
ronquido Ruido sordo y anómalo durante la expiración que indica obstrucción de las vías respiratorias debido a secreciones espesas o a espasmos; ruido seco y continuo en la garganta o en el tubo bronquial debido a una obstrucción parcial.

rider A special provision or group of provisions added to an insurance policy to expand or limit the benefits otherwise payable. It may increase or decrease benefits, waive a condition or coverage, or in any other way amend the original contract.
cláusula adicional Provisión o conjunto de provisiones especiales añadidas a una póliza de seguro para ampliar o limitar los beneficios que de otro modo se pueden pagar. Puede aumentar o disminuir beneficios, anular una condición o cobertura o puede enmendar el contrato original de otra manera.

robotics Technology dealing with the design, construction, and operation of robots in automation.
robótica Tecnología de la automatización que se ocupa del diseño, construcción y operación de robots.

rods Structures located in the retina of the eye that form the light-sensitive elements.
bastoncillos Estructuras que están en la retina del ojo y constituyen los elementos sensibles a la luz.

Roentgen (R) The conventional unit of radiation exposure.
Roentgen (R) Unidad convencional de exposición a radiación.

router A device used to connect any number of LANs which communicate with other routers and determine the best route between any two hosts.
direccionador Dispositivo usado para conectar cualquier cantidad de LAN que se comunican con otros direccionadores para determinar la mejor ruta entre dos computadoras conectadas a una red.

sagittal plane The plane that divides the body into right and left halves.
plano sagital Plano que divide el cuerpo en la mitad derecha y la mitad izquierda.

salutation Word or gestures expressing greeting, good will, or courtesy.
saludo Expresión de saludo, buenos deseos o cortesía por medio de palabras o gestos.

sanitization Reducing the number of potentially harmful **microorganisms** to a relatively safe level.
saneamiento Reducción del número de **microorganismos** a un nivel relativamente seguro.

sarcasm A sharp and often satirical response or ironic utterance designed to cut or give pain.
sarcasmo Respuesta aguda y frecuentemente satírica o declaración irónica destinada a burlarse o a lastimar.

scanner A device that reads text or illustrations on a printed page and translates the information into a form that the computer can understand.
escáner Dispositivo que lee texto o ilustraciones de una página impresa y traduce esa información a un formato comprensible para la computadora.

sclera The wite part of the eye that encloses the eyeball.
esclerótica Parte blanca del ojo que encierra el globo ocular.

scleroderma An autoimmune disorder that affects the blood vessels and connective tissue, causing fibrous degeneration of the major organs.
escleroderma Trastorno autoinmune que afecta a los vasos sanguíneos y los tejidos conectivos provocando degeneración en las fibras de los órganos principales.

sclerotherapy The injection of sclerosing (hardening) solutions to treat hemorrhoids, varicose veins, or esophageal varices.
escleroterapia Inyección de soluciones de esclerosis (endorecedores) para tratar hemorroides, venas varicosas o varices esofágicas.

scoliosis Abnormal lateral curvature of the spine.
escoliosis Curvatura lateral anómala de la columna.

scored tablet A drug tablet manufactured with an indentation that allows it to be broken or cut into equal parts.
tableta con hendidura Tableta que se fabrica con una hendidura que permite dividirla o romperla en partes iguales.

screen Something that shields, protects, or hides; to select or eliminate products or applicants by comparing them to a set of desired criteria.
pantalla Algo que actúa como escudo, que protege u oculta para permitir un proceso de selección.

search engines Computer programs that search documents for keywords and return a list of documents containing those words.
buscadores Programas de computadoras que buscan documentos a partir de palabras clave y proporcionan una lista de los documentos que contienen esas palabras.

seborrhea Excessive discharge of sebum from the sebaceous glands, forming greasy scales on the skin or cheesy plugs in skin pores.
seborrea Descarga excesiva de sebo de las glándulas sebáceas, formando escamas de grasa en la piel o tapones con aspecto de queso en los poros de la piel.

secondary hypertension Elevated blood pressure caused by another medical condition.
hipertensión secundaria Presión sanguínea elevada causada por otra enfermedad o afección médica.

"see also" An instruction to the coder to look elsewhere if the main term or subterm(s) for an entry are not sufficient for coding the information. If a code number follows, "see also" is enclosed in parentheses; there is no code number, "see also" is preceded by a dash.
"ver también" Instrucción que se le da a la persona encargada de la codificación para que consulte en algún otro lugar si el término o subtérminos principales para una entrada no son suficientes para codificar la información. Si "ver también" va seguido por un número de código, dicho código va entre paréntesis; si no hay número de código, "ver también" va precedido por un guión.

"see category" An instruction to the coder to refer to a specific category (three-digit code); it must always be followed.
"ver categoría" Instrucción que se le da a la persona encargada de la codificación para que consulte una categoría específica (código de tres dígitos); Siempre debe seguirse.

"see" An instruction to the coder to look in another place. This instruction must always be followed and is found in the Alphabetic Index, volumes 2 and 3.
"ver" Instrucción que se le da a la persona encargada de la codificación para que consulte en otro lugar. Siempre debe seguirse esta instrucción; la expresión se encuentra en el Índice alfabético, tomos 2 y 3.

self-insured plans Insurance plans funded by organizations having a big enough employee base that they can afford to fund their own insurance program.
planes de autoaseguración Planes de seguros implementados por organizaciones con un número de empleados lo suficientemente grande como para permitirles financiar su propio programa de seguros.

sequentially Happening in relation to or by arrangement in a sequence.
secuencial Aquello que ocurre relativo a una secuencia o que es ordenado en secuencia.

serous Pertaining to thin, watery, serumlike drainage.
seroso Perteneciente o relativo a una materia poco espesa, acuosa, parecida al suero.

serum The portion of whole blood that remains liquid after the blood has clotted.
suero La porción de la sangre que queda líquida después de la coagulación.

service benefit plan A plan that provides benefits in the form of certain surgical and medical services rendered, rather than in cash. A service benefit plan is not restricted to a fee schedule.
plan de beneficios de servicio Plan que proporciona beneficios en forma de ciertos servicios médico-quirúrgicos en vez de con dinero en metálico. Un plan de servicio de beneficio no está restringido por una escala de cargos.

sheath The covering surrounding the axon of the nerve cell that acts as an electrical insulator to speed the conduction of nerve impulses.
película Recubrimiento que rodea los axones de la célula nerviosa y que se comporta como aislante eléctrico para aumentar la velocidad de conducción del impulso nervioso.

shingling A method of filing whereby each new report is laid on top of the next older report, resembling the shingles of a roof.
laminado Método de archivo en el cual cada informe nuevo se coloca encima del informe anterior, del mismo modo que se colocan las tejas en un techo.

Sievert (Sv) International unit of radiation dose equivalent.
Sievert (Sv) Unidad internacional de dosis equivalentes de radiación.

sinoatrial (SA) node The pacemaker of the heart, located in the right atrium.
nódulo sinoauricular (SA) Marcapasos del corazón que se halla en la aurícula derecha.

sinus arrhythmia Irregular heartbeat originating in the sinoatrial (pacemaker) node.
arritmia de seno Ritmo cardiaco irregular que tiene su origen en el nódulo sinoauricular (marcapasos).

socioeconomic Relating to a combination of social and economic factors.
socioeconómico Perteneciente o relativo a una combinación de factores sociales y económicos.

sociological Oriented or directed toward social needs and problems.
sociologico Que se orienta o dirige hacia las necesidades y problemas sociales.

sonography An imaging modality that uses sound waves to produce images of soft tissues; also called diagnostic ultrasound.
sonografía Modalidad de formación de imágenes que usa ondas sonoras para producir imágenes de los tejidos blandos; también se conoce como ultrasonido de diagnóstico.

sound card A device that allows a computer to output sound through speakers that are connected to the main circuitry board (motherboard).
tarjeta de sonido Dispositivo que le permite a una computadora emitir sonido a través de altavoces conectados a la tarjeta principal del circuito.

specimen A sample of body fluid, waste product, or tissue that is collected for analysis and diagnosis.
espécimen Muestra de un fluido corporal, residuo o tejido que se usa para análisis y diagnósticos.

spirometer An instrument that measures the volume of inhaled and exhaled air.
espirómetro Instrumento que sirve para medir el volumen del aire inhalado y exhalado.

spores Thick-walled reproductive cells formed within bacteria and capable of withstanding unfavorable environmental conditions; thick-walled dormant forms of bacteria that are very resistant to **disinfection** measures.
esporas Células reproductoras de paredes gruesas que se forman dentro de las bacterias y son capaces de resistir condiciones ambientales adversas; tipos de bacterias letárgicas de paredes gruesas que son muy resistentes a las medidas de **desinfección**.

staff privileges Authorization for a healthcare professional to practice within a specific facility.
privilegios del personal Autorización para un profesional de atención sanitaria, para ejercer la práctica dentro de unas instalaciones específicas.

standards Items or indicators used to measure quality or compliance with a statutory or accrediting body's policies and regulations.
estándares Artículos o indicadores usados para medir la calidad o cumplimiento de las pólizas y regulaciones de un cuerpo normativo o acreditativo.

stat Medical abbreviation for immediately or at this moment; an order found on a laboratory requisition indicating that the test must be done immediately (from the Latin word *statin*, meaning "at once"); immediately.
stat Abreviatura usada en medicina que significa inmediatamente o ahora mismo. Orden encontrada en un pedido de laboratorio que indica que el análisis debe llevarse a cabo inmediatamente (de la palabra latina *statin*, que significa "ahora"); inmediatamente.

stationers Sellers of writing paper.
dependientes de papelería Vendedores de artículos de papelería.

statute A law enacted by the legislative branch of a government.
estatuto Ley sancionada por la rama legislativa de un gobierno.

stereotactic An x-ray procedure to guide the insertion of a needle into a specific area of the breast.
estereotáctico Procedimiento de rayos X para guiar la inserción de una aguja en zonas específicas del pecho.

stereotype Something conforming to a fixed or general pattern; a standardized mental picture that is held in common by many and represents an oversimplified opinion, prejudiced attitude, or uncritical judgment.
estereotipo Algo que se ajusta a un patrón fijado o general; imagen mental estandarizada que tienen en común muchas personas y que representa opiniones simplificadas, actitudes con prejuicios o razonamientos carentes de sentido crítico.

sterilization Complete destruction of all forms of microbial life.
esterilización Destrucción total de toda forma de vida microbiana.

stertorous Describing strenuous respiratory effort that has a snoring sound.
estertóreo Esfuerzo respiratorio penoso que tiene el sonido de un ronquido.

stipulate To specify as a condition or requirement of an agreement or offer; to make an agreement or covenant to do or forbear something.
estipular Especificar como condición o requisito de un acuerdo u oferta; establecer un acuerdo o prometer hacer, o dejar de hacer, algo.

stock option Offer of stocks for purchase to a certain individual or to certain groups, such as employees of a for-profit hospital.
opción sobre acciones Oferta de venta de acciones que se le hace a un ciertos individuos o grupos, como a los empleados de un hospital.

stressors Stimuli that cause stress.
estresantes Dícese de los estímulos que causan estrés.

stridor A shrill, harsh respiratory sound heard during inhalation during laryngeal obstruction.
estridor Sonido respiratorio estridente que se oye durante la inhalación en los casos de obstrucción laríngea.

stroke Sudden paralysis and/or loss of consciousness caused by extreme trauma or injury to an artery in the brain.
apoplejía Súbita pérdida de conocimiento y parálisis causada por una lesión o daño grave de una arteria del cerebro.

stylus A metal probe inserted into or passed through a catheter, needle, or tube that is used for clearing purposes or to facilitate passage into a body orifice.
punzón Sonda metálica que se inserta o pasa por medio de un catéter, aguja o tubo y que se usa para limpiar o para facilitar el paso a un orificio del cuerpo.

subjective information Information gained by questioning the patient or taking it from a form.
información subjetiva Información obtienida haciendo preguntas al paciente o tomándola de un formulario.

subluxation Incomplete dislocation of a bone from its normal anatomical location
subluxación Dislocación incompleta de un hueso desde su posición anatómica normal.

subluxations Slight misalignments of the vertebrae, or a partial dislocation.
subluxaciones Alineamientos ligeramente defectuosos o dislocaciones parciales de las vértebras.

subordinate Submissive to or controlled by authority; placed in or occupying a lower class, rank, or position.
subordinado Que está sometido a una autoridad o controlado por ella; que ostenta un cargo u ocupa una clase, rango o puesto inferior.

subpoena A writ or document commanding a person to appear in court, under penalty for failure to appear.
subpoena Documento escrito ordenando a una persona comparecer en el juzgado bajo penalidad en caso de no comparecencia.

substance number A number based on the weight of a ream of paper containing 500 sheets.
número de sustancia Número basado en el peso de una resma de papel de 500 hojas.

subtle Difficult to understand or perceive; having or marked by keen insight and the ability to penetrate deeply and thoroughly.
sutil Difícil de comprender o percibir; que tiene perspicacia y la capacidad de penetrar a fondo y en toda su extensión en un asunto.

succinct Marked by compact, precise expression without wasted words.
sucinto Caracterizado por una expresión precisa y concisa sin palabras inútiles.

superfluous Exceeding what is sufficient or necessary.
superfluos Que exceden aquello que es suficiente o necesario.

suppurative Forming and/or discharging of pus.
supuración Formación o emisión de pus.

surrogate A substitute; put in place of another.
subrogado Sustituto; puesto en lugar de otro.

switch In networks, a device that filters information between LAN segments, decreases overall network traffic, and increases speed and bandwidth usage efficiency.
conmutador En las redes de comunicación, dispositivo que filtra información entre segmentos de LAN y disminuye el tráfico global de la red, aumentando la velocidad y la eficacia en el uso del ancho de banda.

syncope Fainting; a brief lapse in consciousness
síncope Desmayo; lapso breve en estado de consciencia.

syndrome A group of signs and symptoms related to a common cause or presenting a clinical picture of a disease or an inherited abnormality.
síndrome Conjunto de signos y síntomas relacionados con una causa común o que presentan el cuadro clínico de una enfermedad o una anomalía heredada.

synopsis A condensed statement or outline.
sinopsis Declaración resumida; resumen.

synovial fluid Clear fluid found in joint cavities that facilitates smooth movements and nourishes joint structures.
fluido sinovial Fluido claro que se halla en las cavidades de las articulaciones y que facilita los movimientos suaves y nutre las estructuras articulatorias.

tachycardia Rapid but regular heart rate exceeding 100 beats per minute.
taquicardia Ritmo cardiaco rápido pero regular que sobrepasa los 100 latidos por minuto.

tachypnea Respiration that is rapid and shallow; hyperventilation.
taquipnea Respiración rápida y profunda; hiperventilación.

tactful Having a keen sense of what to do or say in order to maintain good relations with others or avoid offense.
tacto Tener un sentido de lo que se debe hacer o decir para mantener buenas relaciones con los demás y evitar ofenderlos.

target organ The organ that is affected by a particular hormone.
órgano objetivo Órgano afectado por una hormona específica.

target tissue A group of cells that are affected by a particular hormone.
tejido objetivo Grupo de células afectadas por una hormona específica.

targeted to Directed or used toward a target; directed toward a specific desire or position.
dirigido a Dirigido a un fin o meta específico, usado hacia un fin; dirigido hacia un deseo o un puesto específico.

TCP/IP Abbreviation for Transmission Control Protocol/Internet Protocol; a suite of communications protocols used to connect users or hosts to the Internet.
TCP/IP Abreviatura de protocolo de control de transmisión/protocolo Internet; conjunto de protocolos de comunicación que se usa para conectar usuarios o computadoras a Internet.

tedious Tiresome because of length or dullness.
tedioso Que cansa porque es demasiado largo o aburrido.

telecommunications The science and technology of communication by transmission of information from one location to another via telephone, television, telegraph, or satellite.
telecomunicaciones Ciencia y tecnología de la comunicación basada en la transmisión de información de un lugar a otro por teléfono, televisión, telégrafo o satélite.

telemedicine The use of telecommunications in the practice of medicine, allowing great distances between healthcare professionals, colleagues, patients, and students.
telemedicina Uso de las telecomunicaciones en la práctica médica, permitiendo la comunicación entre profesionales de atención sanitaria, colegas, pacientes y estudiantes que se hallan a grandes distancias.

teleradiology The use of telecommunications devices to enhance and improve the results of radiological procedures.
telerradiología Uso de dispositivos de telecomunicación para mejorar y perfeccionar los resultados de procedimientos radiológicos.

tendon A tough band of connective tissue connecting muscle to bone.
tendón Banda resistente de tejido conectivo que conecta los músculos con los huesos.

teratogen Any substance that interferes with normal prenatal development.
teratógeno Cualquier sustancia que interfiere con el desarrollo prenatal normal.

teratogenic A substance that is known to cause birth defects.
teratogénico Sustancia que se sabe que provoca defectos de nacimiento.

testimony A solemn declaration usually made orally by a witness under oath in response to interrogation by a lawyer or authorized public official.
testimonio Declaración solemne, por lo general oral, hecha por un testigo bajo juramento como respuesta a una pregunta (o preguntas) de un abogado o un funcionario público autorizado.

thanatology The description or study of the phenomena of death and of psychological methods of coping with death.
tanatología Descripción o estudio del fenómeno de la muerte y de los métodos psicológicos para hacerle frente.

third-party payer An entity (usually an insurance company) that makes a payment on an obligation or debt but is not a party to the contract that created the debt.
pagador mediador Entidad (por lo general una compañía aseguradora) que hace un pago de una obligación o deuda pero que no es parte del contrato que ha creado dicha deuda.

third-party payer Someone other than the patient, spouse, or parent who is responsible for paying all or part of the patient's medical costs.
pagador mediador Alguien ajeno al paciente, cónyuge, padre o madre que es responsable del pago de todo o parte de los gastos médicos del paciente o de parte de ellos.

thixotropic gel A material that appears to be a solid until subjected to a disturbance such as centrifugation, when it becomes a liquid.
gel tisotrópico Material que parece ser sólido hasta el momento en que se somete a una alteración como la centrifugación, cuando se convierte en líquido.

thoracic Pertaining to the region of the back containing 12 thoracic vertebrae, between the neck and low back.
torácica Perteneciente o relativo a región de la espalda entre el cuello y la región lumbar inferior en la que hay 12 vértebras torácicas.

thready pulse Pulse that is scarcely perceptible.
pulso débil Pulso que es apenas perceptible.

thrombus Blood clot.
trombo Cóagulo de sangre.

thyroid stimulating hormone (TSH) A hormone secreted by the anterior lobe of the pituitary gland that stimulates the secretion of hormones produced by the thyroid gland.
hormona estimulante de la tiroides (TSH) Hormona que segrega el lóbulo anterior de la glándula pituitaria y que estimula la secreción de hormonas producidas por la glándula tiroides.

tickler file A chronological file used as a reminder that something must be taken care of on a certain date.
archivo cronológico Archivo que se usa para recordar que algo que debe llevarse a cabo en una fecha determinada.

tinea Fungal skin disease that results in scaling, itching, and inflammation.
tinea Enfermedad de la piel causada por hongos y que produce descamación, picazón e inflamación.

tissue culture The technique or process of keeping tissue alive and growing in a culture medium.
cultivo de tejidos Técnica o proceso de mantener un tejido vivo y en fase de crecimiento en un medio de cultivo.

toxemia An abnormal condition of pregnancy characterized by hypertension, edema, and protein in the urine.
toxemia Característica anómala del embarazo, con presencia de hipertensión, edema y proteínas en la orina.

tracer A radioactive substance administered to a patient undergoing a nuclear medicine imaging procedure.
trazador Sustancia radioactiva que se administra al paciente para someterlo a procedimientos de formación de imágenes en medicina nuclear.

tracheostomy A surgical opening through the neck into the trachea, to facilitate breathing.
traqueotomía Abertura realizada quirúrgicamente en el cuello a la altura de la tráquea para facilitar la respiración.

transaction An exchange or transfer of goods, services, or funds.
transacción Intercambio o transferencia de bienes, servicios o fondos.

transcription A written copy made either in longhand or by machine.
transcripción Copia escrita de algo, hecha a mano, o con la ayuda de una máquina.

transducer The part of the sonography machine in contact with the patient that sends high frequency sound waves and receives the sound echoes that return from the patient's body.
transductor Parte de una máquina de sonografía que está en contacto con el paciente envía ondas sonoras de alta frecuencia y recibe los ecos de los sonidos que regresan del cuerpo del paciente.

transection A cross-section, division by cutting across.
sección transversal División cortando a través.

transient ischemic attack Temporary neurological symptoms caused by gradual or partial occlusion of a cerebral blood vessel.
ataque isquémico transitorio Síntomas neurológicos temporales causados por una oclusión gradual o parcial de un vaso sanguíneo del cerebro.

transillumination Inspection of a cavity or organ by passing light through its walls.
diafanoscopia Inspección de una cavidad u órgano haciendo pasar luz a través de sus paredes.

transport medium A medium used to keep an organism alive during transport to the laboratory.
medio para transporte Medio usado para mantener un organismo vivo durante el transporte al laboratorio.

transverse plane Plane that divides the body into superior and inferior parts.
plano transversal Plano que divide el cuerpo en parte superior e inferior.

trauma Physical injury or wound caused by an external force or violence.
trauma Lesión física o herida causada por una fuerza externa o violencia.

treatises Systematic expositions or arguments in writing, including methodical discussion of the facts and principles involved and the conclusions reached.
tratados Exposiciones sistemáticas o argumentos escritos que incluyen una descripción metódica de los hechos y principios involucrados y las conclusiones a las que se ha llegado.

triage Responding to requests for immediate care and treatment after evaluating the urgency of the need and prioritizing the treatment; the sorting and allocation of treatment to patients according to a system of priorities designed to maximize the number of survivors and treat the sickest patients first.
criterio de selección Responder a peticiones de atención y tratamiento inmediato tras evaluar la urgencia de la necesidad y establecer prioridades de tratamiento. Clasificación y asignación de tratamiento a pacientes según un sistema de prioridades destinado a maximizar el número de sobrevivientes y tratar primero a los pacientes más enfermos.

triglycerides Fatty acids and glycerols that are bound to proteins and form high- and low-density lipoproteins.
triglicéridos Ácidos grasos y gliceroles que se unen a las proteínas y forman lipoproteínas de alta y baja densidad.

truss An elastic, canvas, or metallic device for retaining a reduced hernia within the abdominal cavity.
braguero Malla elástica o dispositivo metálico para retener una hernia reducida dentro de la cavidad abdominal.

turgor Resistance of the skin to being grasped between the fingers and released; normal skin tension that is decreased in dehydration and increased with edema.
turgor Resistencia de la piel a ser pellizcada; tensión normal de la piel que disminuye con la deshidratación y aumenta con el edema.

type and cross match Tests performed to assess the compatibility of blood to be transfused.
prueba de tipo y RH Análisis que se realizan para evaluar la compatibilidad de la sangre que va a ser usada en una transfusión.

unequal pulses Pulses in which the beats vary in intensity.
pulso desigual Pulso en el cual los latidos varían en intensidad.

Uniform Commercial Code A unified set of rules covering many business transactions; often referred to simply as the UCC, it has been adopted in all 50 states, the District of Columbia, and most U.S. territories.
Código de Comercio Uniforme (UCC) Conjunto de normas unificadas que cubren muchas transacciones comerciales; se conoce simplemente como UCC y ha sido adoptado en los 50 estados, el Distrito de Columbia y la mayoría de los territorios estadounidenses.

unique identifiers A method of anonymous HIV testing in which a code is used, instead of names, to protect the confidentiality of the patient.
identificadores únicos Método de prueba de VIH (HIV) anónimo en el cual se usa un código en lugar de nombres, para proteger la confidencialidad del paciente.

unit dose A method used by the pharmacy to prepare individual doses of medications. **dosis unitaria** Método usado por la farmacia para preparar dosis individuales de medicamentos.

universal claim form The form developed by the Health Care Financing Administration (HCFA, now known as the Centers for Medicare and Medicaid Services, or CMS) and approved by the AMA for use in submitting all government sponsored claims.
formulario de reclamación universal Formulario desarrollado por la Administración financiera de la atención sanitaria (HCFA, ahora conocida como Centros de servicios de Medicare y Medicaid, o CMS) y aprobado por AMA para usarse al someter todas las reclamaciones subvencionadas por el gobierno.

upper GI series Fluoroscopic examination of the esophagus, stomach, and duodenum using oral administration of barium sulfate as a contrast medium.
serie GI superior Examen fluoroscópico del esófago, estómago y duodeno usando una administración oral de sulfato de bario como medio de contraste.

urea The major nitrogenous end-product of protein metabolism and the chief nitrogenous component of the urine.
urea Principal producto final nitrogenado del metabolismo de las proteínas y el principal componente nitrogenado de la orina.

urease An enzyme that catalyzes the hydrolysis of urea to form ammonium carbonate.
ureasa Enzima que cataliza la hidrólisis de la urea para formar carbonato de amonio.

uremia A toxic renal condition characterized by an excess of urea, creatinine, and other nitrogenous end-products in the blood.
uremia Enfermedad renal tóxica que se caracteriza por un exceso de urea, creatinina y otros productos finales en la sangre.

urgency A sudden, compelling desire to urinate and the inability to control its release.
urgencia Deseo repentino y apremiante de orinar y la incapacidad de controlarlo.

URL Abbreviation for Uniform Resource Locator; the global address of documents or information on the Internet. The URL provides the IP address and the domain name for the web page, such as "*microsoft.com.*"
URL Abreviatura de localizador universal de recursos; la dirección a nivel mundial, de documentos o de información en Internet.
El URL proporciona la dirección IP y el nombre del dominio de una página web, como por ejemplo: "*microsoft.com.*"

urticaria A skin eruption creating inflamed wheals; hives.
urticaria Erupción cutánea que produce ampollas imflamadas.

"use additional code" This term appears only in volume 1 in those subdivisions where the user should add further information by means of an additional code to give a more complete picture of the diagnosis. In some cases you will find "if desired" following the term. For the purpose of coding in military medical treatment facilities, the "if desired" phrase will not be used. Therefore when the term "use additional code ... if desired" appears, you will disregard "if desired" and assign the appropriate additional code.
"usar código adicional" Esta expresión aparece sólo en el tomo 1, en aquellas subdivisiones en las que el usuario debe añadir más información por medio de un código adicional para proporcionar un cuadro más completo del diagnóstico.
En algunos casos, se verá "si se desea" tras el término. En la codificación en establecimientos militares de tratamiento médico, no se usará la expresión "si se desea". Por lo tanto, cuando aparezca el término "usar código adicional ... si se desea", no se tendrá en cuenta "si se desea" y se asignará el código adicional correspondiente.

utilization review The review of individual cases by a committee to make sure that services are medically necessary and to study how providers use medical care resources.
revisión de utilización Revisión de casos individuales por un comité, para asegurarse de que los servicios son médicamente necesarios y estudiar cómo los proveedores usan los recursos de cuidados de salud.

Valsalva's maneuver Occurs when one strains to defecate and urinate, uses the arms and upper trunk muscles to move up in bed, or strains during laughing, coughing, or vomiting. It causes a trapping of blood in the great veins, preventing it from entering the chest and right atrium, which may cause heart attack and death.
maniobra de Valsalva Ocurre cuando uno hace fuerza para defecar y orinar, usa los brazos y los músculos de la parte superior del tronco para levantarse de la cama, o hace fuerza al reír, toser o vomitar. Causa una retención de sangre en las venas mayores, impidiendole que entre en el pecho y la aurícula derecha y puede provocar un ataque al corazón y la muerte.

vasodilation Increase in the diameter of a blood vessel.
vasodilatación Aumento en el diámetro de un vaso sanguíneo.

vector An organism, such as an insect or tick, that transmits the causative organisms of disease.
vector Organismos, tales como un insecto o garrapata, que transmite los organismos que provocan enfermedades.

ventricles The two lower chambers of the heart.
ventrículos Las dos cavidades inferiores del corazón.

veracity Devotion to or conformity with the truth.
veracidad Compromiso o conformidad con la verdad.

verdict The finding or decision of a jury on a matter submitted to it in trial.
veredicto Conclusión o decisión de un jurado en un asunto sometido a juicio.

versatile Embracing a variety of subjects, fields or skills; having a wide range of abilities.
versátil Que abarca diferentes sujetos, campos o destrezas; que tiene una amplia gama de destrezas.

vertigo Dizziness; a sensation of faintness or an inability to maintain normal balance.
vértigo Mareo; sensación de desmayo o de incapacidad de mantener el equilibrio normal.

vested Granted or endowed with a particular authority, right, or property; having a special interest in something.
conferirido Concedido o dotado con una autoridad, derecho o propiedad particular; que tiene un interés especial en algo.

viable Capable of living, developing, or germinating under favorable conditions.
viable Capaz de vivir, desarrollarse o germinar bajo condiciones favorables.

virtual reality An artificial environment, experienced by a computer user often using special gloves, earphones, and goggles to enhance the experience, that feels as if it were a real environment.
realidad virtual Entorno artificial que experimenta el usuario de una computadora, muchas veces usando guantes especiales, audífonos y lentes para mejorar la experiencia, y que parece ser un ambiente real.

virulent Exceedingly pathogenic, noxious, or deadly.
virulento Excesivamente patógeno, nocivo o mortal.

viscosity The quality of being thick and lacking the capability of easy movement.
viscosidad Cualidad de espeso e incapaz de moverse con facilidad.

vocation The work in which a person is regularly employed.
profesión Trabajo en el que una persona está empleada regularmente.

volatile Referring to a flammable substance's capacity to vaporize at a low temperature. Easily aroused; tending to erupt in violence.
volátil Referente a la capacidad de una sustancia flamable para evaporarse a baja temperatura. Que reacciona con facilidad y tiene tendencia a entrar en erupción de forma violenta.

vulva The external female genitalia, which begins at the mons pubis and terminates at the anus.
vulva Zona genital exterior femenina que comienza en el monte púbico y termina en el ano.

watermark A mark in paper resulting from differences in thickness usually produced by pressure of a projecting design in the mold or on a processing roll, and visible when the paper is held up to the light.
filigrana Marca en un papel que resulta de diferencias de espesor, por lo general se produce presionando un diseño en relieve en el molde o en un rodillo de procesamiento, y es visible por transparencia.

wet mount A slide preparation in which a drop of liquid specimen for example, protected by a coverslip and observed with a microscope.
montaje húmedo Preparación de una lámina en la que una gota de espécimen líquido por ejemplo, se protege con una cubierta de vidrio y se observa con un microscopio.

wheal Localized area of edema, or a raised lesion.
roncha Área localizada de un edema o una lesión protuberante.

"with " In the context of ICD-9-CM, the terms "with," "with mention of," or "associated with" in a title dictates that both parts of the title must be present in the statement of the diagnosis in order to assign the particular code.
"con " En el contexto de la ICD-9-CM, las expresiones "con", "con mención de" y "asociado con" en un título exigen que ambas partes del título estén presentes en la descripción del orden de diagnóstico para asignar el código específico.

workers' compensation Insurance against liability imposed on certain employers to pay benefits and furnish care to employees injured, and to pay benefits to dependents of employees killed, in the course of or arising out of their employment.
compensación laboral Seguro contra la responsabilidad impuesta a ciertos patronos para pagar beneficios y proporcionar atenciones a los trabajadores lesionados, y pagar beneficios a las personas que dependan de trabajadores que mueran en el trabajo o a causa de él.

Zip drive A small and portable disk drive that is primarily used for backing up information and archiving computer files; a 100 megabyte zip disk will hold the equivalent of about 70 floppy disks.
Unidad zip Unidad de un disco pequeño y portátil que se usa principalmente para hacer copias de seguridad de información y para guardar archivos electrónicos. Un disco zip de 100 megabytes tiene una capacidad equivalente a la de unos 70 disquetes.

Credits

Page 935-936 constitute an extension of the copyright page. The illustrations that appear on the pages listed below are from the following sources.

From Barkaukas VH, Baumann, LC, and Darling-Fisher, CS: *Health and Physical Assessment,* 3rd ed., St. Louis, 2002, Mosby.
Pages 179-181, 210, 211, 224-226, 228-229, 232, 238, 248, 255-256, 260, 266, 270, 275-276, 285, 288-292, 298-299, 319, 322

From Buck CJ: *Saunders 2002 ICD-9-CM volumes 1, 2, & 3 and HCPCS level II,* Philadelphia, 2002, WB Saunders.
Pages 230-231, 242, 254, 264, 274, 293, 302, 311, 323-324, 332, 340

From Davis N, Lacour M: *Introduction to health information technology,* Philadelphia, 2002, WB Saunders.
Pages 51, 56, 76-81, 120-122, 131-132, 415-418

From Doucette LJ: *Basic mathematics for the health-related professions,* Philadelphia, 2000, WB Saunders.
Pages 207, 209-210, 212, 363-364, 367-368, 388

From Hunt SA, Zonderman JH: *Saunders fundamentals of medical assisting: student mastery manual,* Philadelphia, 2002, WB Saunders.
Pages 58-59, 67, 70, 73, 85-89, 100, 104, 113-116, 118, 136-137, 139, 357, 364, 380-381, 403-406

From Hunt SA, Zonderman JH: *Saunders medical assisting pocket pal,* Philadelphia, 2002, WB Saunders.
Pages 162

From Kinn ME, Woods, M: *The medical assistant: administrative and clinical,* 8th ed., Philadelphia, 1999, WB Saunders.
Pages 176-179, 346, 421

From Lilly AL, Kinn ME, Woods, M: *Student mastery manual for the medical assistant: administrative and clinical,* 8th ed., Philadelphia, 1999, WB Saunders.
Pages 289, 469

From Young T, Kennedy D: *Kinn's the medical assistant: an applied learning approach,* 9th ed., Philadelphia, 2003, Elsevier Science (USA).
Pages 29, 94, 97-98, 101-103, 142, 163, 169

From Sole ML, Lamborn ML, Hartshorn JC: *Introduction to critical care nursing,* 3rd ed., Philadelphia, 2001, WB Saunders.
Pages 319, 321, 328, 345-348

From Swisher L: *Study guide to accompany Thibodeau and Patton the human body in health & disease,* 3rd ed., 2002, Mosby.
Pages 345, 355, 372-373, 375-376, 387, 389, 393-396